STRUCTURE–ACTIVITY RELATIONSHIPS
OF ANTI–TUMOUR AGENTS

DEVELOPMENTS IN PHARMACOLOGY

VOLUME 3

1. J.M. Boeynaems and A.G. Herman, eds.: Prostaglandins, prostacyclin, and thromboxanes measurement. 1980. ISBN 90 247 2417 1.
2. R.M. Berne, Th.W. Rall and R. Rubio, eds.: Regulatory function in adenosine. 1983. ISBN 90 247 2779 0.

STRUCTURE-ACTIVITY RELATIONSHIPS OF ANTI-TUMOUR AGENTS

Edited by

D.N. Reinhoudt
Department of Organic Chemistry
Technical University Twente, Enschede, The Netherlands

T.A. Connors
MRC Toxicology Unit
Medical Research Council Laboratories
Carshalton, Surrey, Great Britain

H.M. Pinedo
Department of Biochemistry
Antonie van Leeuwenhoekziekenhuis
Amsterdam, The Netherlands

K.W. van de Poll
Koningin Wilhelmina Fonds
The Netherlands Cancer Foundation
Amsterdam, The Netherlands

1983
MARTINUS NIJHOFF PUBLISHERS
THE HAGUE / BOSTON / LONDON

Distributors:

for the United States and Canada

Kluwer Boston, Inc.
190 Old Derby Street
Hingham, MA 02043
USA

for all other countries

Kluwer Academic Publishers Group
Distribution Center
P.O. Box 322
3300 AH Dordrecht
The Netherlands

Library of Congress Cataloging in Publication Data

Main entry under title:

Structure-activity relationships of anti-tumour
    agents.

    (Developments in pharmacology ; v. 3)
    Papers presented at a workshop held Mar. 11-13,
1982.
      1. Cancer--Chemotherapy--Congresses. 2. Anti-
neoplastic agents--Congresses. 3. Structure-activity relationship (Pharmacology)--Congresses.
I. Reinhoudt, D. N. II. Series. [DNLM: 1. Structure
-activity relationship--Congresses. 2. Anti-
neoplastic agents--Congresses. Wl DE998NK v. 3 /
QV 269]
RC271.C5S77 1983   616.99'4061   82-19101

ISBN 90-247-2783-9 (this volume)
ISBN 90-247-2435-X (series)

PRINTED IN THE NETHERLANDS

CONTENTS

VI

LIST OF AUTHORS — PARTICIPANTS

ARCAMONE, F., Farmitalia Carlo Erba, Gruppo Montedison, Ricerca & Sviluppo Chimico, Viale E. Bezzi 24, 20146 Milano, ITALY

AUCLAIR, C., Laboratoire de Biochimie-Enzymologie de l'Institut Gustave-Roussy, U 147 CNRS, U 140 INSERM, 94800 Villejuif, FRANCE

BERNADOU, J., Laboratoire de Pharmacologie et Toxicologie fondamentale, CNRS, 205 Route de Narbonne, 31078 Toulouse, FRANCE

BROCK, N., Abteilung Tumorforschung der Asta-Werke Aktiengesellschaft, Postfach 140129, D-4800 Bielefeld 14, WEST-GERMANY

CLEARE, M.J., Johnson Mattey Research Center, Blount's Court, Sonning Common, Reading RG4 9NH, GREAT-BRITAIN

CONNORS, T.A., MRC Toxicology Unit, Medical Research Council Laboratories, Woodmansterne Road, Carshalton, Surrey SM5 4EF, GREAT-BRITAIN

CROS, S., Laboratoire de Pharmacologie et Toxicologie fondamentale, CNRS, 205 Route de Narbonne, 31078 Toulouse, FRANCE

CZERNIAK, R., Department of Chemistry, University of California, Irvine, CA 92717, U.S.A.

DRISCOLL, J.S., Acting Associate Director, Developmental Therapeutics Program, Division of Cancer Treatment, National Cancer Institute, Blair Bldg., Rm. 5A03, 8300 Colesville Road, Silver Spring, MD 20910, U.S.A.

MAFTOUH, M., Laboratoire de Pharmacologie et Toxicologie fondamentale, CNRS, 205 Route de Narbonne, 31078 Toulouse, FRANCE

MEUNIER, B., Laboratoire de Pharmacologie et Toxicologie fondamentale, CNRS, 205 Route de Narbonne, 31078 Toulouse, FRANCE

MEUNIER, G., Laboratoire de Pharmacologie et Toxicologie fondamentale, CNRS, 205 Route de Narbonne, 31078 Toulouse, FRANCE

MONSARRAT, B., Laboratoire de Pharmacologie et Toxicologie fondamentale, CNRS, 205 Route de Narbonne, 31078 Toulouse, FRANCE

MONTGOMERY, J.A., Southern Research Institute, P.O. Box 3307-A, Birmingham, AL 35255, U.S.A.

MOORE, H.W., Department of Chemistry, University of California, Irvine, CA 92717, U.S.A.

NARAYANAN, V.L., Chief Drug Synthesis & Chemistry Branch, Department of Health Education & Welfare, National Cancer Institute, Bethesda, MD 20205, U.S.A.

PAOLETTI, C., Laboratoire de Biochimie-Enzymologie de l'Institut Gustave-Roussy, U 147 CNRS, U 140 INSERM, 94800 Villejuif, FRANCE

PINEDO, H.M., Antoni van Leeuwenhoekhuis, Afdeling Biochemie H-3, Plesmanlaan 121, 1066 CX Amsterdam, THE NETHERLANDS

POLL, K.W. van de, Koningin Wilhelmina Fonds (The Netherlands Cancer Foundation), Sophialaan 8-10, 1075 BR Amsterdam, THE NETHERLANDS

REINHOUDT, D.N., Department of Organic Chemistry, Technical University Twente, P.O. Box 217, 7500 AE Enschede, THE NETHERLANDS

REKKER, R.F., Vrije Universiteit, Vakgroep Pharmacochemie, Subfaculteit der Scheikunde, De Boelelaan 1083, 1081 HV Amsterdam, THE NETHERLANDS

SRINIVASACHER, K., Department of Chemistry, University of California, Irvine, CA 92717, U.S.A.

STEVENS, M.F.G., The University of Ason in Birmingham, Department of Pharmacy, Gosta Green, Birmingham B4 7ET, GREAT-BRITAIN

UMEZAWA, H., Yamanouci International Ltd., 12 Hannover Street, London WIR-9 WB, GREAT-BRITAIN

WEST, K.F., Department of Chemistry, University of California, Irvine, CA 92717, U.S.A.

INTRODUCTION

The Workshop series of the "Koningin Wilhelmina Fonds" is a feature of the interest of this Foundation to promote research and education in the field of cancer, aiming to improve prognosis of the cancer patient. For almost a century, surgery has now been the main treatment modality for the cancer patient. During the past 50 years radiation therapy has developed as a second important modality of treatment. However, neither of the two modalities are able to cure the majority of cancer patients, as the disease is so often metastasized at presentation.

Cancer chemotherapy is a modality which does have the potential to cure patients with this advanced stage of disease. In recent years the three modalities have been combined more and more, and here is one of the reasons why the prospectives for the cancer patient have improved so much. In addition, certain types of cancers, such as testicular carcinoma, childhood tumors, choriocarcinoma, non Hodgkin lymphomas and others, can now indeed often be cured by chemotherapy alone, even if the disease is advanced. The combination of drugs and the use of new drugs have greatly contributed to this development. There are two main groups of new drugs: analogs and new structures. A great number of analogs of conventional structures have been developed during the past ten years. A typical example of this group is adriamycin, which is an analog of daunomycin. The development of new structures, which is probaly even more important, is presently a main field of interest of the "Koningin Wilhelmina Fonds".

Prior to reach the stage of clinical use any new structure has to pass through a sequence of events, which may be referred to as drug development. These events include the isolation, synthesis or other ways of acquisition of the material. Thereafter, the main phase is that in which anti-tumor activity is indentified. For this purpose op to now, the animal screening models have been used. In case an agent proves to

D.N. Reinhoudt, T.A. Connors, H.M. Pinedo & K.W. van de Poll (eds.), Structure-Activity Relationships of Anti-Tumour Agents.
© *1983, Martinus Nijhoff Publishers, The Hague/Boston/London. ISBN 90-247-2783-9.*

have anti-tumor activity it needs to be formulated. Following this phase
preclinical toxicology studies on the drug are essential to establish
a safe starting dose for clinical trial in man. Finally, Phase I clinical
trials are performed to establish safe doses and schedules for new drugs.

The field of drug development has been triggered in Europe by the
activities of the European Organisation on Research and on Treatment of Cancer.
The "Koningin Wilhelmina Fonds" and the Cancer Research Campaign have
stimulated drug development vigorously. There has been a close cooperation
between scientists in this field of cancer research in the Netherlands
and the United Kingdom.

In the past, the first step of drug development, the design and
acquisition of new drugs, has relied mainly on an empirical approach.
Unfortunately, often the agents which were developed appeared to be either
inactive or too toxic. It is evident that clinical studies with such
agents were not justifiable. Fortunately, the biochemical basis for drug
action is now somewhat better understood. New targets in the cell are
being identified. However, more knowledge on biochemical differences
between tumor cells and normal cells is required. This brings me back
to the term selective toxicity, which may be defined as that property
of a drug that enables it to kill tumor cells while leaving normal cells
undamaged. With our present knowledge it appears desirable to develop
and select new chemical structures on a more rational basis. This holds
also for the development of analogs with less toxicity to normal cells.

In order to stimulate research on structure activity relationship
it is essential that tumor biochemists and biologists share their knowledge with the numerous excellent chemists interested in developing new
anti-cancer agents. For this reason the creation of multidisciplinary
working parties, such as that on Pharmacology of anti-neoplastic agents,
has been encouraged by the "Koningin Wilhelmina Fonds".

The limited knowledge on structure-activity relationship of anticancer agents has been holding up drug development. For this reason the
"Koningin Wilhelmina Fonds" and the Cancer Research Campaign have orga-
nised a Workshop on "Structure activity relationship" aiming to dissemi-
nate the knowledge in this field of research among the many excellent
chemists in the Netherlands and the United Kingdom. This Conference was
held from March 11 - 13, 1982. The world's leading experts in the field
were invited to present papers on the most important agents presently

being used in Cancer Chemotherapy. Ample time was allotted for the lively discussion which followed each presentation, which I will briefly summarize.

In the first lecture Dr. Narayanan discussed the strategy for the discovery of new anti-cancer drugs which is presently being followed at the National Cancer Institute in the U.S.A.

Thereafter Dr. Rekker presented the concepts of quantitative structure-activity relationships (QSAR). These relationships can be formulated for congeneric groups of antineoplastic agents, and may be of great value in guiding the investigator's decision- making in the synthesis of new and more effective congenus.

Dr. Connors discussed the structure-activity relationships of alkylating prodrugs. Examples were given of how selectivity can be achieved by the design of latent drugs which would be activated at least to a large extent, by tumor cells and to a much lesser extent by normal cells, particularly by those sensitive to alkylating agents. He also discussed the alternative which is the synthesis of very reactive alkylating agents which could be quickly metabolized to less reactive and non-toxic products in normal cells by enzymes lacking in malignant cells.

A most topical subject was that presented by Dr. Cleare. He discussed the structure activity relationship of various platinum analogs which are presently being studied preclinically and clinically in Europe and the U.S.A.

Dr. Moore presented a simple scheme for identification of naturally occurring quinones with appropriate structural features required to allow them to function as potential bioreductive alkylating agents.

Dr. Driscoll gave data on quinone families which are being studied in clinical trials. He reviewed in particular the aziridinylquinones and anthracene diones.

The interesting field of the doxorubicin analogs has been covered by Dr. Arcamone who has developed the parent compound in the past. He discussed various groups of analogs of doxorubicin with modifications on ring A, the sugar moiety or the anthraquinone moiety.

Dr. Paoletti presented evidence for the theory that 9-hydroxy ellipticine derivatives exert their cytotoxic effects through at least 3 types of interactions with the cell components: 1) generation of free radicals; 2) generation of covalent adducts with molecules carrying nucleophilic centers; and 3) catalytic consumption of NADH.

4

The mechanism of action of DTIC has been discussed by Dr. Stevens who concluded that DTIC most probably is a pro-drug of which the active drug is the monomethyl metabolite which either methylates DNA or inter-acts with enzyme targets. Evidence which supports this hypothesis is given. He also discussed a series of molecules which could be considered second-generation triazenes.

One of the pioneers in the field of structure activity relationship, Dr. Montgomery, gave a lecture on his main field of interest, the nitro-soureas. The relationship of the chemistry , chemical reactivity, water lipid solubility, nature of the carrier group, and metabolism to the biologic active form of these compounds, as well as their possible macro-molecular targets have been presented.

Another pioneer in the field, Dr. Brock, elucidated the structure activity relationship of the oxazaphosphorines and their relative selec-tivity.

Last but not least, Dr. Umezawa, the discoverer of the bleomycins presented studies on antitumor antibiotics, low molecular weight immuno-modifiers and their analogs and derivatives.

It is evident that we were most fortunate to have such a selection of guest speakers at this workshop who are the most knowlegeable and experienced scientists in this particular field of cancer research. The participants and speakers have had a unique opportunity for ample scientific discussions and exchange of ideas.

We wish to thank all participants for their contribution in the discussion and hope that the conference will have contributed to the creation of the scientific basis which is necessary for the development of new active antineoplastic structures.

Finally, we thank the "Koningin Wilhelmina Fonds" and the Cancer Research Campaign both of which have created the possibility for orga-nising this succesful workshop.

H.M. Pinedo

STRATEGY FOR THE DISCOVERY AND DEVELOPMENT OF NOVEL ANTICANCER AGENTS

V.L. NARAYANAN

1. INTRODUCTION

The task of new anticancer drug discovery is particularly difficult because of two main reasons: (a) the lack of adequate knowledge of the biochemistry of the tumor cell types and the way in which tumor cells differ from normal cells; and (b) the low predictability of animal tumor models, especially for solid tumors. The strategy for new drug discovery involves two key steps: lead identification and structure-activity/toxicity fine tuning. A small but significant number of new drug discoveries stem from "rational drug design" and "analog synthesis." We have adopted a pragmatic approach to new anticancer drug discovery which is in essence a combination of both the "rational" and "random" processes, the "selective-random approach." This strategy for the discovery and development of new anticancer agents, currently in place at the National Cancer Institute (NCI), will be discussed as outlined in Figure 1.

PROGRAM STRATEGY

Discovery and Development of New Anticancer Agents

- Multidisciplinary System

- Conceptual Frame-works
  - Structure-Activity Analysis
  - Mathematical Modelling
  - Sub-structure Analysis

  Uniqueness ⟨ ⟩ Computer Assisted

  - Selected-Random Approach

- Operational Logic

- Results
  - Examples of Unique Compounds Under Development

FIGURE 1. Strategy for new drug discovery.

D.N. Reinhoudt, T.A. Connors, H.M. Pinedo & K.W. van de Poll (eds.), Structure-Activity Relationships of Anti-Tumour Agents.
© 1983, Martinus Nijhoff Publishers, The Hague/Boston/London. ISBN 90-247-2783-9.

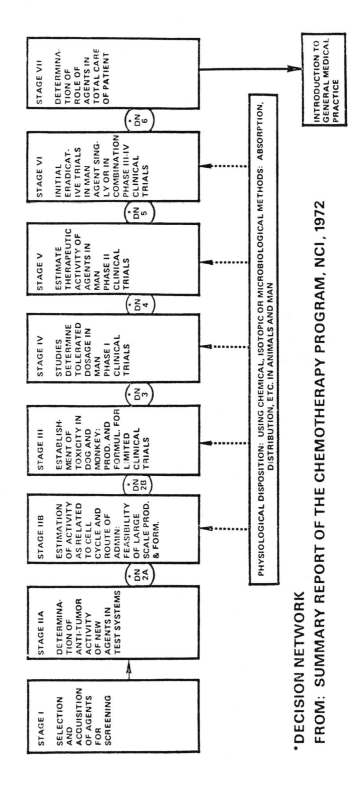

FIGURE 2. Linear Array for drug development.

We have adopted a multidisciplinary systems approach for new drug discovery and development based on continuous interactions and feedback between medicinal chemists, biologists, pharmacists, and clinicians. The various stages of drug development and the logic which guides the program is called the Linear Array and is outlined in Figure 2. It delineates the steps which must take place to assure the flow of compounds through the experimental systems and into the clinic (1). It also spells out the criteria for moving candidate compounds from one stage of development to another.

The program has undergone many changes and refinements over the years. Our discussions will focus on the input side: (a) selection and acquisition of compounds, expecially of synthetic origin (Stage I); and (b) biological evaluation (Stage IIA). Finally, we will describe the novel compounds that are in various stages of development.

The flow of synthetic compounds occurs in three distinct stages as outlined in Figure 3: the acquisition phase, the preselection phase and the anticancer evaluation phase. Several mechanisms are available for the input of unique compounds to the program; namely, voluntary submissions, active solicitations, contracts and grants. The vast majority of compounds are acquired from industries, both domestic and foreign, on a voluntary basis under provisions of confidentiality. Continuous literature surveillance is also employed to select compounds on the basis of relevant chemical, biochemical, pharmacological and biological criteria. These compounds encompass a large variety of structural types prepared as synthetic or iso-

SYNTHETIC COMPOUNDS FLOW CHART

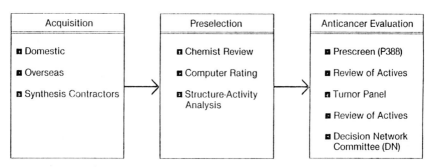

Acquisition	Preselection	Anticancer Evaluation
◘ Domestic	◘ Chemist Review	◘ Prescreen (P388)
◘ Overseas	◘ Computer Rating	◘ Review of Actives
◘ Synthesis Contractors	◘ Structure-Activity Analysis	◘ Tumor Panel
		◘ Review of Actives
		◘ Decision Network Committee (DN)

FIGURE 3. Flow of synthetic compounds.

lated from plants or fermentation broths. The details of the acquisition process are outlined in Figure 4.

2. SCREENING

Before describing the preselection process, it is appropriate
to summarize the biological systems that are used to evaluate new
compounds (Figure 5) (2). The mouse P388 leukemia model is used a
a prescreen to select new compounds for tumor panel evaluation.
Occasionally, the P388 prescreen is bypassed for compounds that
have shown either (a) activity in antitumor screens not available
at NCI or (b) pertinent biochemical or biological activities. The
current tumor panel consists of eight cancer models in mice--five
transplanted mouse tumors (L1210 leukemia, B16 melanoma, colon,
breast and lung) and three human tumor xenografts (colon, breast
and lung) implanted under the kidney capsules of mice. Two different parameters are used for evaluating the activity of a compoun
namely; either the increase in life span of the treated mice versu
the control or the reduction in tumor weight. The route and shed-
ule of administration of the compound and activity criteria that
are used to evaluate new agents are outlined in Table 1.

3. PRESELECTION

The objective of preselection is to enhance the cost-effectiv
ness of the drug discovery process by decreasing the number of com
pounds acquired for screening while improving the quality and the
quantity of potentially active input to the tumor panel. We currently utilize a two-stage selection process, namely; (a) a computerized model and (b) structure-activity analysis and chemist
review (see Figure 6).

3.1. Computerized Model

In 1975 Dr. Louis Hodes at NCI initiated a new statistical-
heuristic method for selecting compounds for screening using molecular structure features as predictors of biological activity (3).
The method has been refined over the years and the main characteristics of the model are outlined in Figure 7. The features used
are those routinely generated as keys for the substructure inquiry
system. The system incorporates an open-ended feature set as
opposed to a dictionary (>5000 structural features). The main

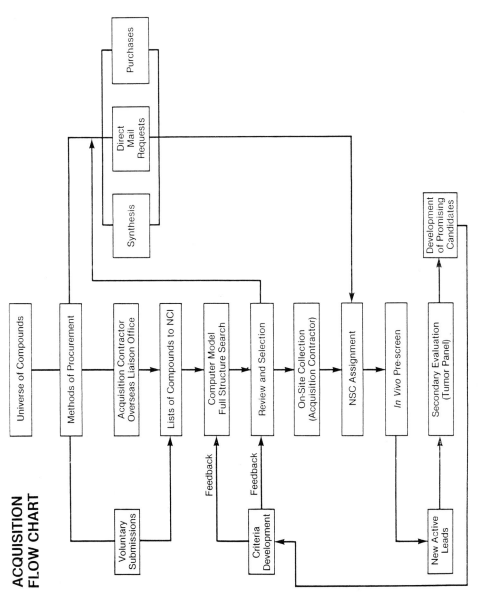

FIGURE 4. Details of the acquisition process.

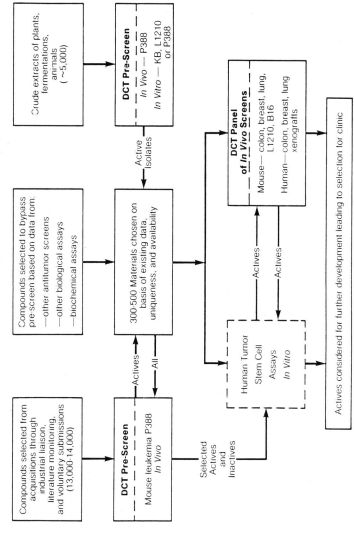

Flow of Drugs Through DCT Screens, 1980

Crude extracts of plants, fermentations, animals (~5,000)

DCT Pre-Screen

In Vivo — P388

In Vitro — KB, L1210 or P388

Active Isolates

Compounds selected to bypass pre-screen based on data from:
—other antitumor screens
—other biological assays
—biochemical assays

300-500 Materials chosen on basis of existing data, uniqueness, and availability

Compounds selected from acquisitions through industrial liaison, literature monitoring, and voluntary submissions (13,000-14,000)

DCT Pre-Screen

Mouse leukemia P388
In Vivo

Actives

All

Selected Actives and Inactives

Human Tumor Stem Cell Assays *In Vitro*

DCT Panel of *In Vivo* Screens

Mouse— colon, breast, lung, L1210, B16

Human—colon, breast, lung xenografts

Actives

Actives

Actives considered for further development leading to selection for clinic

FIGURE 5. Summary of biological systems used to evaluate new compounds.

SCREENING SCORECARD

Model	Code	Drug Rt./Sched.	Parameter	Active T/C%	
				DN1(+)	DN2(++)
Prescreen					
IP P388 Leukemia	3PS31	IP/Q1D×5	med survival time	≥120	≥175
Transplanted Mouse Tumors					
*IP B16 Melanoma	3B131	IP/Q1D×9	med survival time	≥125	≥150
SC B16 Melanoma	3B132	IP/Q1D×9	med survival time	≥140	≥150
*SC CD8F$_1$ Mammary	3CDJ2	IP/Q1D×1	med tumor wt change	≤20	≤0
	3CD72	IP/Q7D×5	med tumor wt	≤42	≤10
IP Colon 26	3C631	IP/Q4D×2	med survival time	≥130	≥150
*SC Colon 38	3C872	IP/Q7D×2	med tumor wt	≤42	≤10
IC Ependymoblastoma	3EM37	IP/Q1D×5	med survival time	≥125	≥150
*IV Lewis Lung	3LL39	IP/Q1D×9	med survival time	≥140	≥150
*IP L1210 Leukemia	3LE31	IP/Q1D×9	med survival time	≥125	≥150
	3LE21	IP/Q1D×9	mean survival time	≥125	≥150
SC M5 Ovarian	3M572	IP/Q2D×11	med tumor wt	≤42	≤10
Human Tumor Xenografts					
*SRC CX-1 Colon	3C2G5	SC/Q4D×4	mean tumor wt change	≤20	≤10
SC CX-1 Colon	3C2H2	IP/Q4D×3	mean tumor wt change	≤20	≤10
*SRC LX-1 Lung	3LKG5	SC/Q4D×3	mean tumor wt change	≤20	≤10
SC LX-1 Lung	3LKH2	IP/Q4D×3	mean tumor wt change	≤20	≤10
*SRC MX-1 Mammary	3MBG5	SC/Q4D×3	mean tumor wt change	≤20	≤10
SC MX-1 Mammary	3MBH2	IP/Q4D×3	mean tumor wt change	≤20	≤10

Table 1. Screening information.

*denotes system that is routinely used.

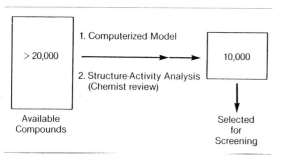

PRE-SELECTION 1982

> 20,000

1. Computerized Model

⟶ 10,000

2. Structure-Activity Analysis
(Chemist review)

Available
Compounds

Selected
for
Screening

COMPUTERIZED MODEL

- Evaluates Broad Range of Compounds
- Utilizes Structural Fragments (Keys)
- Utilizes Total Screening Experience
- Integrates Massive Volume of Structural
  Data and Screening Experience
  to Predict:

  Novelty
  and
  Activity

FIGURE 6.   Selection process.

FIGURE 7. Characteristics of
computerized model.

types of keys are (see Figure 8):

1).   Augmented atom keys (AA)

2).   Ganglia augmented atom keys (GAA)

3).   Ring keys

4).   Two kinds of nucleus keys

5).   Individual element keys.

The method assigns weight to each feature according to the statistical significance of its contribution to activity using the P388
test data.   An unknown compound is scored by adding the weights of
its dozen or so structure features.   The score is not intended to
estimate the strength of activity, but only provide some measure o
the likelihood that the compound is active.

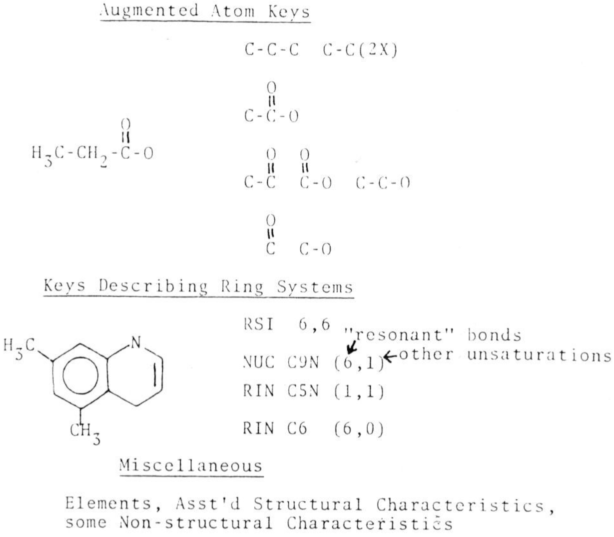

Augmented Atom Keys

C-C-C   C-C(2X)

$$C-\overset{\overset{O}{\|}}{C}-O$$

$H_3C-CH_2-\overset{\overset{O}{\|}}{C}-O$

$C-\overset{\overset{O}{\|}}{C}$ $\overset{\overset{O}{\|}}{C}-O$ C-C-O

$\overset{\overset{O}{\|}}{C}$ C-O

Keys Describing Ring Systems

RSI   6,6   "resonant" bonds
NUC C9N (6,1)←other unsaturations
RIN C5N (1,1)
RIN C6   (6,0)

Miscellaneous

Elements, Asst'd Structural Characteristics,
some Non-structural Characteristics

FIGURE 8. Types of keys.

Another useful measure supplied by the computer is an indication of novelty based on the more than 100,000 compounds tested in P388 regardless of activity. Compounds are flagged as unique if they have a key which never occurred in all P388 testing. For each new compound, the feature that occurs least often in P388 testing is printed along with its frequency of occurrence. If the least-occurring key in the compound occurred more than 50 times, the compound is considered adequately studied. Novelty score is even more useful in selecting compounds for acquisition.

The method has undergone a great deal of development and testing. As a result of two prospective experiments, the method became operational as of March 1980. All potential acquisitions are rated for novelty and activity (see Tables 2 and 3). A recent analysis

Novelty Rating	Decision
U = Unique Key	Select
N = Common Key	Deselect

Activity Rating	Decision
J = Highest Rating	Select
A = Lowest Rating	Deselect
B-I = Intermediate Ratings	Chemist Judgement

Tables 2 and 3. Novelty and activity ratings.

14

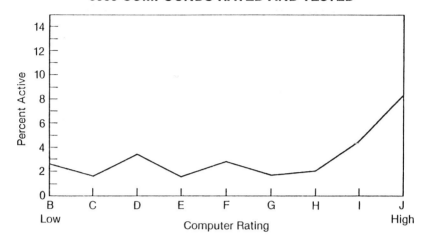

(Compounds Acquired from March, 1980, to October 1980)
(Test Data current to August, 1981)
FIGURE 9. Analysis of the performance of the computer
model.

of the performance of the model is illustrated in Figure 9.

It must be emphasized that although this method is computerized, it is not designed to automatically pass or reject compounds
Rather, it is proposed as a tool to aid the medicinal chemist in
selecting compounds. Although its assumption of feature indepen-
dence is a strong limitation, the unbiased use of much data should
make the scores useful. The best way to use the computer lies in
eliminating compounds from screening. It supplements the intuitio
of the chemist.

3.2. Structure-activity analysis

Detailed structure-activity analyses based on our large chem-
ical-biological data bsse are an essential part of acquisition and
synthesis activities. Compounds are coded as they are selected fo
screening. The performance of particular sets of compounds can
then be evaluated and structure-activity relationships determined.
Some of the codes used include bioactivity, structural fragments
and computer model rating codes (Table 4). Such large-scale
analyses of NCI data files have become feasible because of the
development of the chemistry-biology interlink and its active
implementation during this year.

STRUCTURE-ACTIVITY ANALYSIS

General Category	Codes	Examples
Bioactivity	X00R	Anthelmintics
	X02W	Antivirals
Structure Fragments	X18A	$-S-\overset{R}{\underset{\|}{C}}=N-N$
	X11H	$-O-\overset{N}{\overset{\|\|}{C}}-S-S-$
	Z0004	
Computer Model Ratings	X73J	Highest Activity Rating

Table 4. Codes used in structure-activity
analysis.

Two examples of such structure-activity analyses are tin compounds (Table 5) and cyclic methylene ketones, lactones and lactams (Tables 6 and 7). Such structure-activity studies allow us to select compounds maximizing structural uniqueness and anticancer potential.

4. RESULTS

Figures 10 through 12 illustrate some examples of the unique compounds that are currently under active development at NCI. The spectrum of activity of each compound, as well as its stage of development, is indicated. Specific details on several compounds will be provided by other speakers on the symposium and hence will not be detailed here. In particular, we would like to draw your attention to 2-β-D-ribofuranosylthiazole-4-carboxamide (NSC-286193) (Figure 10) whose activity against the Lewis lung carcinoma is exceptional for both its degree of activity and its range of

EVALUATION OF TIN COMPOUNDS

Description	No. of Compds. Tested	No. Tested in P388	% Activity in P388	No. Tested in L1210	% Activity in L1210
Tin Compounds	1554	680	25	696	1.0
C—Sn(—HT)(—HT)(C)	327	129	48	136	1.0
SN (Coordinated)	160	143	50	35	0.0
C—Sn(C)(C)—C	358	132	9	203	0.0
C—Sn(C)(C)—C	339	166	2	144	0.4
C—Sn(HT)(HT)—HT	33	11	9	11	0.0
HT—Sn(HT)(HT)—HT	45	15	7	10	0.0

*HT = Any atom except C or H (Mainly N, S or halogen)   —— = Another bond may or may not exist

Table 5. Evaluation of tin compounds.

CYCLIC METHYLENE KETONES, LACTONES AND LACTAMS

R	R$_1$	Y	Ring Sizes	Number in P388	% Act. P388	Number in L1210	% Act. L1210
Any	Element	C	All Sizes	292	6	272	1
H	H	C	All Sizes	38	15	6	0
H	H	O	All Sizes	240	23	140	1
H	H	N	All Sizes	10	0	36	0
H	H	S	— —	—	—	—	—
H	H	P	— —	—	—	—	—
H	H	O	5*	220	24	126	1
H	H	O	5**	12	22	17	3
H	H	N	5*	—	—	—	—
H	H	HT	6*	14	36	21	0
H	H	HT	7*	4	0	—	—
Any	Ring	HT	All Sizes	98	18	127	1

HT = Any element except C or H;　　* = Fusion allowed　　** = No fusion

Table 6. Evaluation of cyclic methylene ketones, lactones, lactams

Compounds Which Incorporate a "Proximal" Oxygen to the Methylene Group

Y	No. of Compounds Tested	No. in P388	Activity % P388	No. in L1210	Activity % L1210
HT	233	129	29	91	1
O	203	129	29	62	2
N	28	None	—	29	0
C	8	6	44	3	0

Table 7. Compounds which incorporate a "proximal" oxygen to the methylene group.

18

PROMISING NEW LEADS
SYNTHETIC COMPOUNDS IN TOXICOLOGY

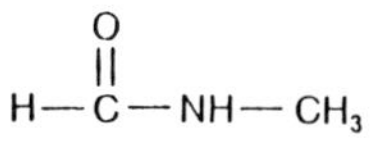

N-Methylformamide
NSC-3051

Tumor Model	Activity
P388	+
L1210	+
CX1	+ +
LX1	+ +
MX1	+ +

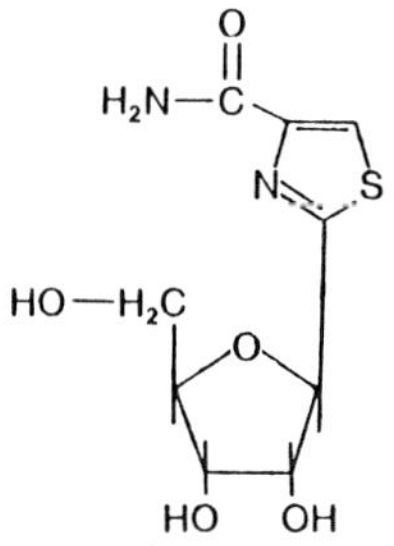

TCAR
NSC-286193

Tumor Model	Activity
P388	+ +
L1210	+ +
Lewis Lung	+ +

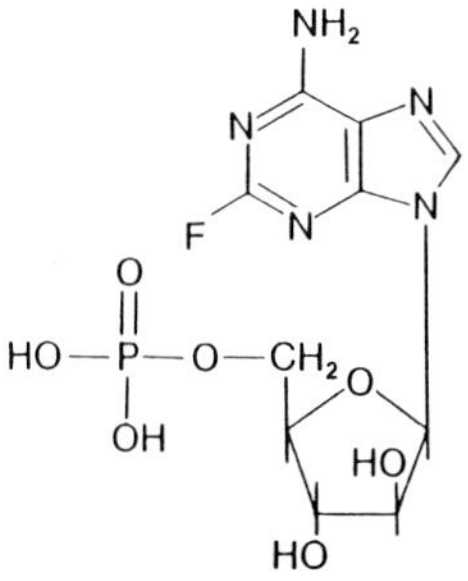

2-Fluoro-Ara-AMP
NSC-312887

Tumor Model	Activity
P388	+ +
L1210	+ +
LX1	+ +

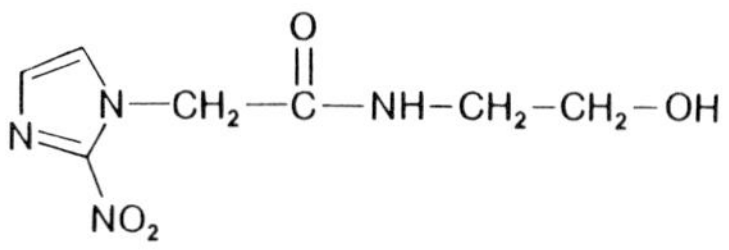

SR-2508
NSC-301467

Radiosensitizer

FIGURE 10. Promising new synthetic compounds in toxicology.

PROMISING NEW LEADS
SYNTHETIC COMPOUNDS EXPECTED TO
ENTER TOXICOLOGY DURING 1981

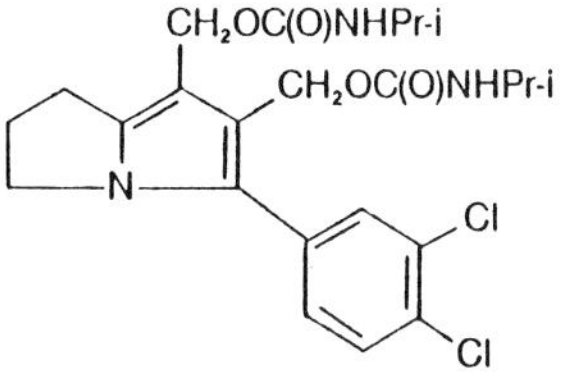

CH$_2$OC(O)NHPr-i
CH$_2$OC(O)NHPr-i

Cl
Cl

NSC-278214

Tumor Model	Activity
P388	+ +
B16	+ +
CD8F$_1$	+ +
Colon 38	+
L1210	+
MX1	+ +

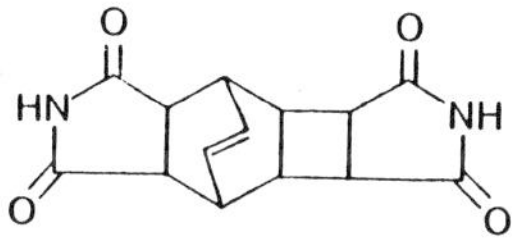

NSC-284356

Tumor Model	Activity
P388	+ +
B16	+
CD8F$_1$	+ +
Colon 38	+
L1210	+ +

· HCl

Me

HN

Me—N—Ac

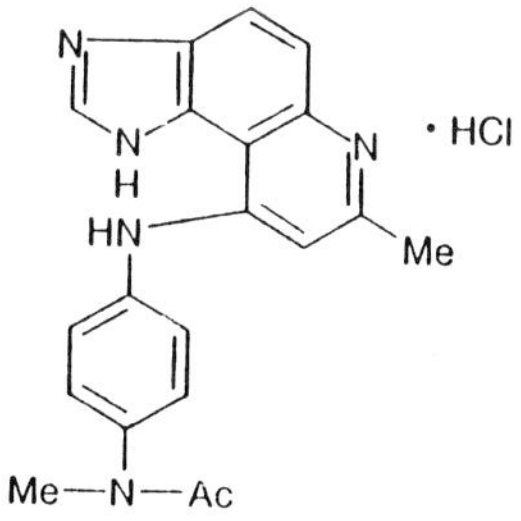

NSC-305884

Tumor Model	Activity
P388	+ +
B16	+ +

Me—O— —S—NH—N=CH—C—OH

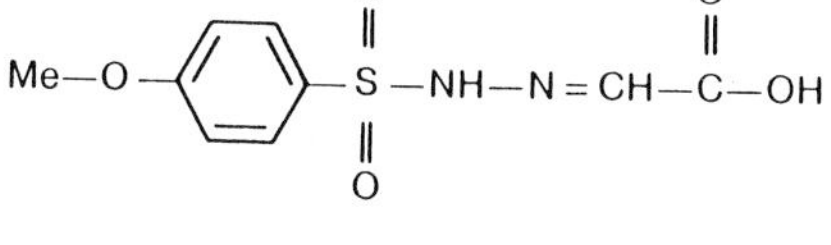

NSC-267213

Tumor Model	Activity
P388	+
L1210	+ +
B16	+
CD8F$_1$	+
MX1	+ +

FIGURE 11. Promising new synthetic compounds entering toxicology in 1981.

**PROMISING NEW LEADS
SYNTHETIC COMPOUNDS EXPECTED TO
ENTER TOXICOLOGY DURING 1981 (Continued)**

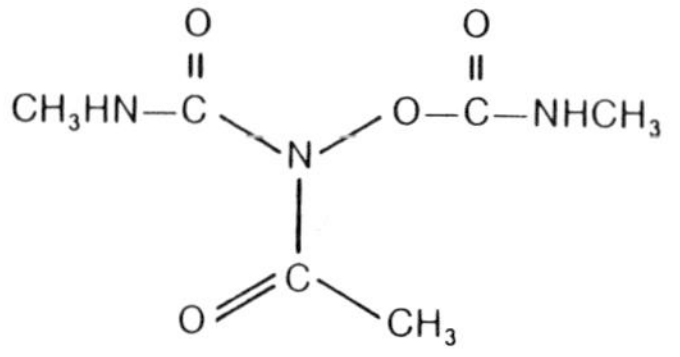

Tumor Model	Activity
P388	+
CX 1	+
MX 1	+ +

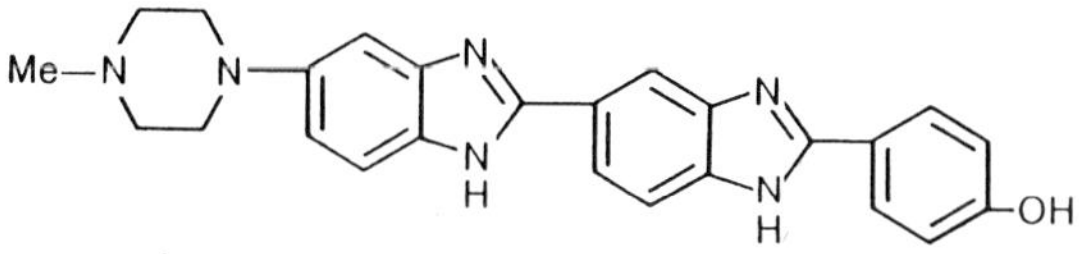

NSC-253272

• 3 HCl

Tumor Model	Activity
P388	+
L1210	+ +
MX 1	+ (?)

NSC-322921

FIGURE 11. Cont'd.

INVESTIGATIONAL NEW DRUG APPLICATIONS — 1975 TO 1981

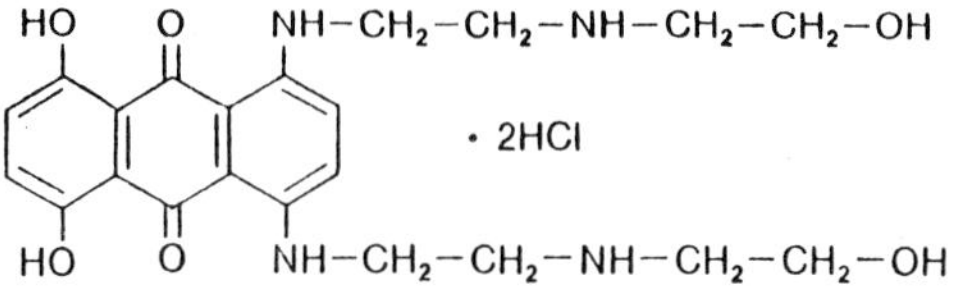

• 2HCl

Mitoxantrone
NSC-301739

Tumor Model	Activity
P388	+ +
B16	+ +
CD8F₁	+
Colon 38	+ +
L1210	+ +

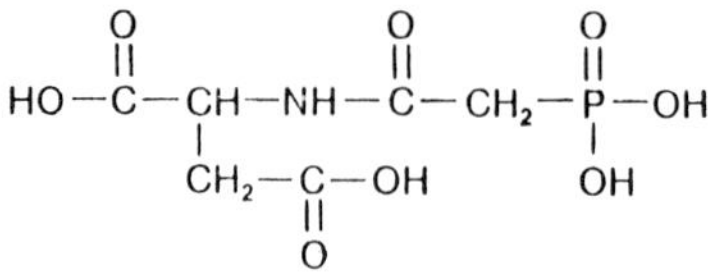

• 4Na

PALA
NSC-224131

Tumor Model	Activity
P388	+
B16	+ +
CD8F₁	+ +
Colon 38	+
Lewis Lung	+ +

FIGURE 12. Compounds with Investigational New Drug Applications.

INVESTIGATIONAL NEW DRUG APPLICATIONS
1975 TO 1981 (Cont'd)

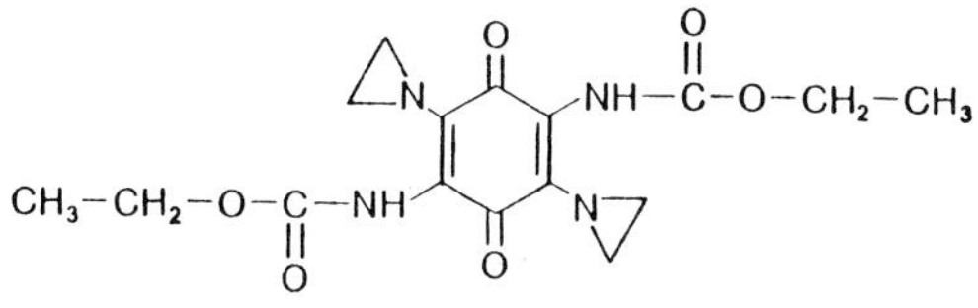

Tumor Model	Activity
P388	+ +
B16	+
CD8F,	+
Colon 38	+
L1210	+ +
MX1	+ +

AZQ
NSC-182986

Tumor Model	Activity
P388	+ +
B16	+ +
CD8F,	+ +
Colon 38	+
L1210	+ +

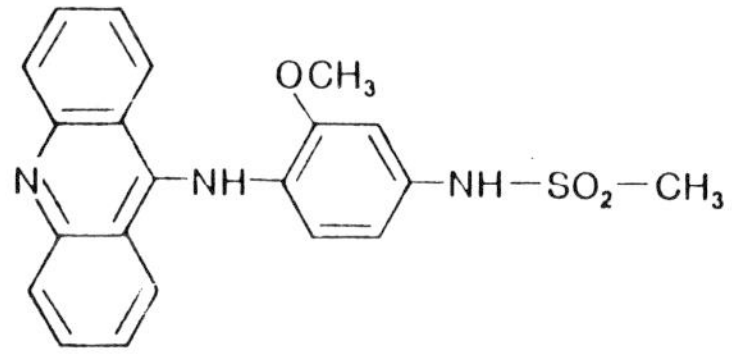

AMSA
NSC-249992

Tumor Model	Activity
P388	+ +
B16	+ +
CD8F,	+ +
Colon 38	+
L1210	+ +
Lewis Lung	+ +
LX1	+ +
MX1	+ +

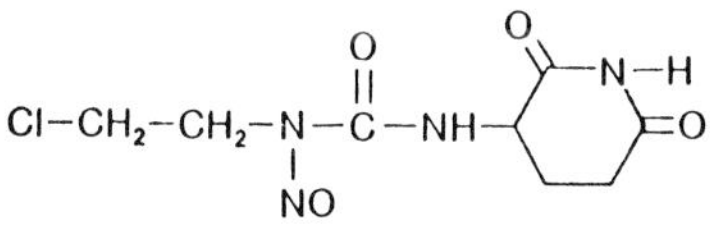

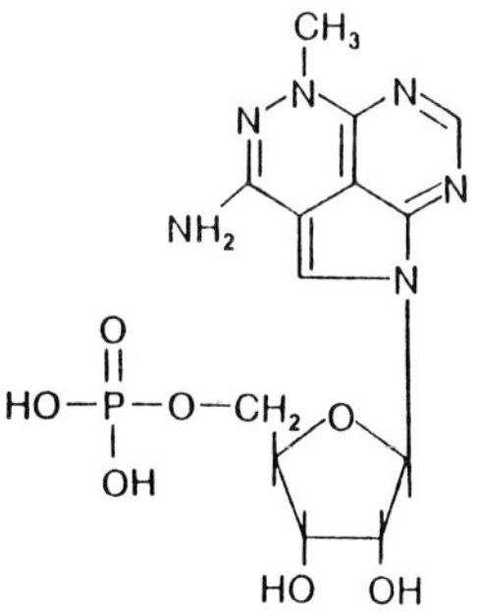

PCNU
NSC-95466

Tumor Model	Activity
P388	+
CD8F,	+
L1210	+ +
MX1	+ +

Tricyclic Nucleotide
NSC-280594

FIGURE 12. Investigational New Drug Applications, cont'd.

EFFECT OF NSC-286193 ON LIFE-SPAN OF MICE INOCULATED
I.V. WITH LEWIS LUNG CARCINOMA

Lewis lung tumor cells (10^6) were implanted i.v. in groups of 10 BDF$_1$ mice (experiment 1) or B6C3F$_1$ mice (experiment 2) (40 mice in untreated control groups) 24 hr. before initiation of therapy. An aqueous solution of NSC-286193 was administered daily on days 1 to 9.

NSC 286193 Dose (mg/kg/injection)	Survival Time (Days) Median	Range *	ILS (%)	60-Day Survivors
Untreated Controls	25	18-35	—	0/40
800	60	7-18	140	6/10
400	60	7-12	140	7/10
200	60	—	140	10/10
100	60	17	140	9/10
50	60	—	140	10/10
25	60	—	140	10/10

*Dying mice only.

Table 8.   Range of activity of NSC-286193.

effective doses (Table 8). (4). We are currently pursuing NSC-286193 as a high-prioity candidate for clinical trials with potential importance for treatment of lung tumors and metastases.

5. CONCLUSION

In summary, our strategy for the development of new anticancer agents has been productive in identifying novel synthetic compounds active against a spectrum of solid tumors; melanoma, mammary, colon and lung. Because of the long lead time, none of the newer compounds have yet received New Drug Applications (NDA's). Some of these compounds are in Phase II clinical trials, some are in toxicology, and others are in earlier stages and are actively being developed toward the clinic. Thus the future looks promising.

REFERENCES

1. deVita VT, Oliverio VT, Muggia FM, Wiernik PW, Ziegler J, Goldin A, Rubin D, Henney J, Schepartz SA. 1979. Cancer Clin. Trials 2, 195.
2. Goldin A, Venditti JM. 1980. In "Recent Results in Cancer Research" (S.K. Carter and Y. Sakurai, eds.), Vol. 7, pp 5-20, Spring-Verlag, Berlin.
3. Hodes L, Hazard GF, Geran RI, Richman S. 1977. J.Med. Chem. 20, 469.
4. Robbins RK, Srivastava DC, Narayanan VL, Plowman J, Paull KD. 1931. J.Med. Chem. 25, 107.

QUANTITATIVE STRUCTURE – ACTIVITY RELATIONSHIP STUDIES AROUND CYTOTOXIC DRUGS

R.F. REKKER

Summary: The aim of a common QSAR (Quantitative Structure – Activity Relationship) approach is the correlation of a set of biological test-data with a set of appropriately quantified structural features.

These test-data should be obtained from (a) well-defined interactions between chemical substances belonging to (b) congeneric series of structures and (c) an active site in a biological system.

In general, toxicological phenomena do not fulfil this requirement since they are not in the least representing a well-defined interaction. Test-data obtained on carcinogenic structures probably belong to the same category, being reflections of extensively complex and incomprehensible interactions between chemical structures and bio-systems.

Anti-tumor activities, on the contrary, look much more promising for a successful attack by QSAR approaches.

A detailed overview will be given of the HANSCH and FREE – WILSON approaches including a discussion on the most important physicochemical parameters in use in HANSCH-type QSAR models.

Due emphasis is given to lipophilicity, apparently one of the most important among the parameters in QSAR studies.

Examples for illustration are selected from both categories of compounds: carcinogenic and anti-tumor active structures.

1. INTRODUCTION

One may make as heavy work of the problems around the theme QSAR of cancerogenic and antitumor activities as one wishes to do. This is shown up clearly by a recent publication by Von HOFF et al (1) in Cancer Chemother. Pharmacol. with the arresting title: "Does Color of an Anti-tumor Agent Predict for Clinical Antitumor Activity?"

For statistical reasons, a certain parallelism between colour and clinical antitumor activity seems undeniable (see Table 1). It would be quite unwise, however, to consider the method as a serious tool in finding new active compounds. Only in cases where rapid decisions have to be made in a group with established activities, it might facilitate a choice.

D.N. Reinhoudt, T.A. Connors, H.M. Pinedo & K.W. van de Poll (eds.), Structure-Activity Relationships of Anti-Tumour Agents.
© 1983, Martinus Nijhoff Publishers, The Hague/Boston/London. ISBN 90-247-2783-9.

Table 1. Classification of Antitumor Active Agents (Von HOFF et al)

	Totals	Insufficient clin.inform.	Classified	Classification
Coloured	21	5	16	13 / 16
White or clear	50	10	40	20 / 40
Total	71	15	56	33 / 56

Our final conclusion: a relatively easily excitable electronic system seems to be a necessary though insufficient prerequisite for clinical antitumor activity.

A few years ago (2) I described QSAR as a kind of manipulation between "drop and lock". This description has been borrowed from a lecture given by MAUTNER in Jeruzalem in 1974 (3) and it shows striking resemblance with the Rube GOLDBERG constructions which were quite popular in the thirties (4). MAUTNER's concept shows a black box with a locked door and, on top, a handle. By turning this handle a tap is opened (which appears, of course, only later) and the running water collects dropwise in a beaker kept in balance by a burning candle and located under a string stretched through the box. Suspended from this string, a key is hanging over a monkey's head. One will easily understand what happens: the burning candle is put out of balance and rises, the string burns through, the key falls and the monkey, clever as it is, grabs the key and unlocks (see Fig. 1).

The most frequently used models for describing structure – activity relationships are those of FREE – WILSON and HANSCH. They will receive due attention in next section.

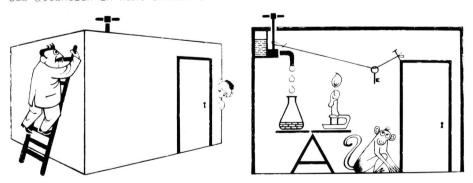

FIGURE 1. Black box; closed and open.

2. QSAR MODELS

2.1. FREE-WILSON Model

The FREE-WILSON model (5) describes structure-activity relation-ships by associating the biological activity of a molecule with the ac-tivity of a basic structure along with the total of the contribu-tions of the various substituting groups to the overall activity:

$$BR = \mu + \sum AB_n \qquad \text{(eqn 1)}$$

In this formula BR represents the biological response, which, on the basis of the original concept and as the occasion demands, can be intro-duced either as a linear or as a logarithmic value. Later work (6,7,8) has revealed, however, that the use of non-logarithmic BR-values is ac-tually incorrect.

Fig. 2a schematizes the most salient points of the FREE-WILSON model; the centrally drawn circle denotes the basic structure with ac-

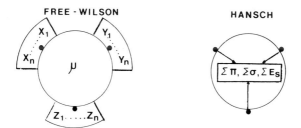

FIGURE 2. Schematized FREE-WILSON (a) and HANSCH (b) models

tivity μ and round about the three (or more) segments X, Y and Z indi-cate the three (or more) regions of the molecule where substitution has taken place. The various substituents in each of these regions have been consecutively numbered from 1 to n and their proper contributions (B) to total activity have been incorporated in the term $\sum AB_n$ of eqn 1; factor A has a value 0 or 1, depending on the absence or presence of a given group in the position indicated, whereas if this group is attached to an asymmetrical centre, A becomes 0, 1 or 0.5. In the latter case, the fi-nal choice depends on whether one of the optical isomers or a racemic product is involved. It will be clear, that both μ and the various B's function as unknowns in eqn 1, so that a set of equations is actually required to obtain a proper solution of the FREE-WILSON model. Such solution - in order to have significance - needs the availability of a

sufficiently extended set of structures with a well-balanced distribution pattern of the applied substituents over the substitution regions.
Many cases are known where these conditions were grossly neglected.

A striking example — though outside the context of the present themes —
is the FREE – WILSON treatment performed by BERKOFF et al (9) on the
antimycoplasmal activity (against M. salivarium) in a series of quinoline hydrazones.

with

R_1 = 3-pyrrolyl, 2-pyrrolyl, 6-methyl-2-
        pyrrolyl, 5-nitrofuranyl, 3-pyridyl,
        2-pyridyl or 4-pyridyl;
R_2 = H, CH_3 or C_6H_5;
R_6 = H, F, CH_3, CH_3O or CF_3;
R_7 = H, F, CH_3, CH_3O or CF_3;
R_8 = H, F, CH_3, CH_3O or CF_3;

Five substitution regions were used and this transformed eqn 1 into
eqn 2:

$$\log BR = \mu + \sum AB(R_1) + \sum AB(R_2) + \sum AB(R_6) + \sum AB(R_7) + \sum AB(R_8) \qquad (\text{eqn }2)$$

For 108 quinoline hydrazones eqn 2 could be worked out to a set of equations with 26 unknowns, which yielded a final solution with correlation
coefficient r = 0.69 and a standard error of the estimate s = 0.813.
Altogether a very bad result, which made the authors decide to repeat
the computation procedure on a reduced set of 22 derivatives, with the
underlined substituents given above missing and deminishing the total
number of unknowns to 19. The solution of this reduced set yielded a
statistics with r = 0.897 and s = 0.476. The authors considered these
results satisfying enough although they admitted that the correlation
failed to pass a proper F-test; F appeared to be 2.55 and at the 5%
confidence level it requires a value of 3.25.

In this example of FREE – Wilson application a serious omission was
made, however; the number of parameters in this quinoline hydrazone study
are approaching to saturation, i.e., the ratio between available data
points and degrees of freedom is on the verge of becoming critical.
And this means that due corrections on behalf of this critical situation are urgently required. Proper adjustments of r and s can be a-
chieved by (10,11,12,13,14):

$$r_{adj.} = \sqrt{1 - [(1 - r^2)(n - 1)/(n - k)]} \qquad (\text{eqn }3)$$

$$s_{adj.} = s\sqrt{(n - 1)/(n - k)} \qquad \text{(eqn 4)}$$

which replace the normally used expressions:

$$r = \sqrt{1 - SS_2/SS_1} \qquad \text{and} \qquad s = \sqrt{SS_2/(n - k')}$$

Application of the formulae given by (3) and (4) reveales $r_{adj.}$ and $s_{adj.}$ values of 0.604 and 0.858, respectively; and this proves in a convincing way the poor quality of the FREE – WILSON solution obtained by BERKOFF et al. Actually, their solution tends to non-correlation.

In accordance with these poor qualities is the result of the HANSCH approach applied by BERKHOFF et al. to the same data-set. The best correlation is the following:

$$\log BR = -0.564(\pm 0.776)\,\pi^2 + 1.886(\pm 2.302)\,\pi - 0.457(\pm 0.769)\,\sigma$$
$$+ 2.996(\pm 1.673) \qquad \text{(eqn 5)}$$

$n = 22 \quad r = 0.468 \quad s = 0.289$

A poor balance between the number of data points and the number of variables is frequently encountered in FREE – Wilson analyses and, besides, it will be seen accompanied in many cases by so-called single occurrence of substituents. The latter will escape proper statistical control.

2.2. HANSCH Model

The HANSCH equation was derived by HANSCH and FUJITA (15). It differs from the FREE – WILSON model in that it connects to the various substituents attached to the basic structure a series of parameter values which adequately describe the physical chemical properties of these substituents.

Thinking about structure – activity was actually started by CRUM – BROWN and FRASER as early as 1870, i.e. at a time that the synthesis of a product with biological activity had hardly been realized. The authors viewed upon biological activity as being dependent on the chemical structure of a compound, thus fully disposing of the then prevailing vitalistic concepts (16).

Vitalism may be compared with an extremely tough weed, which time and again rears its head. It was certainly useful for HOPKINS (17) to re-emphasize in 1932 that only an approach in which living organism

---

*) In these expressions: n = number of data points, k = number of independent variables, k' = number of degrees of freedom, r = unadjusted correlation coefficient, s = unadjusted standard error, $r_{adj.}$ = adjusted r, $s_{adj.}$ = adjusted s, SS_1 = sum of squares around the averaged dependent variable and SS_2 = sum of squares obtained in the regression.

is thought of as the seat of <u>chemical events</u> may advance biological
sciences.

Three of these properties have appeared to be of extreme importance in
QSAR studies; lipophilic, electronic and steric behaviour, indicated by
π (or f), σ and E_s, respectively, so that a simple version of the HANSCH
model can be formulated by means of the following equation:

$$\log BR = a\,\pi + \rho\,\sigma + b\,E_s + c \tag{eqn 6}$$

where BR = biological response, π, σ and E_s represent lipophilic, electronic and steric effects, respectively, of the various substituents and
a, ρ, b and c are constants to be generated by a regression analysis.

In many series of compounds tested in biological systems, one observes
as lipophilicity increases an activity rise to a maximum, followed by a
fall off which finally ends in an activity value zero. This phenomenon
can be connected with the idea that low lipophilic compounds – high
water-solubilities – have a low probability to reach some distant receptor system due to rapid excretion as a strongly competitive factor;
lipophilicity increase, however, will favour transport and activity will
increase consequently but a too extreme lipophilicity will be so unfavourable for transport through aqueous phases that activity will drop to
extremely low or even zero values.

HANSCH proposed a <u>parabolic</u> lipophilicity pattern for a proper de-
sciption of the above denoted facts, although surprisingly correct de-
scriptions of observed data can be given by KUBINYI's <u>bi-linear</u> model
as well (18,19,20,21,22).

The introduction of a squared lipophilicity factor will change eqn 6
into eqn 7:

$$\log BR = a\,\pi + b\,\pi^2 + \rho\,\sigma + c\,E_s + d \tag{eqn 7}$$

and the previously given eqn 5 may serve as a practical example of such
correlation types.

The HANSCH approach differs from the FREE – WILSON model in that it:

a) operates with physicochemical parameters assigned to all substituents;

b) applies a <u>summation</u> of all parameter-values regardless of the region
in which they appear. See the schematized picture given in Fig.2b;

c) it meets the want of applying incidentally squared parameters, a treatment which is not directly applicable to the FREE – WILSON model. As

soon as the activity pattern points towards a squared parameter, it
is recommended to separate it from the basic FREE – WILSON model and
to continue the normal computation procedure. This modified FREE –
WILSON equation will then look as follows:

$$\log BR = \mu + a \pi^2 + \sum AB_n \qquad \text{(eqn 8)}$$

d) the predictive merits of the FREE – WILSON approach are highly limited,
since any novel substituent will have no known substituent constant
(B-value) – this is even true for the transfer of a a known substituent from one region to another where its appearance is new – ;

e) The B-values from a FREE – WILSON analysis have no immediately apparent basis in well-defined physico-chemical terms;

3. PARAMETRIZATION OF LIPOPHILICITY IN THE HANSCH APPROACH
3.1. Lipophilicity; the hydrophobic parameter

Of the various parameters available for HANSCH approaches of structure-activity problems, those used to express lipophilicity, electronic
properties and steric factors are by far the most important, and among
those three the one for lipophilicity ranks first.

In eqn 7, which describes a biological event with the aid of four
substituent parameters with two of them connected through a squared relationship, one may use as well the partition coefficient of the complete molecule:

$$\log BR = a' \log P + b (\log P)^2 + \rho \sigma + c E_s + d' \qquad \text{(eqn 9)}$$

The relationship between $\log P$ and π was proposed by HANSCH (23) by
analogy of the HAMMETT equation for describing the dissociation of benzoic acids (24,25,26):

HAMMETT: $\quad \log K_s = \log K_o + \sigma \qquad \text{(eqn 10)}$

HANSCH: $\quad \log P_s = \log P_H + \pi \qquad \text{(eqn 11)}$

where K_s and K_o denote dissociation constants for a substituted and non-
substituted benzoic acid, respectively; P_s and P_H are partition coeffi-
cients of a substituted compound and its basic structure, respectively.

In eqn 9 the transfer of π-values into $\log P$'s is accompanied by an
appropriate change of the original constants a and d of eqn 7:

$$a' = a - 2b \log P_H \qquad\qquad d' = d + b (\log P_H)^2 - a \log P_H$$

As a rule, the lipophilic aspects in eqn 9 are described by means of log P values determined in or calculated from the octanol-water partition system. The two log P terms in our equation can in point of fact, however, be regarded as being composed of:

$$b \left(\log P\right)^2 + a_1' \log P + a_2' \log P \qquad \text{(eqn}$$

where the first two terms are concerned with the transport of the drug molecule between locus of administration and site of binding and the third term with the hydrophobic features of that binding process.

Eqn 12 is based on the assumption that only one solvent system, preferably that of octanol-water, is sufficient for a correct description of all that happens to a structure after introduction into a biological system. One should, however, not rule out the possibility that an adequate description of drug transport may require lipophilicity parameters different from those needed to describe hydrophobic interactions in the receptor area. In the latter case, the following equation would fulfil conditions far better:

$$\log BR = b \left(\log P^*\right)^2 + a_1' \log P^* + a_2' \log P^{**} + \rho \sigma + c E_s + d' \qquad \text{(eqn}$$

Eqn 13 indicates that hydrophobic interaction is described by a log P determined in or calculated from a solvent system different from that used to approach transport problems including those related to membrane passages.

The essentials of the hydrophobic interaction between a drug (D) and

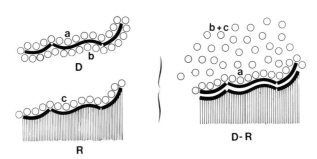

FIGURE 3. Schematic representation of hydrophobic interaction.
R = hydrophobic part of receptor covered by c water molecules;
D = approaching drug enveloped by a+b water molecules;
D-R = drug-receptor interaction complex with a representing ordered water covering D-R and b+c are the displaced, disordered water molecules;
(Reprinted from (27) with permission of the copyright owner)

a receptor (R) are a reduction of the number of water molecules which are in direct and mutually ordered contact with the hydrophobic surfaces of D and R (see Fig.3).

In a simplified equation we may write:

$$D\left[(a+b)\right]H_2O_{\text{ord.}} + R\left[c\ H_2O\right]_{\text{ord.}} \longrightarrow D-R\left[a\ H_2O\right]_{\text{ord.}} + (b+c)\ H_2O_{\text{disord.}} \qquad \text{(eqn 14)}$$

This disordening in the water structure causes an entropy increase in the D-R system and this implies a decrease in free energy ultimately resulting in a stabilization of the contacts between non-polar parts of D and R.

Transfer of a compound from water into a hydrophobic solvent (i.e.,the normal solvent-solvent partitioning procedure) or onto a hydrophobic receptor surface (hydrophobic interaction) can energetically be described by following simple expression.

$$\Delta G = -RT \ln P = -1.4 \log P \text{ kcal.mol}^{-1} \qquad \text{(eqn 15)}$$

where ΔG denotes the change in free energy of the system, R = gas constant, T = absolute temperature and P = partition coefficient. For a CH_2 group with a proper amount of lipophilicity of 0.52 (measured in the octanol-water system), we calculate ΔG = 0.73 kcal.mol^{-1} and for the C_6H_5 group with an amount of lipophilicity of 1.84, the result is 2.58 kcal.mol^{-1} or 0.43 kcal per CH-unit.

The above denoted stabilization is called hydrophobic interaction or hydrophobic binding(28,29,30). The great importance of hydrophobic binding finds reflection in the biological activities observed in many classes of structures. And both carcinogenic and antitumor active structures seem to share this property.

3.1.1. Calculation of log P values. Application of eqn 11 offers the possibility to estimate π values of a great varity of groups, especially when use is made of the following extension of eqn 11:

$$\log P\left(X_1,X_2,\ldots X_n\right) = \log P\left(H_n\right) + \sum_1^n \pi\left(X_n\right) \qquad \text{(eqn 16)}$$

where $P\left(X_1,X_2,\ldots X_n\right)$ denotes the partition coefficient of a compound in which n groups have to be replaced by H to arrive at the basic structure with log $P\left(H_n\right)$ and $\pi\left(X\right)$ representing the hydrophobic substituent constant of group X.

The π - concept can be used to estimate unknown log P's provided that the log P of some basic or parent structure is known and the proper π-values are available.

Severe objections to the π-system are:

1) Most values arise from simple 'pair-subtractions':

$$\pi(F)_{ar} = \log P (C_6H_5-F) - \log P (C_6H_6) \qquad \text{(eqn 17)}$$
$$\pi(NH_2)_{ar} = \log P (C_6H_5-NH_2) - \log P(C_6H_6) \qquad \text{(eqn 18)}$$
$$\pi(OH)_{ar} = \log P (C_6H_5-OH) - \log P(C_6H_6) \qquad \text{(eqn 19)}$$

so that the ultimate reliability of the system will heavily rely on the accuracy of the log P determinations for these 'pairs'.

2) In practice the system easily leads to unjustified modifications. Two examples: IUPE proposed the usage of a 'fully' additive procedure (31):

$$\log P = \sum_1^n \pi_n \qquad \text{(eqn 20)}$$

which completely abandons the original substitution concept.

PENG et al calculate log P of an antitumor agent with structural form A as follows (32):

(A)

$$\log P (A) = \log P (5,5-\text{diphen.hydantoin}) + \log P (Et_3N) + 2\,\pi(Cl) \qquad \text{(eqn 21)}$$

a calculation typical for an incorrect application of the concept which requires that in any equation used for the calculation of a log P value the left-hand member of the equation must contain exactly the same number of log P terms as the right-hand member.

3) It needs the concept of folding of structures of the $C_6H_5-CH_2-CH_2-CH_2-X$ type, where X denotes an electronegative functional group. Log P determinations would reveal that lipophilicity in this series is about 0.60 lower than calculations indicate.

In 1972 REKKER started the development of the hydrophobic fragmental system (33,34,35).

Basis for the new approach is the following equation:

$$\log P = \sum_1^n a_n f_n \qquad \text{(eqn 22)}$$

where f represents the hydrophobic fragmental constant, the lipophili-

city contribution of a constituent part of a structure to the total lipophilicity, and a is a numerical factor indicating the incidence of a
given fragment in the structure.

Since 1979 the system was extended to a series of about 100 f-values
in all, based on a data file consisting of about 1000 log P values from
the octanol-water system (36).

Some advantages of the f-system over the π-system are:
1) Fragment values have high statistic evidence since they were drawn
from a great number of data points. To restrict ourselves to the examples
given above (eqns 17, 18 and 19):

	F	NH$_2$	OH
abundance	150	80	199
f-value	−0.476	−1.420	−1.470
stand. dev.	0.009	0.014	0.011

For more detailed information on the f-system reference is made
to (36).

Since the envisaged data-set represents a good arbitrary cross-section
of organic comounds and assuming that both fragmentation procedure and
fragment computation were performed correctly, the obtained f-values
will be suited for log P predictions with comparably accurate results.
2) There is no longer a need for any folding correction. All structures
needing the above-mentioned correction of −0.60 in the π-system can be
treated without any complication when using f-constants:

$$\log P \ (C_6H_5-CH_2-CH_2-CH_2-Cl) = f(C_6H_5) + 3\ f(CH_2) + f(Cl)$$
$$= 1.840 + 3 \times 0.519 + 0.057 = 3.45 \ (obs.: 3.55)$$

$$\log P \ (C_6H_5-CH_2-CH_2-CH_2-CONH_2) = f(C_6H_5) + 3\ f(CH_2) + f(CONH_2)$$
$$= 1.840 + 3 \times 0.519 + (-1.975) = 1.42 \ (obs.: 1.41)$$

whereas the calculations in the π-system run as follows:

$$\log P \ (C_6H_5-CH_2-CH_2-CH_2-Cl) = \log P \ (C_6H_6) + 3\ \pi(CH_3) + \pi(Cl)$$
$$= 2.13 + 3 \times 0.50 + 0.39 - 0.60 = 3.42$$

$$\log P \ (C_6H_5-CH_2-CH_2-CH_2-CONH_2) = \log P \ (C_6H_6) + 3\ \pi(CH_3) + \pi(CONH_2)$$
$$= 2.13 + 3 \times 0.50 + (-1.71) - 0.60 = 1.32$$

3) The f-concept lends itself for an easily performable calculation of
fragmental values which are of importance in a specified investigation
but are not yet available in the f-file . A good example is the

Table 2. Lipophilic behaviour of N-nitrosamines

Nitrosamine	log P		
	obs.	est.	Δ
octanol - water partitining system			
N-nitrosodimethylamine	-0.57	-0.71	0.14
N-nitrosopyrrolidine	-0.19	-0.03	-0.16
N-nitrosomorpholine	-0.44	-0.47	0.03
N,N'-dinitrosopiperazine	-0.85	-0.92	0.07
N-nitrosodiethylamine	0.48	0.33	0.15
N-nitrosopiperidine	0.63	0.49	0.14
2-methyl-N,N'-dinitrosopiperazine	-0.28	-0.37	0.09
2,5-dimethyl-N-nitrosopyrrolidine	0.86	1.00	-0.14
3-methyl-N-nitrosopiperidine	0.99	1.00	-0.01
4-methyl-N-nitrosopiperidine	1.05	1.00	0.05
N-nitrosohexamethyleneimine	0.92	1.00	-0.08
2,5-dimethyl-N,N'-dinitrosopiperazine	0.15	0.10	0.05
2,6-dimethyl-N,N'-dinitrosopiperazine	0.08	0.10	-0.02
2,6-dimethyl-N-nitrosopiperidine	1.36	1.52	-0.16
3,5-dimethyl-N-nitrosopiperidine	1.53	1.52	0.01
N-nitrosoheptamethyleneimine	1.48	1.52	-0.04
N-nitrosodipropylamine	1.36	1.37	-0.01
N-nitrosooctamethyleneimine	2.04	2.04	0.00
2,3,5,6-tetramethyl-N,N'-dinitrosopiperazine	0.91	1.00	-0.09
2,2,6,6-tetramethyl-N-nitrosopiperidine	2.49	2.56	-0.07
hexane - water partitioning system			
N-nitrosodimethylamine	-1.52	-1.56	0.04
N-nitrosomethylethylamine	-0.92	-0.95	0.03
N-nitrosodiethylamine	-0.28	-0.33	0.05
N-nitrosodipropylamine	0.97	0.90	0.07
N-nitrosodi-isopropylamine	0.77	0.90	-0.13
N-nitrosoethylbutylamine	1.00	0.90	0.10
N-nitrosomethylamylamine	0.99	0.90	0.09
N-nitrosodibutylamine	2.07	2.13	-0.06
N-nitrosomethylheptylamine	2.02	2.13	-0.11
N-nitrosobutylamylamine	2.65	2.74	-0.09

Table 2. (continued)

diethylether-water partitioning system

N-nitrosopyrrolidine	-0.43	-0.29	-0.14
N-nitrosodiethylamine	0.32	0.10	0.22
N-nitrosopiperidine	0.49	0.28	0.21
N-nitrosomethylbutylamine	0.65	0.68	-0.03
N-nitrosodipropylamine	1.34	1.25	0.09
N-nitrosodi-isopropylamine	1.28	1.25	0.03
N-nitrosoethylbutylamine	1.41	1.25	0.16
N-nitrosomethylamylamine	1.43	1.25	0.18
N-nitrosodibutylamine	2.46	2.39	0.07

Note: Observed log P values are from ref.(37).

$\gtrsim$N-NO group. This fragment is present in the carcinogenic series of N-nitrosamines and its value can easily be obtained via

$$f\left(\gtrsim N\text{-NO}\right) \;=\; \log P\,\left(R_1R_2N\text{-NO}\right) \;-\; \sum f\left(R_1 + R_2\right) \qquad \text{(eqn 23)}$$

$$\begin{array}{c} R_1 \\ \diagdown \\ \diagup \quad N\text{-NO} \\ R_2 \qquad \underline{N\text{-nitrosamines}} \end{array}$$

Table 2 collects the lipophilicity data obtained on a number of N-nitrosamines in three different solvent-systems: octanol-water, hexane-water and diethylether-water. The $\gtrsim$N-NO fragmental values are given in Table 3. Those for the octanol-water system have been obtained by application of eqn 23 and the other values stem from direct regression analysis of a more extended data-set.

Table 3. Hydrophobic fragmental values of $\gtrsim$N-NO

Partitioning system	f	st.dev.
octanol-water	-2.110	0.030
hexane-water	-3.163	0.035
diethylether-water	-2.576	0.065

The practical utility of the fragmental constants may be exemplified by log P calculations on 2,5-dimethyl-N,N'-dinitrosopiperazine (B) and N-nitrosodiethanolamine (C) of which especially the latter becomes increasingly important on account of its formation from diethanolamine, which is used as an additive in many cosmetic preparations.

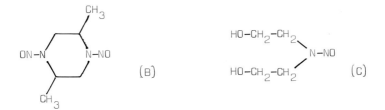

(B)

(C)

Table 4. Lipophilicities of N-nitrosamines (calculated)

Compound	Partitioning system	log P estim.	obs.
B	octanol-water	0.15	0.10
	hexane-water	-1.39	n.m.
	diethylether-water	-0.60	n.m.
C	octanol-water	-1.82	n.m.
	hexane-water	-6.58	n.m.
	diethylether-water	-2.10	n.m.

Note: n.m. = not measured

An analogous treatment can be given for partitioning data of anti-tumor active structures. A small collection of log P values determined in the octanol-water system on some members of the class of substituted nitrosoureas is represented in Table 5. They were taken from ref. (37).

$$R_1 - N - C - N - NO$$
$$\quad\ \ R_2\ \ O\ \ R_3 \qquad \text{nitrosoureas}$$

Table 5. Lipophilic behaviour of nitrosoureas

R_1	R_2	R_3	log P obs.	est.	Δ
H	H	CH_3	-0.16	-0.41	0.25
			-0.03	-0.41	0.38
CH_3	CH_3	CH_3	0.36	0.05	0.31
CH_3	CH_3	C_2H_5	0.71	0.57	0.14
C_2H_5	C_2H_5	CH_3	1.11	1.09	0.02
C_2H_5	C_2H_5	C_2H_5	1.54	1.61	-0.07
$ClCH_2CH_2$	H	FCH_2CH_2	0.96	1.35	-0.39
FCH_2CH_2	H	$ClCH_2CH_2$	0.95	1.35	-0.40
$ClCH_2CH_2$	H	$ClCH_2CH_2$	1.53	1.77	-0.24

The material lends itself for an estimation of -2.05 as the most consistent f value for the $\geq$N – CO – N –NO unit. The standard deviation is pretty high: 0.29 and is probably connected with decomposition problems during the partitioning procedure. Especially bis(halogenethyl) derivatives would seem suspect (32).

4) The f-concept lends itself extremely well for the computation of hydrophobic fragmental sets in solvent-systems other than the most frequently used octanol-water partitioning pair. Table 6 exemplifies a few data in giving a small overview of f-values in the systems octanol-water, aliphatic hydrocarbon-water, aromatic hydrocarbon-water, diethylether-water, butanol-water and chloroform-water.

Table 6. The influence of the partitioning system on the magnitude of the hydrophobic fragmental constant.

Fragment	oct	al.hc	ar.hc	ether	BuOH	CHCl$_3$
C	0.155	0.179	0.184	0.179	0.100	0.192
H	0.182	0.218	0.181	0.196	0.169	0.210
OH(al)	−1.470	−3.560	−2.779	−1.964	−0.920	−2.274
COOH(al)	−0.938	−3.862	−2.608	−1.253	−0.597	−2.409
O(al)	−1.595	−1.668	−1.671	−1.810		
NH(al)	−1.814	−2.648	−2.576	−2.970	−1.517	−2.274
COO(al)	−1.251	−1.669	−0.995	−1.432	−0.970	
Cl(ar)	0.924	0.882	0.985	(1.01)		
NO$_2$(al)	−0.920	−1.634	−0.537			
$\geq$N–NO(al)	(−2.11)	−3.163		−2.576		

Remarks: oct = octanol-water;
   al.hc = aliphatic hydrocarbon-water: within the range of measuring errors no significant differences could be found between log P values obtained in systems with the organic phase: pentane, hexane, cyclohexane, 2-methylpentane, heptane, methylcyclohexane, octane, isooctane, nonane, decane, dodecane, hexadecane or decahydronaphthalene, the practical consequence being that all these log P values can be pooled at wish;
   ar.hc = aromatic hydrocarbon-water; the log P measurements available from literature sources as far as they were concerned to the systems benzene-water, toluene-water and xylene-water were pooled; here too – at least in those cases where a due comparison was possible – no significant difference could be observed;
   BUOH = butanol-water; data used consisted of measurements performed in n.butanol-water and in isobutanol-water;

Many of the consequences of these f -computations for the medicinal chemical and pharmaceutical practice have not yet been fully explored.

3.2. Constituent components of the hydrophobic fragmental constant

An interesting attack on the problems around meaning and significance of the hydrophobic fragmental constant was made by TESTA and SEILER (38). They construed a graph in which the hydrophobic values of a great number of aromatic fragments were plotted versus their appropriate volume values, the latter calculated from ALLINGER's compilation of Van der WAALS radii (39) and average interatomic distances (40). Their plot is reproduced in Fig.4; it shows an almost random distribution of the various data-

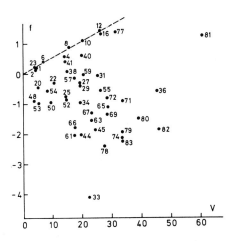

FIGURE 4. Plot of f versus V for aromatic fragments (reproduced by kind permission of the copyright owners from ref.38)

points. An exception are the apolar fragments H (no 1), C (No 2), F (No 6), Cl (No 8), Br (No 10), I (No 12) and CF_3 (No 16), which can be connected in a correct way by a straight line (see Fig.4) with a perfect correlation:

$$f = 0.0534(\pm 0.0035) \ V \qquad \qquad (eqn \ 2$$
$$n = 7 \quad r = 0.998 \quad s = 0.067$$

The other fragments have, without exceptions, lower f-values than would be expected from their volumes. TESTA and SEILER name these negative increments lipophobicity effects; they are related to hydration effects and symbolized by Λ.

From not yet published computations in our department (41) it appeared that these Λ values are multiples of 0.289. This factor is used to loqm up unintentionally in many of our lipophilicity studies.

A successful incorporation of the varied collection of outlying data-
points into the above given eqn 24, applying a proper fitting procedure,
would require that the new equation have

a) an unchanged slope;

b) absence of a significant intercept;

c) an incidence factor (we are used to denote it as 'key number' – kn)
which is accompanied by a regressor value not significantly different
from 0.289;

d) acceptable statistics;

Eqn 25 excellently fulfils all these requirements:

$$f = 0.0535(\pm 0.001) \; V - 0.2951(\pm 0.003) \; kn + 0.0029(\pm 0.035) \qquad \text{(eqn 25)}$$

$$n = 68 \quad r = 0.9985 \quad s = 0.075 \quad F = 11320$$

In a more generalized form latter equation will look as follows:

$$f_a = \rho \times 0.0535 \, V - \rho \times 0.289 \, kn_a \qquad \text{(eqn 26)}$$

where index a denotes an arbitrarily chosen solvent-system and the factor ρ is identical to the slope of the so-called COLLANDER equation
(42,43) used to transfer partition data from one system (for instance
octanol-water) to another solvent-system:

$$\log P_a = \rho \log P_{oct} + q \qquad \text{(eqn 27)}$$

Tentative summarization makes clear that lipophilicity is build up
from a relatively constant bulk-factor (all ρ values were found so far
between 0.6 and 1.2) and a hydration-sensative factor which is largely
dependent on the specific merits of the solvent-system chosen for partitioning. In biological systems the role of the solvent-system is partly taken over by membranes and receptor-sites, so that we may conclude
that the ultimate lipo-hydro-philic behavioural pattern of a molecule,
as far as its functional groups are concerned, depends on the hydrating
properties of the bio-system.

Table 7 gives the kn values of three frequently occurring simple functional groups in two solvent-systems. They indicate an approximatively

Table 7. Examples of hydration differences

functional group	octanol-water	aliphatic hc-water
OH(al)	kn = 7	kn = 13
COOH(al)	8	17
CONH$_2$(al)	12	21

two-fold factor for these systems, i.e., the most non-polar system of
the two endures the considered functional groups as 'two times stronger
hydrated'.

   Although for a closely reasoned characterisation of membrane systems
and the correct understanding of drug passage through these systems much
more material is needed, the schematized set-up in Fig.5 will definitely
be of help in marshalling some facts.

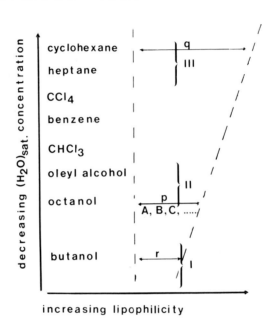

FIGURE 5. Graphical representation of the discriminating properties
          of a number of solvent-systems (only indicated by their or-
          ganic phases) as a function of the water-saturation concen-
          tration of the organic phases; p, q and r denote the discrim-
          inating powers of the octanol-water, cyclohexane-water and
          butanol-water systems, respectively, towards a set of parti-
          tioned structures A, B, C .... I, II and III denote approxi-
          mate locations of three membrane systems.
          (Reprinted from (44) with permission of the copyright owner)

   The graph visualizes the _discriminative_ behaviour of a number of
solvent-systems. From the above given considerations it became clear
that this discrimination – we may speak as well of susceptibility or
more simply of spread – is slightly dependent on the factor ρ and heavily dependent on the nature of the partitioned functional group. Grosso
modo, the lengths of p, q and r will be indicative for the discrimina-

ting power of the three systems octanol-water, cyclohexane-water and butanol-water.

There are good indications that bio-membrane systems will fit in the
given pattern of Fig.5, so that, for instance, the buccal and sublin-
gual membranes are situated in the region I, the membranes of the gastro-
intestinal tracts and the red cell membranes are found in region II and
the blood-brain barrier can best be modelled in the top-region III.
Transport phenomena go slower and less complete the more we travers the
figure from bottom to top with molecules of comparatively low lipophilicity.

4. CONGENERICITY AND NON-CONGENERICITY

Whenever a series of activities is to be studied on the basis of a QSAR,
it is first of all necessary to find out whether the compounds are congeneric, both with respect to structure and to action. The concept "congeneric series" is not so easy to define correctly; literally it means
'of the same kind, class, or stock'.

In practice one will simply start a QSAR approach and continue the introduction of extra parameters until one is satisfied — and than per definition
the series is congeneric — or satisfaction stays out and the series will
obtain the qualification of non-congenericity.

It seems advantageous to speak of a degree of congenericity, which could
than be coupled to the number of independent variables necessary to bring
the correlation on a sufficiently high level of account.

Actually, the advantages of the proposed concept (2) are two-fold:
a) it would identify all equations with an unduly high number of independent
variables as possibly suspect;
b) it would give us the possibility to label certain parameters as restorers
of non-congenericity;

Two examples will be given for clarification:
1) Non-congenericity comprised in the right-hand part of the equation;
We will not dwell on easily recognizable and adjustable non-congener-
icities such as those caused by differences in basic structure or differences between ortho-substitution and para-meta-substitution.

A not so easily recognizable non-congenericity may be hidden in a series
of compounds consisting of outwardly congeneric looking structures with an
inconsistent partitional behaviour towards solvent-systems with dissimilar

42

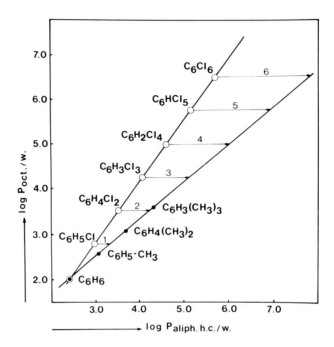

FIGURE 6. Plot of log P values (obtained by f-summation) of methylbenzenes (black dots) and chlorobenzenes (open circles) measured in octanol-water versus those measured in aliphatic hydrocarbon-water. Horizontal lines indicate how chlorobenzenes can be transferred to a closely fitting pattern by applying a constant 'move' for each chlorine-substituent.

organic phase polarities.

Fig.6 visualizes a plot of log P values of a series of 10 compounds consisting of benzene, 3 methylbenzenes and 6 chlorobenzenes. Brought together in one equation of the COLLANDER type:

$$\log P_{aliph.hc} = \rho \log P_{oct} + q \qquad \text{(eqn 28)}$$

the correlation is not so bad (r = 0.969) but it comprises one severe outlier and an intercept value of −1.537.

The set procedure is to continue with the application of an indicator value ('dummy'-parameter) which distinguishes between the two parts of the series: D = 0 for the methylbenzenes including benzene and D = 1 for the chloro-derivatives.

The correlation can be given by:

$$\log P_{aliph.hc} = \rho \log P_{oct} + a \times D + q \qquad \text{(eqn 29)}$$

and we observe a significant improvement: 0.988 instead of 0.969 for the correlation coefficient; the intercept value remains unduly high, however: -1.295.

As soon as we realize that the non-congenericity is not a matter of 'total-structure'-difference but connected with the difference in lipo-philic behaviour of the chlorine-substituents proper, the way out is im-mediately clear and will consist of a constant 'move' for each chlorine as visualized in Fig.6. The final correlation is of the type:

$$\log P_{aliph.hc} = \rho \log P_{oct} + \rho (n \times 0.289) + q \qquad \text{(eqn 30)}$$

and yields a correlation coefficient 1.000, whereas the intercept has become fully insignificant: -0.0017.

2) <u>Non-congenericity comprised in the left-hand part of the equation;</u>

The importance of congenericity was emphasized in the previous section with regard to the structural features parametrized in the right-hand part of the QSAR equation. Perhaps even more important is the demand for congenericity in the left-hand part. The aim of a correct QSAR approach should comprise the correlation of biological test-data obtained from

(a) <u>well-defined interactions</u>
between chemical substances belonging to

(b) <u>congeneric series of structures</u>
and

(c) <u>a proper active site</u>
in the biological system.

Toxicological phenomena and especially oral LD_{50} values are typical examples of biological data which do not in the least fulfil the require-ment of representing a well-defined interaction and as long as no studies are available on the toxic symptomatology and the identification of the target organ (the proper active site of toxic impact) all publications in this field should be examined with due suspicion. The same might be true for work done or to be done on the coupling of carcinogenic data to struc-tural parameters (for additional information on problems around LD_{50} we refer to refs. 45 and 46).

5. ANTITUMOR ACTIVITY AND QSAR

Among the publications delivered during the last years we selected the one by PENG et al (32) which was denoted by MARTIN (47) as a QSAR study with positive predictive results. PENG's publication is devoted to potential

central nervous system agents of the hydantoin type. This investigation
fulfils the requirements for congenericity and starts with the leading
idea, that in order to obtain an antitumor—active compound of the nitrogen
mustard type, it would be recommendable to use as acarrier 5,5—diphenylhydantoin, which on account of its log P of 2.47 easily passes the blood-
brain barrier.

   Their series comprised 13 compounds with structure D.

$$R_2 - \overset{\overset{\displaystyle R_1}{|}}{\underset{\displaystyle HN}{C}} \!\!\!\!\!\!\!\!\!\!\!\!\! \underset{\underset{\displaystyle C}{\diagdown}\underset{\displaystyle \overset{\|}{O}}{}\diagup}{\!\!\!\!-\!\!\!\!} \overset{\overset{\displaystyle }{|}}{\underset{\displaystyle N - R_3}{C = O}}$$

(D)

   All compounds were tested in the lymphoid leukemia L1210 system by
standard NCI protocols and five of them showed enough activity to be further tested in additional tumor systems comprising lymphocytic leukemia
P388, melanocarcinoma B16, LEWIS lung carcinoma and the ependymoblastoma
mouse brain tumor. The antitumor activities are reported in Table 8 as

Table 8. Antitumor Activities − Observed and estimated.

Comp. No.	R_1	R_2	log 1/OD obs.	est.	log P = $\sum f$
16	C_6H_5	C_6H_5	−2.00	−2.04	4.87
17	$CH_2CH_2CH_2CH_2CH_2$		−1.54	−1.52	3.79
18	CH_3	CH_3	−0.78	−0.88	2.50
19	C_2H_5	C_2H_5	−1.40	−1.44	3.64
20	H	C_6H_5	−1.40	−1.24	3.22

Notes: $R_3 = CH_2CH_2N(CH_2CH_2Cl)_2$
   OD = optimum dose (mg/kg/dose); PENG et al report OD values, but
   in behalf of the regression analysis we transformed them into
   log 1/OD;

far as the activities against L1210 lymphoid leukemia are concerned.
Regression analysis of log 1/OD agaainst the summated f values gave an
equation with surprisingly fine statistics:

$$\log 1/OD = -0.489 \sum f + 0.339 \qquad \text{(eqn 31)}$$
$$r = 0.972 \quad s = 0.118 \quad F = 51.5 \quad n = 5$$

   We may conclude: the extra amount of lipophilicity introduced by the
nitrogen mustard moiety into the diphenylhydantoin structure (No. 16) is

redressed by replacing the two phenyl groups by two methyl groups to bring the lipohilicty back on practically the same level as that of the 5,5-diphenylhydantoin, a structure with ideal blood-brain barrier passsage properties.

We suggest that investigations performed in the denoted way could be of great help in designing valuable modifications of antitumor active agents.

REFERENCES

1. Von Hoff, D.D., Kuhn, J. and Clark, G., Cancer Chemother. Pharmacol. 6(1981)93.

2. Rekker, R.F., Actualités de Chimie thérapeutique, 5e série, 1977, pg.75, Société de Chimie Thérapeutique - Châtenay-Malabry.

3. Mautner, H.G., The Jeruzalem Symposia on Quantum Chemistry and Biochemistry, Vol.7: Molecular and Quantum Pharmacology (Editors: E. Bergmann and B. Pullman), D. Reidel Publ. Comp. - Dordrecht, Holland / Boston, U.S.A., 1974.

4. Hansch, C., private communication.

5. Free, S.H. and Wilson, J.W., J. Med. Chem., 7(1964)395.

6. Cammarata, A., J. Med. Chem., 15(1972)573.

7. Kubinyi, H., J. Med. Chem., 19(1976)587.

8. Kubinyi, H. and Kehrhahn, O.-H., J. Med. Chem., 19(1976)1040.

9. Berkoff, C.E., Craig, P.N., Gordon, B.P. and Pellerana, C., Arzneim.-Forsch. (Drug Research), 23(1973)830.

10. Haitovsky, Y., Amer. Stat., 23(1969)20.

11. Edwards, J.B., Amer. Stat., 23(1969)28.

12. Rao, P., Amer. Stat., 30(1976)190.

13. Nauta, W.Th. and Rekker, R.F. (Eds.), Pharmacochemistry of 1,3-Indandiones (Pharmacochemistry Library, Vol. 3), Elsevier Scientific Publishing Comp. - Amsterdam - Oxford - New York, 1981.

14. IBM System 1360 Scientific Subroutine Package, Version III.

15. Hansch, C. and Fujita, T., J. Amer. Chem. Soc., 86(1964)1616.

16. Crum-Brown, A. and Fraser, T.R., Trans. Roy. Soc. Edinburgh, 25(1868-1869)151,693.

17. Gowland Hopkins, F., Problems of Specificity in Biochemical Catalysis, London, Oxford University Press, 1932.

18. Kubinyi, H., J. Med. Chem., 20(1977)625.

19. Kubinyi, H., Arzneim.-Forsch. (Drug Research), 26(1976)1991.

20. Kubinyi, H., Arzneim.-Forsch. (Drug Research), 29(1979)1067.

21. Kubinyi, H., in: Biological Activity and Chemical Structure, p. 239 (Ed. J.A. Keverling Buisman). Elsevier Publishing Company. -Amsterdam - Oxford - New York, 1977.

22. Kubinyi, H., Progr. Drug Res., 23(1979)97.

23. Hansch, C., Muir, R.M., Fujita, T., Maloney, Geiger, F. and Streich, M., Nature, 194(1962)180.

24. Hammett, L.P., Chem. Rev., 17(1935)125.

25. Hammett, L.P., Physical Organic Chemistry, McGraw – Hill Book Comp. New York, 1940.

26. Jaffé, H.H., Chem. Rev., 53(1953)191.

27. Rekker, R.F., in: Biological Activity and Chemical Structure, p. 107 (Ed. J.A. Keverling Buisman). Elsevier Publishing Company. – Amsterdam – Oxford – New York, 1977.

28. Frank, H.S. and Evans, M.W., J. Chem. Phys., 13(1945)507.

29. Breslow, R., Organic Reaction Mechanisms, 2nd ed., Benjamin, New York, 1969.

30. Némethy, G., Ang. Chem., 79(1967)260.

31. Tute, M.S., Advances in Drug Research, 8(1971)1.

32. Peng, G.W., Marquez, V.E. and Driscoll, J.S., J. Med. Chem., 18(1975)846.

33. Nys, G.G. and Rekker, R.F., Chim. Thérap., 8(1973)521.

34. Nys, G.G. and Rekker, R.F., Eur. J. Med. Chem., 9(1974)361.

35. Rekker, R.F. and Nys, G.G., Relations Structure-Activité, Séminaire Paris – 25/26 Mars 1974; Société de Chimie Thérapeutique, Paris 1975.

36. Rekker, R.F. and De Kort, H.M., Eur. J. Med. Chem., 14(1979)479.

37. Hansch, C. and Leo, A.J., Substituent Constants for Correlation Analysi in Chemistry and Biology, John Wiley & Sons – New York, 1979.

38. Testa, B. and Seiler, P., Arzneim.-Forsch. (Drug Research), 31(1981)105.

39. Allinger, N.L., in: Advances in Physical Organic Chemistry, Vol. 13 (Eds.: V. Gold and D. Bethell), Academic Press – London, 1976.

40. Tables of Interatomic Distances and Cofiguration in Molecules and Ions, The Chemical Society, London – 1958; Supplement 1956-1959 (publ. 1965).

41. Rekker, R.F. and Bijloo, G.J., unpublished results.

42. Collander, R., Acta Chem. Scand., 4(1950)1085.

43. Collander, R., Acta Chem. Scand., 5(1951)774.

44. Rekker, R.F., The Hydrophobic Fragmental Constant, Elsevier Scientific Publishing Company. – Amsterdam – Oxford – New York, 1977.

45. Enslein, K. and Craig, P.N., J. Environ. Pathol. Toxicol., 2(1978)115.

46. Rekker, R.F., TIPS 1(1980)383.

47. Martin, Y.C., J. Med. Chem., 24(1981)229.

ALKYLATING PRODRUGS IN CANCER CHEMOTHERAPY

T.A. CONNORS

The concept of the design of latently active drugs (or prodrugs), that is chemicals which are not themselves active but which require conversion to their active form has been well established for many years and has been used with success in many areas of therapy.

In cancer chemotherapy examples of latently active drugs may be found amongst the antimetabolites, antitumour antibiotics and a range of miscellaneous agents. The most systematically investigated prodrugs, however, are the alkylating agents. The reason for this is that in general the chemical reactivity of an alkylating agent is related to its degree of cytotoxicity while small changes in structure, as could occur in vivo, can lead to large changes in chemical reactivity. An unreactive and non-toxic alkylating agent therefore has the possibility of being converted in vivo to a reactive and very toxic metabolite. The rational design of alkylating agents has been reviewed on many occasions (1,2,3,4,5). Figure 1 gives some examples of relatively non-toxic alkylating agents which have been synthesised in the hope that they may be converted in vivo to very reactive alkyl-ating agents acting selectively in tumour cells.

However, only a few such prodrugs have been successful in improving the selectivity of action of alkylating agents because either the expected metabolic activation did not take place in vivo or activation did occur but in normal tissues so that there was no specific antitumour effect. Cyclophosphamide designed as a prodrug has a somewhat greater selectivity (increased thera-peutic index) than most other clinically used nitrogen mustards but is not specifically activated by any tumours. Its increased

D.N. Reinhoudt, T.A. Connors, H.M. Pinedo & K.W. van de Poll (eds.), Structure-Activity Relationships of Anti-Tumour Agents.
© *1983, Martinus Nijhoff Publishers, The Hague/Boston/London. ISBN 90-247-2783-9.*

FIGURE 1

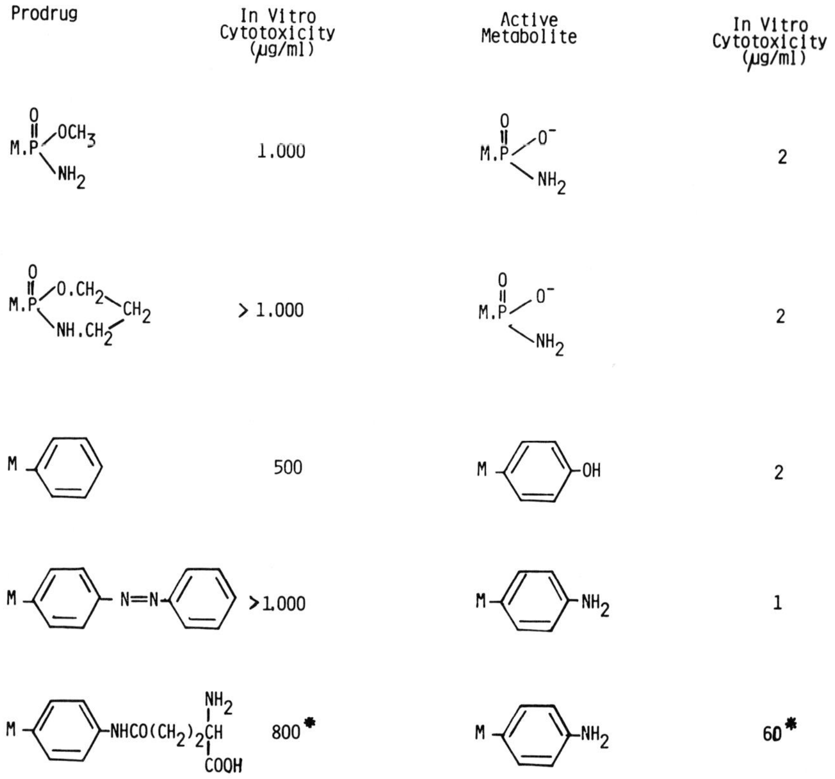

Prodrug	In Vitro Cytotoxicity (μg/ml)	Active Metabolite	In Vitro Cytotoxicity (μg/ml)

M.P (=O)(OCH$_3$)(NH$_2$) 1.000   M.P(=O)(O$^-$)(NH$_2$) 2

M.P(=O)(O.CH$_2$-CH$_2$)(NH.CH$_2$) > 1.000   M.P(=O)(O$^-$)(NH$_2$) 2

M—⟨benzene⟩ 500   M—⟨benzene⟩—OH 2

M—⟨benzene⟩—N=N—⟨benzene⟩ >1.000   M—⟨benzene⟩—NH$_2$ 1

M—⟨benzene⟩—NHCO(CH$_2$)$_2$CH(NH$_2$)(COOH) 800[*]   M—⟨benzene⟩—NH$_2$ 60[*]

$$M = (ClCH_2CH_2)_2N^-$$

[*] Hepatocytes in culture (23)

selectivity is due to a complicated series of metabolic transformations (6). Aniline mustard is converted to a less reactive
O-glucuronide in the liver of mice which then acts as a prodrug,
being selectively hydrolysed in certain tumours high in β-glucur-
onidase, to a very reactive and toxic metabolite (7). However,
it is of little importance clinically because human cancers contain
the activating enzyme only rarely and unpredictably (8).

The starting point in the design of alkylating prodrugs
should ideally be the demonstration of some unique biochemical
property of a tumour. This often, but not always, will be the
finding that a particular class or sub-group of tumours has a very
high activity of an enzyme compared to all other tissues. Since
animal models are not representative of human tumours then this
finding would be more relevant in a human tumour than an animal
tumour. The difficulties involved in studying the biochemistry of
human cancer has meant that few alkylating prodrugs have been
designed from this rational starting point. However, application
of molecular biological techniques to human cancers has already
identified specific proteins produced by different tumour types
(eg 9) and it seems that in the near future a number of human
cancers will be shown to have biochemical properties which may be
exploited in rational drug design.

Once an appropriate prodrug has been synthesised it should
then be shown to be a substrate for the tumour 'specific' enzyme,
certainly in vitro and preferably in vivo. Finally the prodrug
should release in the tumour a metabolite which is extremely
reactive so that all toxic alkylations take place in the malignant
tissue and no reactive metabolite leaves the tumour and reaches
sensitive tissues of the host such as the bone marrow.

Very few latently active alkylating agents have so far been
designed which fulfill all these criteria. There are at least two
areas which might merit more detailed study in the future,
(a) the activation of prodrugs by reduction in tumour ischaemic
zones and (b) the exploitation of enzymes occurring with some
selectivity in human malignancies in general or in some particular
types of cancer.

(a) Activation by Reduction

The low oxygen tension of tumours and their 'reducing' ability has been studied for many years and has been the basis for the design of a number of antitumour prodrugs (3,10,11,12). The reason why some solid tumours may reduce certain substrates more efficiently than other tissues has been worked out in some detail When animals bearing solid tumours are injected with lissamine green, the charged dye does not penetrate cells but maps out the vascularised areas of tissues. Using this technique it has been shown that solid tumours, even when quite small, may develop ischaemic areas containing mainly necrotic tissue (13,14). However, a layer of cells between the dyed region and the ischaemic cells has been shown to be viable although under hypoxic conditions. The ability of these cells to selectively reduce nitroimidazoles has been elegantly demonstrated using radioactive substrate and visualisation of covalently bound material following autoradiography. In both solid tumours and cell spheroids the electrophilic reactants, formed on reduction of the substrate, undergo covalent binding in a zone of cells probably corresponding to the interface between well vascularised and ischaemic zones (15,16). It may well be that these hypoxic cells are resistant to chemotherapy because they take up less of the anticancer agent (because of the poor blood supply) or because they are less sensitive (eg non-proliferating). As in radiotherapy, hypoxic cells may limit the effectiveness of chemotherapy. It is of interest that electron affinic radiation sensitisers such as misonidazole, which also form reactive intermediates in hypoxic tumour cells, have been recently shown to act synergistically with some anticancer agents. It would seem an appropriate time to reconsider some of the earlier attempts to design alkylating agents activated by reduction to determine whether they are (a) selectively activated and undergo co-valent binding in hypoxic cells and (b) if so, are synergistic with clinically used alkylating agents.

One of the first nitrogen mustards designed to be activated by reduction was nitromin (Fig 2;I). Nitromin is the N-oxide of nitrogen mustard (Fig 2;II) in which the lone pair of electrons takes place in bonding and can no longer activate the chloro-ethylamino groups. As a consequence it is 30-40 times less active than HN2. There is already some indication that it may be a useful pro-drug since it is active against well established solid tumours in rats (which may be expected to have a large number of hypoxic cells) and has a higher therapeutic index than HN2 suggesting selective reduction in the tumour (17). The fact that is has little activity against cells in culture also indicates that it is only active after reduction in cells of low oxygen tension. It might be useful to study the effect of nitromin in combination with other anticancer agents or if it is shown that it does not effectively penetrate ischaemic tumour regions to study perhaps more lipid soluble nitrogen mustard N-oxides.

Other nitrogen mustards that might be activated by a similar mechanism include the quinone (Fig 2;III) which could form the very much more toxic hydroquinone (Fig 2;IV), the disulphide (Fig 2;V) which is chemically only half as reactive as its reduction product (Fig 2;IV)(3) and possibly the nitrobenzene (or nitrosobenzene) mustard (Fig 2;VII) which might be selectively reduced in the tumour to the highly toxic p-phenylene diamine mustard (Fig 2;VIII). One drawback with this approach is that the anaerobic bacteria of the large bowel are also very effective in carrying out these reductions and might thus contribute to the systemic toxicity of the prodrug and reduce selectivity.

(b) Selective Enzymatic Activation

(B1) Plasmin

A characteristic feature of many cancers, including human cancers is the production of plasminogen activator. In many cases transformation of cells in vitro by a variety of methods is accompanied by a rise in secretion of plasminogen activator. Plasminogen activator is a protease which converts plasminogen into plasmin, and since serum fairly rapidly inactivates free plasmin then the tumour environment is at any time higher than

FIGURE 2

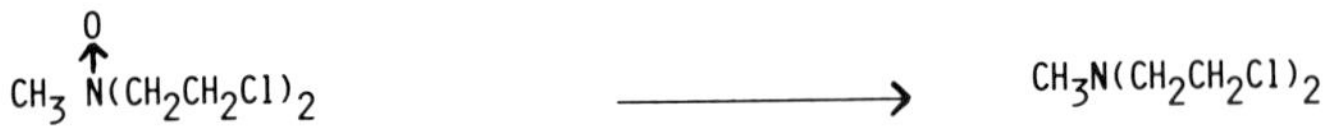

CH3 N(CH2CH2Cl)2
O
CH3N(CH2CH2Cl)2

I — II

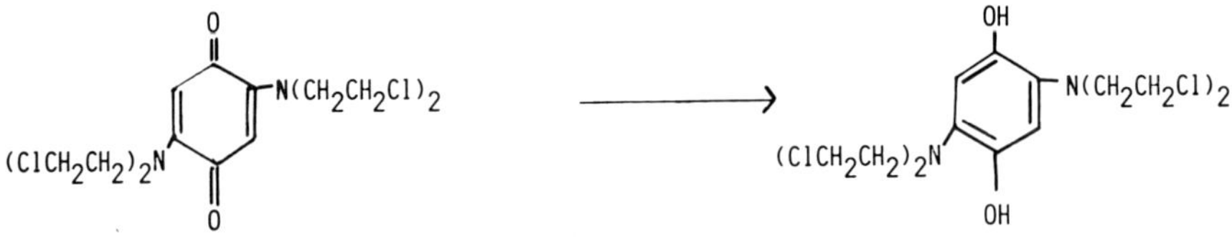
O
N(CH2CH2Cl)2
(ClCH2CH2)2N
O
OH
N(CH2CH2Cl)2
(ClCH2CH2)2N
OH

III — IV

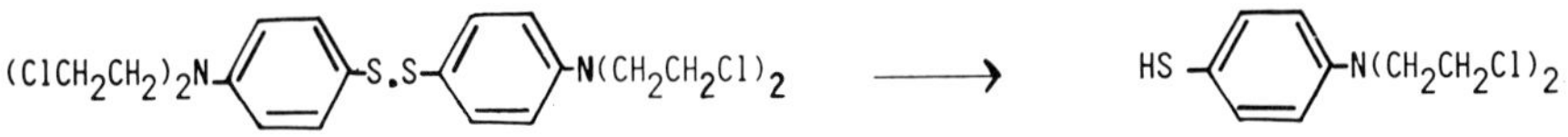
(ClCH2CH2)2N
S.S
N(CH2CH2Cl)2
HS
N(CH2CH2Cl)2

V — VI

O2N
N(CH2CH2Cl)2
H2N
N(CH2CH2Cl)2

VII — VIII

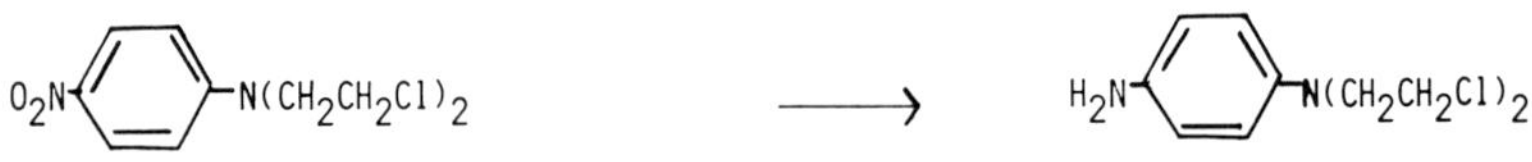

other tissues in its concentration of plasmin. This property
has been exploited by the design of prodrugs activated by plasmin
to release active drugs (18). Plasmin is a protease which
generally cleaves proteins and peptides at lysine and arginine
residues, particularly if they are next to a hydrophobic amino
acid such as leucine. Peptides of the structure D-valyl-leucyl-
lysyl linked to the amine group of an anticancer agent (AT 125
or p-phenylenediamine mustard) have been shown to be specifically
toxic for transformed cells producing plasminogen activator.
The D-valyl group on the peptide prevents breakdown by serum
aminopeptidases and the leucyl-lysyl linkage is split to release
the free drug. This is an interesting approach because it would
appear that many cancers have an environment which is high in
plasmin. Since there are also a number of anticancer agents
which contain primary amine groups, which become inactive when
the amine group is substituted then the way is open to synthesise
many prodrugs which may be improved selectivity. Examples of
anticancer drugs containing an 'essential' amino group would
include besides those already mentioned, cytosine arabinoside,
adriamycin, azaserine, dopamine and 1-aminocyclopentane-1-
carboxylic acid. Other anticancer drugs which contain a primary
amino group which might be essential for antitumour activity
and which might be converted into a prodrug form activated by
plasmin would include 9-aminoellipticine, mytomycin-C,
Sangivamycin, L-alanosine, melphalan, actinomycin bleomycin
and isoguanine. In some cases, such as neocarzinostatin, the
amino groups may not be essential for cytotoxicity but could be
prevented from entering host cells by the attachement of a
relatively large plasmin sensitive polypeptide attached to the
amino group.

   (B2) γ-glutamyltransferase

   A related approach concerns the synthesis of γ-glutamyl
derivatives of anti-cancer agents containing primary amino groups
of the type described above (19). This approach was suggested
by the finding that a consistent feature of liver tumours induced
by aflatoxin is their extremely high level of γ-glutamyl
transferase (20). A high level of the enzyme has also been

found in some human cancers (21,22). As with the design of
plasmin activated prodrugs, γ-glutamyl derivatives of the same
agents might selectively release the drug in the tumour
environment. Since the enzyme is on the cell surface facing
outwards it may also assist in the intracellular concentration
of the agent. The γ-glutamyl derivative of p-phenylene diamine
mustard has been found to be about thirty times more toxic to
a hepatocyte cell line high in the enzyme when compared to
another hepatocyte line lacking the enzyme (23). One problem
with this approach is that other tissues, especially the kidney,
have detectable levels of the activating enzyme which might lower
the selectivity of the prodrug. One way in which this might
be overcome would be in the design of prodrugs of the type shown
in Figure 3. A polypeptide would be synthesised of such a
molecular weight that it would not be readily taken up by cells.
An essential feature of the polypeptide would be a terminal
D-amino acid to reduce hydrolysis in plasma followed by a series
of amino acids terminating in a plasmin sensitive 'specifier'
linked to a γ-glutamyl derivative of an antitumour amine. The
polypeptide would release the γ-glutamyl prodrug in the tumour
environment. The enzyme on the tumour surface would then
concentrate it intracellularly in its active form.

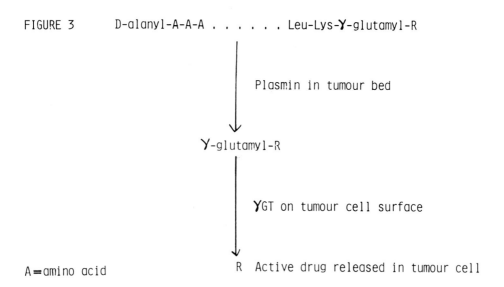

FIGURE 3   D-alanyl-A-A-A . . . . . . Leu-Lys-γ-glutamyl-R

Plasmin in tumour bed

γ-glutamyl-R

γGT on tumour cell surface

A=amino acid   R Active drug released in tumour cell

(B3) Esterase enzymes

Using different substrates a variety of esterases have been detected in different tissues, although in many cases their physiological function is unknown. Over the years there have been reports of unusual 'esterase' activities of different tumours. It would seem appropriate by means of newly developed methods to determine, perhaps by using human tumour xenografts, whether any tumour type has abnormally high levels of esterases of defined substrate activity. If this were the case then different types of prodrug could be synthesised which were activated by the esterase. One type of prodrug could be made from alkylating epoxides. It is known, for example, that the syn isomer of benzpyrene diol epoxide is some 163 times as reactive to 4-nitrothiophenolate than its corresponding anti-isomer (24). The increased electrophilicity of the epoxide in the syn configuration is due to the anchimeric assistance of the cis hydroxyl group, which, possibly by hydrogen bonding, facilitates the opening of the epoxide ring. In the same way triptolide is a good antileukaemic agent because it has a hydroxyl group cis to an epoxide. If the OH group is trans all anti-cancer activity is lost (25). It is also possible that the epoxide group of anguidine may be activated by hydroxylation of a neighbouring group in vivo. Structures of the sort shown in Figure 4 might be prodrugs if the ester group were a substrate for a tumour specific esterase. Hydrolysis of the ester would generate a hydroxyl group which would activate the epoxide and lead to co-valent binding.

FIGURE 4

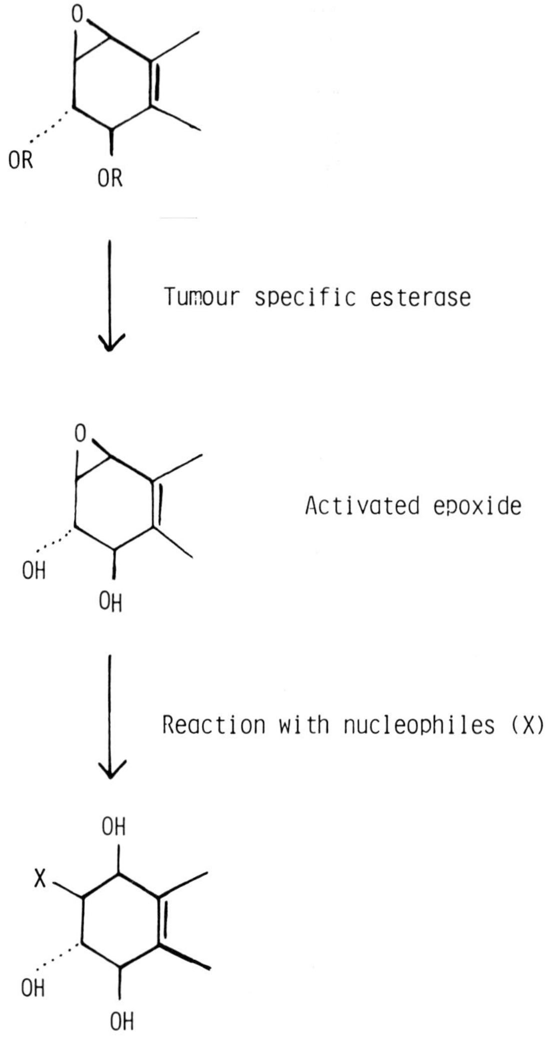
OR
OR
Tumour specific esterase
Activated epoxide
OH
OH
Reaction with nucleophiles (X)
OH
X
OH
OH

There thus seems good reasons for continuing to investigate the suitability of alkylating agents as prodrugs in the treatment of cancer. The main obstacle is still a poor knowledge of the biochemical properties of human cancers and the ways in which they differ from normal tissue. Once a prodrug has been designed on a rational basis it is essential that it is studied in detail rather than 'screened' against tumour systems that happen to be available.

REFERENCES

1. Seligman AM, Nachlas MM, Manheimer LH, Friedman OM, Wolf G. 1949. Ann. Surg. 130, 333.
2. Ishidate M, Sakurai T, Yoshida T, Sato H, Matui E. 1953. GANN 44, 342.
3. Ross WCJ. 1962. Biological Alkylating Agents, London. Butterworth Press.
4. Connors TA. 1976. in Progress in Drug Metabolism, eds Bridges JW, Chasseaud LF. Wiley, New York, pp41-75.
5. Cox PJ, Farmer PB. 1977. Cancer Treatment Reviews, 4, 47 and 119.
6. Connors TA, Cox PJ, Farmer PB, Foster AB, Jarman M. 1974. Biochem. Pharmacol. 23, 115.
7. Connors TA, Whisson ME. 1966. Nature 210, 866.
8. Young CW, Yagoda A, Bittar ES, Smith SW, Grabstald H, Whitmore W. 1976. Cancer 38, 1887.
9. Stanners CP, Lam T, Chamberlain JW, Stewart SS, Price GB. 1981. Cell 27, 211.
10. Cater DB. 1964. Tumori 50. 435.
11. Lin AJ, Cosby LA, Shansky CW, Sartorelli AC. 1972. J. Med. Chem. 15, 1247.
12. Moore HW, Czerniak R. 1981. Med Res. Rev. 1, 249.
13. Goldacre RJ, Sylven B. 1962. Brit. J. Cancer 16, 306.
14. Goldacre RJ, Whisson ME. 1966. Brit.J.Cancer, 20, 801.
15. Chapman JD, Franko AJ, Sharplin J. 1981. Brit. J. Cancer, 43, 546.
16. Franko AJ, Chapman JD. 1982. Brit. J. Cancer, 45, 694.
17. Farber W, Toch R, Sears EM, Pinkel D. 1960. Acta Un. int. Cancr, 16, 611.
18. Carl PL, Chakravarty PK, Katzenellenbogen JA, Weber MJ. 1980. Pro. Natl. Acad. Sci. 77. 2224.
19. Slater TF, White W. Personal Communication.
20. Fiala S, Fiala ES. 1973. J. Natl. Cancer Inst., 51, 151.
21. Rosalki SB. 1975. Adv. Clin. Chem., 17, 53.
22. Peters TJ, Seymour CA, Wells G, Fakunle F, Neale G. 1977. Br. Med. J., i, 1576.
23. Manson MM, Legg RF, Watson JV, Green JA, Neal GE. 1981. Carcinogenesis 2, 661.
24. Politzer P, Trefonas P. 1980. in Carcinogenesis. Fundamental mechanisms and environmental effects. eds. Pullman B, Tso POP, Gelboin H. Dordrecht, Boston, London. D Reidel publishing company, pp67-79.
25. Kupchan SM, Schubert RM. 1974. Science 185, 791.

STRUCTURE–ACTIVITY RELATIONSHIPS FOR ANTI–TUMOUR PLATINUM COMPLEXES

M.J. CLEARE

1. INTRODUCTION

Cis-dichlorodiammineplatinum(II) is now an established member in the armamentarium of anti-neoplastic agents. It is variously known as cisplatin (which is used in this paper) and neoplatin, depending on the country in which it is being sold. It is unique amongst the anti-cancer drugs in that it is based on a heavy metal, namely platinum.

As has been the case in many other medical developments, the discovery of anti-tumour activity in cisplatin and other platinum amine complexes was rather fortuitous. While conducting experiments aimed at studying the effects of electromagnetic fields on cell division, Rosenberg and his co-workers induced filamentous growth in bacteria (1). A long series of control experiments showed that the ac current was causing some 10ppm of platinum to dissolve into the growth medium (C) from the supposedly inert electrodes. The ammonium chloride in the medium led to the formation of $(NH_4)_2[PtCl_6]$ which underwent the following photochemical reaction in the light:-

$$[PtCl_6]^{2-} + 2NH_4^+ \longrightarrow \underline{cis}\text{-}[Pt(NH_3)_2Cl_4] + nH^+ + nCl^-$$

Testing of synthesised cis and trans isomers of $[Pt(NH_3)_2Cl_4]$ and the corresponding platinum(II) species $[Pt(NH_3)_2Cl_2]$ showed that the cis isomers were potent inhibitors of cell division while having only a small inhibitory effect on the growth rate - hence filamentation of the bacteria. The trans isomers were inactive (Figure 1). The property of inhibiting cell division but not cell growth led to the successful demonstration of anti-tumour activity in mice by Rosenberg et al in 1969 for four platinum amine species (2). Testing in several centres, particularly the National Cancer Institute (NCI) in the U.S. and the Chester Beatty Institute in the U.K., indicated that cis-$[Pt(NH_3)_2Cl_2]$ (cisplatin) was the more potent of these original compounds. This

D.N. Reinhoudt, T.A. Connors, H.M. Pinedo & K.W. van de Poll (eds.), Structure-Activity Relationships of Anti-Tumour Agents.
© 1983, Martinus Nijhoff Publishers, The Hague/Boston/London. ISBN 90-247-2783-9.

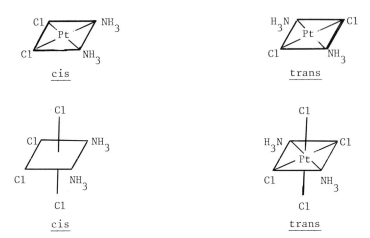

FIGURE 1. Cis and trans isomers of $[Pt(NH_3)_2Cl_2]$ (Pt(II)) and $[Pt(NH_3)_2Cl_4]$ (Pt(IV)).

compound was found to have activity against a wide variety of
transplanted animal tumours and was piloted under sponsorship of the
NCI to initial clinical trials in 1972. In the decade which has
followed the anti-tumour and toxic properties of cisplatin in man have
been fully evaluated and are outlined below.

2. CLINICAL ACTIVITY AND TOXICITY OF CISPLATIN

Cisplatin, either as a single agent or, more usually, in combination
therapy, is active against several human tumours, particularly those of
genito-urinary origin. It has undoubtedly broadened the spectrum of
tumours which are amenable to chemotherapy. This contribution has been
summarised by Durant using the definition of chemotherapeutic sensitivity
shown in Table 1 (3). Thus, while cisplatin has improved responses in
cervix, bladder, prostate and head and neck cancer, it has, to date,
only made a major impact on long term survival for ovarian and,
particularly, testicular tumours (Table 2). One advantage of cisplatin
is that it seems to be effective in combination with a variety of other
agents with different modes of action. Examples include cisplatin –
vinblastin – bleomycin – adriamycin (testicular) (4,5) and cisplatin –
adriamycin – cytoxan (ovarian) (6).

TABLE 1. Classification of chemotherapeutic sensitivity.

Class	Response Rate	CR %[a]	Duration Response	Cures %	Example
Unresponsive	<15%	None	–	None	Kidney
Resistant	15-30%	None	Weeks	None	Colon
Responsive	30-60%	≅5%	Months	0-rare	Breast
Sensitive	50-80%	≅50%	Months	5-20%	AML[b]
Curable	100%	≅100%	Years	>75%	Chorio-carcinoma[c]

[a] CR = complete remissions   [b] AML = acute myeloblastic leukemia

[c] Gestational   Reference : J.R. Durant (3)

TABLE 2. Clinical contributions of cisplatin

Class Change	Major Indications
Unresponsive → Resistant	Cervix, prostate.
Resistant → Responsive	Bladder, Head and Neck.
Responsive → Sensitive	Ovary
Sensitive → Curable	Testicular

Other reported isolated activities : Penile, Endometrial, Lymphoma, Melanoma, Thyroid, Hepatoma, Osteogenic, Sarcoma, Neuroblastoma, Pediatric solid tumours.

The major toxic effects induced by cisplatin in man are nephro-toxicity, myelosuppression, nausea and vomiting and ototoxicity. All toxicities are dose related while nephrotoxicity and ototoxicity appear to be cumulative. Although hydration techniques have reduced nephro-toxicity, which is the major dose limiting factor, higher doses have resulted in some cases in the appearance of peripheral neuropathy symptoms after several treatments (7). Also nausea and vomiting is so severe as to limit the number of courses that some patients will tolerate. Myelosuppression, involving all three blood elements, is another limiting factor on dose schedules, although this toxicity is low compared to many of the other classes of anti-tumour drug.

Thus, although it exhibits good activity as indicated above, cisplatin's therapeutic efficacy is somewhat compromised by the occurrence of severe, dose limiting side effects. This has stimulated a widespread effort to identify alternative platinum complexes which retain the useful anti-tumour properties of cisplatin while having reduced toxicity. Progress to date on "second generation" platinum drugs is discussed in the following sections.

3. STRUCTURE ACTIVITY STUDIES

Not surprisingly, since Rosenberg et al first reported the activity of cisplatin and [Pt(en)Cl$_2$] (and their Pt(IV) analogues) (2), structure-activity studies have largely concentrated on complexes of the type [PtA$_2$X$_2$] (where A$_2$ = two monodentate or one bidentate amine ligand and X$_2$ = two monodentate or one bidentate anionic ligand). The chemistry of such species has been discussed in detail elsewhere (8,9,10) but it is sufficient here to emphasise that the strength of the Pt-N (amine) bond is a dominating feature which means that the X groups are relatively reactive compared to the A groups which are inert to substitution.

Early studies by Cleare and Hoeschele (11,12) and Tobe, Connors et al (13) clearly established two simple criteria for anti-cancer activity, namely the requirements for a neutral complex with adjacent (cis) reactive (X) groups. These criteria have held for all compounds tested to date. At the same time these early studies confirmed that such systematic variations were likely to lead to cisplatin analogues with superior properties in terms of activity and toxicity. A wide range of complexes have since been synthesised and studied over the last ten years. For example, by 1979, the U.S. NCI alone had screened 1,055 platinum complexes, of which anti-tumour activity had been demonstrated in 18% (14). These studies are summarised below with reference to changes in A and X groups respectively, although it should be appreciated that the most successful compounds are combinations of effective A and X groups.

3.1. A Groups

Although the A groups are relatively inert to substitution they have a primary effect on the anti-tumour property of the [PtA$_2$X$_2$] complexes. The pioneering studies in this area were made by Tobe, Connors et al

working in association with Johnson Matthey Company Limited and
Rustenburg Platinum Mines (13). They showed that heterocyclic, alicyclic
(Table 3) and straight and branched chain alkylamines (Table 4) all give
compounds with appreciable anti-tumour activity against the ADJ/PC6A
tumour which proved to be very sensitive to platinum. Relatively minor
structural changes can lead to major changes in the therapeutic index
(TI). Interestingly most of the TI changes were associated with toxicity
rather than potency. The highest TI's were found in compounds of
extremely low solubility (injected in suspension), which may have
involved a slow release system, making true comparisons of toxicity
impossible. However, these plasma cell tumour results indicated that
toxicity might not be so closely related to activity as to preclude the
existence of active complexes with significantly lower toxicities than
cisplatin.

TABLE 3. Activity of complexes cis-[PtA$_2$Cl$_2$]

A = Alicyclic or heterocyclic amine.   Tumour = ADJ/PC6 in BALB/$\bar{\text{C}}$ mice.
a = Arachis oil   Data of Connors et al (13)

A	Solvent	Dose Range (mg/kg)	Dose Response	LD$_{50}$	ID$_{90}$	TI
NH$_3$	Ar^a	0.1–40	+	13.0	1.6	8.1
(aziridine) NH	A	2.5–160	+	56.5	2.6	21.7
(piperidine) NH	A	3–200	+	141	10.8	13.1
(aziridine) N–C$_2$H$_4$OH	A		–	90	>90	<1.0
(morpholine) O N H	A		–	18	>18	<1.0
(cyclopropyl) NH$_2$	A	1–80	+	56.5	2.3	24.6
(cyclobutyl) NH$_2$	A	6–750	+	67	<6	>11.1
(cyclopentyl) NH$_2$	A	1–3200	+	480	2.4	200
(cyclohexyl) NH$_2$	A	1–3200	+	>3200	12	>267
(cycloheptyl) NH$_2$	A	5–625	+	>625	18	>35

TABLE 4. Changes in activity on varying A in cis-[PtA$_2$Cl$_2$]

A = straight and branched chain alkylamines
Tumour = ADJ/PC6A in BALB/C mice

A[a]	ID$_{90}$	LD$_{50}$	TI
i-propylamine	0.9	33.5	37
i-butylamine	6.2	83	13
i-pentylamine	5.8	1150	198
2-aminohexane	27.5	730	26.5
ethylamine	<12	26.5	>2.2
n-propylamine	12	26.5	2.2
n-butylamine	<10	110	>11
n-pentylamine	37	92	2.5

[a] Compounds given i.p. as a suspension in arachis oil
Data of Connors et al (13)

It is interesting to note that the earliest studies (11,13,14) initiated interest in chelating diamines which have been the main focus of recent activities in synthesising and testing new Pt complexes. Most notable of these is 1,2-diaminocyclohexane which has subsequently been studied in detail in combination with a wide variety of X groups by Gale and co-workers (15).

Studies by Bradner et al using the L1210 tumour have confirmed the activity of straight and branched chain alkylamines, particularly those with C$_3$-C$_4$ carbon chains (Table 5) (16), with the best results being obtained on a daily dose schedule. Estimates of blood urea nitrogen (BUN) levels and total white blood cell (WBC) count indicated that most of the compounds were less nephrotoxic than cisplatin in this test system. Branched chain compounds appeared to be more active than the corresponding straight chain isomers. Alicyclic amine complexes were also active against the L1210 (22), but all these amines were less active against the leukemia than the ADJ/PC6 (Table 6). This underlines a persistent problem when attempting to identify platinum cogeners possessing anti-tumour activity superior to that of cisplatin, namely considerable inconsistency in structure-activity comparisons across different tumour systems. Indeed some tumours, such as Sarcoma 180 used in the earliest studies (11,12), seem to be rather insensitive to variations in the amine (A) ligand.

TABLE 5. Changes in activity on varying A in cis-[PtA$_2$Cl$_2$]

A = alkylamine (n, iso, t)
Tumour = L1210 in BDF$_1$ mice (10^6 cells)

A	Optimum Dose (i.p. mg/kg)	Schedule	ILS (%)
CISPLATIN (NH$_3$)	8	d1	164-229
	2	d1-9	157-285
MeNH$_2$	16	d1	129
EtNH$_2$	6	d1	142
n-PrNH$_2$	8	d1	157
i-PrNH$_2$	32	d1	171
	8	d1-9	179
n-BuNH$_2$	8	d1	114
i-BuNH$_2$	64	d1	171
	16	d1-9	193
t-BuNH$_2$	64	d1	100

Data of Bradner et al (16)

TABLE 6. Changes in activity on varying A in cis-[PtA$_2$Cl$_2$]

A = cycloalkylamine
Tumour = L1210 in BDF$_1$ mice (10^6 cells)

A	Optimum Dose (i.p. mg/kg)	Schedule	ILS (%)
NH$_3$	8	d1	164-229
	2	d1-9	157-285
cyclopropylamine	16	d1	157
	8	d1-9	164
cyclobutylamine	32	d1	157
	16	d1-9	221
cyclopentylamine	128	d1	121
	32	d1-9	143

Data of Bradner et al (16)

Recent studies have concentrated on bidentate amine ligands, particularly those containing saturated or aromatic hydrocarbon rings. For example, the 1,2-diaminocyclohexane nucleus (1,2-dac) has proved to be a prolific structure for active complexes in combination with a variety of leaving groups (see below). Tests by Gale et al against the L1210 tumour identified the malonate, hydroxymalonate, nitrate and sulphate as of potential interest (15). Macquet and Armand extended this to include citrato and isocitrato species (18).

Researchers in the Netherlands reported the value of ligands based on substituted 1,3-diaminopropane systems (17), particularly those involving cycloalkanes in the 2-carbon position (e.g. 1,1-diaminomethylcyclohexane - 1,1-damcha). Complexes with various X groups show good activity against L1210 (24) and B16 melanoma (Tables 7 and 23).

TABLE 7. Variation of activity for $[PtACl_2]$ species

A = bidentate amine
Tumour = L1210 in BDF_1 mice (10^6 cells)

A	Optimum Dose (i.p. mg/kg)	Schedule	ILS (%)
1,1-diaminomethyl-cyclohexane	15 3	d1 d1-9	208 292
1,1-diaminomethyl-cyclopentane	12.5	d1	148
2,2-dimethyl-1,3-diaminopropane	12.5	d1	323
2,2-diethyl-1,3-diaminopropane	9 1.5	d1 d1-9	325 (2/6) 242
2-methyl-2-ethyl-1,3-diaminopropane	12.5	d1	289

Data of Bradner et al (16)   National Cancer Institute (17)

Kidani et al have demonstrated good activity for 1-aminomethyl-2-aminocyclohexane (amcha) complexes in racemic and resolved forms (see section 3.3). Totani et al have reported good ILS figures against L1210 (10^5 cells) for exocyclic amine complexes based:-

(exo-cis-2,3-diaminobicyclo(2,2,1)heptane)
(Table 8, Reference 20)

TABLE 8. Activity of complexes of type $[PtAX_2]$ where A = exo, cis-2,3-diaminobicyclo(2,2,1)heptane[a] and X_2= mono- and bidentate anionic ligands

Tumour = L1210 in BDF_1 mice (10^5 cells)[b]

X_2	Optimum Dose (mg/kg)	ILS (%)
CISPLATIN	10	184 (1)
$[Pt(1,2-dac)Cl_2]$[c]	10	229 (2)
Cl_2	10	243 (3)
$(NO_3)_2$	10	251 (4)
$SO_4(H_2O)$	10	321 (5)
oxalate	20	249 (4)
malonate	50	184 (1)
glucuronate	20	226 (2)

a   b Doses i.p. d1 only. Test groups 4-7 mice - 30 day.

c 1,2-dac = 1,2-diaminocyclohexane

Data of Totani et al (BP 2,074,567 A) (20)

Amino acid based complexes have also shown activity against the P388 tumour (21) (Table 9).

Rosenberg and Van Camp had originally reported cis-$[Pt(NH_3)_2Cl_4]$ and $[Pt(en)Cl_4]$ to be equally active as their Pt(II) dichloro complexes against Sarcoma 180 (2). Thus Tobe, Connors et al extended their study of different amine systems to include Pt(IV) complexes, particularly those of type $[PtA_2Cl_2(OH)_2]$ in order to obtain improved water solubility (13). The latter was achieved in some cases whilst maintaining activity, however, the general order of activity was:-

$[Pt(II)A_2Cl_2]$ > $[Pt(IV)A_2Cl_4]$ > $[Pt(IV)A_2Cl_2(OH)_2]$ (Table 10)

This technique has been adopted by Verbeck et al for bidentate amines

based on 1,3-diaminopropane (23). Bradner et al confirmed that
alkylamine alicyclic amines and the bidentate systems also gave Pt(II)
species active against the L1210 with bidentate amines > alkyl/alicyclic
amines and $[PtA_2Cl_2(OH)_2] \geq [PtA_2Cl_4]$ (Tables 11, 12 and 13) (22).

TABLE 9. Activity of Species

$$R - C(NH_2)(NH_2) - Pt \left< {Cl \atop Cl} \right.$$

Tumour = P388 in CDF$_1$ mice $(10^6$ cells$)$[a]

R	Optimum Dose (mg/kg)	ILS (%)	Aqueous Solubility	Nephrotoxicity (Rabbit)
CH$_3$OOC–	5	210	Soluble[b]	++
HOOC–	5	220	High	+
NaOOC–	5	230	Very high	+
KOOC–	5	225	Very high	+
CISPLATIN	5	180	Low	++++
[Pt(1,2-dac)Cl$_2$][c]	–	–	Very low	++++

[a] Doses i.p. d1-5   [b] At elevated temperature
[c] 1,2-dac = 1,2-diaminocyclohexane   Data of Yoshikumi et al (21)

TABLE 10. Activity of Pt(II) and Pt(IV) amine complexes

Tumour = ADJ/PC6 in BALB/C̄ mice

Amine	Pt(II)Cl$_2$			Pt(IV)Cl$_4$			Pt(IV)Cl$_2$(OH)$_2$		
	LD$_{50}$	LD$_{90}$	TI	LD$_{50}$	LD$_{90}$	TI	LD$_{50}$	LD$_{90}$	TI
NH$_3$	13.0	1.6	8.1	–	(a)	–	135	4.8	28.1
⟩–NH$_2$	33.5	0.9	37	132	>60	<2.0	90	7.5	12,0
⬡–NH$_2$ / –NH$_2$	22.5	10	2.25	–	–	–	135	60	2.2
–NH$_2$	83	6.2	13.4	111	<10	>11.1	410	19.5	21
⬠–NH$_2$	556	2.4	236	141	3.0	48	83	(b)	–

(a) Active against other systems   (b) 89% inhibition obtained
Data of Connors et al (13)

TABLE 11. Changes in activity for species $[Pt(IV)A_2X'_2X''_2]$

A = alkylamine (up to C_3) X' or X" = Cl and OH
Tumour = L1210 in BDF_1 mice (10^6 cells)

A	X'	X"	Optimum Dose (i.p. mg/kg)	Schedule	ILS (%)
NH_3	Cl	OH	120	d1	164
			20	d1-9	193
$MeNH_2$	Cl	Cl	5	d1	142
	Cl	OH	112	d1	143
$EtNH_2$	Cl	Cl	45	d1	114
	Cl	OH	104	d1	143
$n-C_3H_7NH_2$	Cl	Cl	3	d1	121
	Cl	OH	45	d1	129
			22.5	d1-9	157
$i-C_3H_7NH_2$	Cl	Cl	24	d1	129
	Cl	OH	32	d1	171
			16	d1-9	207

Data of Bradner et al (16)

TABLE 12. Changes in Activity for species $[PtA_2X'_2X''_2]$

A = alkyl- or cycloalkylamine (C_4) X' or X" = Cl and OH
Tumour = L1210 in BDF_1 mice (10^6 cells)

A	X'	X"	Optimum Dose (i.p. mg/kg)	Schedule	ILS (%)
$n-C_4H_9NH_2$	Cl	Cl	26	d1	129
			6.5	d1-9	129
	Cl	OH	104	d1	179
			26	d1-9	157
$i-C_4H_9NH_2$	Cl	Cl	18	d1	136
			9	d1-9	157
	Cl	OH	120, 160	d1	150, 200
			40	d1-9	200, 171 (3/6)[a]
$C_4H_8NH_2$	Cl	OH	20	d1	133
			10	d1-9	150

[a] 171% ILS for dying mice; 3 mice alive on day 30.

Data of Bradner et al (16)

TABLE 13. Changes in activity for species $[PtA_2Cl_2X_2]$

A = Bidentate chelating amine
Tumour = L1210 in BDF_1 mice (10^6 cells)

A	X	Optimum Dose (i.p. mg/kg)	Schedule	ILS (%)
NH_3	OH	120	d1	164
		20	d1-9	193
1,1-diaminomethyl-cyclohexane	Cl	12	d1	236
		2	d1-9	229
1,1-diaminomethyl-cyclohexane	OH	16	d1	214 (3/6)
		12	d1-9	417
2,2-diethyl-1,3-diaminopropane	Cl	8	d1	229 (1/6)
		2	d1-9	264
1,1-diaminomethyl-cyclobutane	Cl	8	d1	207
		1.5	d1-9	236
1,1-diaminomethyl-cyclopentane	Cl	6	d1	257
		1.5	d1-9	257

Data of Bradner et al (16)

Several studies indicate that the nature of the A group has only a secondary effect on the overall reactivity (unless it is very bulky when steric hindrance can reduce substitution rates (10)). Variation in activity probably owes more to differences in biophysical properties such as membrane transport and possibly steric influences on enzyme repair processes. Effective A groups tested to date are summarised in Table 14.

TABLE 14. Effective A groups

A	Examples
n-alkylamines	C_2-C_4
i-alkylamines	C_3-C_5 [a]
Alicyclic amines	C_3-C_8 [a]
Diamino alkanes	Ethylenediamine, substituted 1,3-propylene diamines
Diamino cycloalkanes	1,2-diaminocyclohexane 1,1-diaminomethylcyclohexane
Heterocyclic amines	Ethyleneimine pyrolidine
Diamino acids	1,2-diamino-1,2-dicarboxylatoethane
Exocyclic amines	

[a] Aqueous solubility very low with long carbon chain.

3.2. X Groups

Initial studies concentrated on ammine species $[Pt(NH_3)_2X_2]$ and demonstrated that labile (easily replaced groups) such as NO_3^- and H_2O gave rise to highly toxic species while strongly bound ligands such as NO_2^- and SCN^- formed inactive complexes (11,12). Since this several groups have reported on the complex nature of cis-$[Pt(NH_3)_2(H_2O)_2]^{2+}$ solutions which tend to polymerise on standing via the formation of hydroxo bridges (24,25); the monomers and oligomers have widely different toxicities and activities with the dimer being particularly toxic.

A major outcome of the early studies was the discovery that chelating dicarboxylate ligands, particularly malonates and substituted malonates, give rise to a wide variety of active species (Table 15).

Subsequent studies have shown that complexes with these ligands, in combination with many of the amine types described above, have comparable or superior activity against L1210 and some solid tumours to corresponding chloride and other monodentate anions (Tables 16 and 17) (17,24). Malonates tend to be less effective against leukemias than solid tumour test systems (Table 18). Malonates substituted in the 2-position are abbreviated Etmal (ethylmalonate), OHmal (hydroxymalonate), etc.

TABLE 15. Activity of Pt(II) amine malonato species

Tumour = ADJ/PC6 in BALB/$\overline{\text{C}}$ mice

Malonato complexes	LD_{50} (mg/kg)	ID_{90} (mg/kg)	TI	Aqueous solubility (mM)
[Pt(NH$_3$)$_2$mal]	225	18.5	12.2	1.0
[Pt(NH$_3$)$_2$Memal]	112	4.5	24.9	7.0
[Pt(NH$_3$)$_2$Etmal]	132	12	11	160.0
[Pt(NH$_3$)$_2$OHmal]	150	4.9	30.6	-
[Pt(NH$_3$)$_2$Benzmal]	150	1.85	81.1	-
[Pt(NH$_3$)$_2$(1,1-CBDCA)]	180	14.5	12.4	50.0
[Pt(en)mal]	220	18.5	12	-
[Pt(en)Memal]	200	50	4	-
[Pt(en)Etmal]	450	49	9.2	-
[Pt(MeNH$_2$)$_2$mal]	670	56	12	-

Data of Cleare et al (8)

TABLE 16. Activity of malonato complexes [PtA$_2$mal] where mal = malonate or 2-substituted malonate and A = NH$_3$ or alkylamine.

Tumour = L1210 in BDF$_1$ mice (10^6 cells)

A	mal	Optimum Dose (i.p. mg/kg)	Schedule	ILS (%)
NH$_3$	Etmal	128	d1	150
		64	d1-9	157
NH$_3$	OHmal	64	d1	150
		32	d1-9	200
NH$_3$	CBDCA	128	d1	150
		64	d1-9	157
CH$_3$NH$_2$	Etmal	400	d1	179
		100	d1-9	207
CH$_3$NH$_2$	OHmal	400	d1	143
		100	d1-9	164
C$_2$H$_5$NH$_2$	Etmal	400	d1	150
		200	d1-9	179
C$_2$H$_5$NH$_2$	OHmal	256	d1	143
		64	d1-9	143
n-C$_3$H$_7$NH$_2$	mal	104	d1	113
		8.5	d1-9	142
i-C$_3$H$_7$NH$_2$	mal	256	d1	121
i-C$_3$H$_7$NH$_2$	Etmal	120	d1	114

Data of Bradner et al (16,22)   CBDCA = 1,1-cyclobutanedicarboxylate

TABLE 17. Activity of malonato complexes [PtAmal] where mal = malonate or
2-substituted malonate and A = bidentate amine

Tumour = L1210 in BDF$_1$ mice (10^6 cells)

A	mal	Optimum Dose (i.p. mg/kg)	Schedule	ILS (%)
ethylenediamine	mal[a]	34	d1	129
		25	d1-9	196
ethylenediamine	OHmal	120	d1	129
		40	d1-9	136
1,2-diamino-propane	mal	60	d1	143
		15	d1-9	136
1,2-diamino-cyclohexane	mal	32	d1	154
		16	d1-9	254
1,2-diamino-cyclohexane	OHmal	100	d1	183
		40	d1-9	243
1,1-diaminomethyl-cyclohexane	CHDCA[b]	120	d1	129
		60	d1-9	136

[a] Results from U.S. NCI   [b] CHDCA = 1,1-cyclohexanedicarboxylate
Data of Bradner et al (16,22)

TABLE 18. Activity of malonato complexes [PtA$_2$mal] where mal = malonate
or 2-substituted malonate and A = NH$_3$ or alkylamine

Tumour = Lewis Lung Carcinoma[a] and B16 Melanoma[b]

A	mal	Lewis Lung		B16 Melanoma	
		Optimum Dose (mg/kg/day)[c]	ILS (%)[d]	Optimum Dose (mg/kg/day)[c]	ILS (%)[d]
CISPLATIN		0.8-1.6	144-343 (0-8/10)	0.8-1.6	157-230 (0-1/10)
NH$_3$	Etmal	32	124 (3/10)	16	173
NH$_3$	OHmal	24	231 (8/10)	32	124 (6/10)
NH$_3$	CBDCA	–	–	16	174
MeNH$_2$	OHmal	–	–	60	182
MeNH$_2$	Etmal	–	–	65	183 (3/10)
EtNH$_2$	OHmal	–	–	96	178
EtNH$_2$	Etmal	–	–	150	213 (1/10)
n-C$_4$H$_9$	OHmal	–	–	40	148
i-C$_4$H$_9$	OHmal	–	–	40	141

[a] 10^6 cells i.p.   [b] 0.5ml of 10% tumour brei, i.p.
[c] All treatments q.d1-9 i.p.   [d] Dying mice only. Tumour free mice on
day 60 in parentheses.

Data of Bradner et al (16,22)

Gale et al showed that simple anions such as sulphate and nitrate could be used with advantage in the 1,2-diaminocyclohexane complexes and with no excessive toxicity as in the NH_3 system (26,27). This was extended to include chlorocarboxylates and phthalates (28,29) and used in conjunction with other amines, particularly 1,1-diaminomethylcyclohexane and derivatives of 1,3-diaminopropane (17,24,30).

Effective X groups are summarised in Table 19. The chemistry of the X groups has been discussed in detail elsewhere (8,9,31) but it is important here to emphasise that three classes of active species can be identified on a kinetic basis.

1. Reactive species that are rapidly hydrolysed and which would be quickly converted to chloro species in the presence of physiological concentrations of saline. Examples would be sulphato and nitrato complexes.

2. Species with intermediate reactivity towards water and chloride and half life of around 1-3 hours. Cisplatin falls into this category for hydrolysis, although reactions of chloro complexes are somewhat suppressed in the presence of chloride ion which serves to protect them in the serum. Compounds containing chloroacetate undergo replacement at an intermediate rate.

3. Bidentate carboxylate complexes are kinetically inert. These are so non-reactive in vitro in comparison with other anti-tumour active species that we have previously suggested the involvement of an in vivo activation mechanism.

Examples of all three classes of agent are currently on clinical trial. Preliminary evidence suggests that short term toxicity is somewhat lower for the less reactive species (see section 5.2).

TABLE 19. Structure-activity studies on cis-[PtA$_2$X$_2$] species
           - Effective X groups

X	Examples
Halide	Chloro, bromo
Oxyanions	Sulphate, nitrate
Carboxylates	Halogeno-acetates
Dicarboxylates	Oxalate, malonate, substituted malonates, phthalates

3.3. Isomers involving different forms of cyclic diamines

The diaminocyclohexane nucleus has proved a prolific amine structure for active complexes and Kidani et al investigated the possibility of optimising its activity by purifying the ligand as three different isomers (32). Two are geometrical (cis and trans) while the trans can be resolved into two optical isomers (trans-d and trans-1-)

cis   trans-d   trans-1

Chloro complexes with the trans ligand (i.e. [Pt(1,2-dac)Cl$_2$]) were more effective against the L1210 tumour, with trans-1 somewhat more superior to trans-d (Table 20). However, the distinction in activity was not apparent for malonate and oxalate species (Table 21) although the trans-1 seemed to have a better therapeutic index. However, some workers have preferred the trans-1 isomer in subsequent tests. A similar study on isomers of 2-aminomethylcyclohexane (2-amcha) by the same workers indicated that generalised extrapolations for trans over cis ligands could not be made. In this case both cis and trans isomers can be resolved to give four possibilities, cis-d, cis-1, trans-d and trans-1. Here cis isomers seemed somewhat more effective and selective against L1210 and P388 with cis-1 ≥ cis-d. It remains to be seen if the fairly narrow differences are maintained against solid animal tumours and in human clinical trials.

TABLE 20. Activity of 1,2-dac isomers[a] in species [Pt(1,2-dac)Cl$_2$]
Tumour = L1210 in CDF$_1$ mice (10^5 cells)[b]

Isomer	Optimum Dose (mg/kg)	ILS (%)
CISPLATIN	12.5	278
cis-dac	12.5	211
trans-d-dac	12.5	291
trans-1-dac	12.5	392

[a] 1,2-dac = 1,2-diaminocyclohexane   [b] Doses i.p. on d1 and d5
Data of Kidani et al (32)

TABLE 21.   Activity of 1,2-dac isomers[a] in species [Pt(1,2-dac)X] where
X - dicarboxylate

Tumour = P388 leukemia in CDF_1 mice (10^6 cells)[b]

Isomer	X	Optimum Dose (mg/kg)	ILS (%)
cis-dac	oxalate	25	200
	malonate	50	155
	methylmalonate	80	133
trans-d-dac	oxalate	20	198
	malonate	50	155
	methylmalonate	100	154
trans-l-dac	oxalate	6.25	188
	malonate	75	202
	methylmalonate	100	141

[a] 1,2-dac = 1,2-diaminocyclohexane   [b] Doses i.p. on d1 and d5
Data of Kidani et al (32)

4. PRECLINICAL STUDIES ON CISPLATIN ANALOGUES : IDENTIFICATION OF CANDIDATES FOR CLINICAL TRIALS

The major targets for a second generation platinum based drug would be
any of the following properties and preferably all three:-

1. Reduced toxicity with activity at least comparable to
   cisplatin - particularly nephrotoxicity which is dose
   limiting.

2. An improved spectrum of activity.

3. Activity against cisplatin resistant tumours.

It can be deduced from the last section that an almost bewildering range
of active platinum complexes have been identified by testing against
primary screens such as the ADJ/PC6, L1210 and P388 tumours. Thus it has
been necessary to employ a combination of further criteria in order to
identify candidates for Phase 1 clinical trials. These criteria have
included anti-tumour activity against a variety of solid animal tumours
and xenografted human tumours in immune deprived mice. Lack of cross
resistance with cisplatin against the L1210 has also been used as a basis
for selection (33). Such advanced activity tests have usually been
coupled with various types of preclinical toxicological
investigations.

4.1. Anti-tumour studies

The U.S. National Cancer Institute selected compounds from their initial screen to compare with cisplatin against a comprehensive tumour panel (Table 22) (14). Although this revealed some qualitative differences in activity in some of the tumour systems, few differences were observed in the general spectrum of activity. Toxicity studies were required to identify clinical trial candidates (40). Bradner and his colleagues at Bristol Laboratories examined a series of complexes, with comparable L1210 activity to cisplatin, against two solid tumours, namely the Lewis Lung Carcinoma and the B16 Melanoma (16,22). While no analogue displayed clear superiority over cisplatin against the Lewis Lung tumour several compounds showed comparable effects, i.e.

$[Pt(OHmal)(NH_3)_2]$ and $[Pt(Etmal)(NH_3)_2]$ - Table 18

$[Pt(1,2-dac)(mal)]$ and $[Pt(1,2-dac)(SO_4)(H_2O)]$ - Table 23

cis-$[Pt(i-C_3H_7NH_2)_2(NO_3)_2]$ and cis-$[Pt(n-C_3H_7NH_2)_2(ClAc)_2]$ - Table 24

$[Pt(i-C_3H_7NH_2)_2Cl_2(OH)_2]$ (hereafter called CHIP) (16)

(ClAc = chloroacetate)

In the B16 Melanoma case $[Pt(OHmal)(NH_3)_2]$ was clearly superior to cisplatin while others were closely comparable, i.e.

$[Pt(CH_3NH_2)_2(Etmal)]$ - Table 18

$[Pt(C_2H_5NH_2)_2(Etmal)]$ - Table 18

$[Pt(ethylenediamine)(mal)]$ - Table 23

The promising activity of $[Pt(OHmal)(NH_3)_2]$ was somewhat compromised by its limited aqueous solubility and it has yet to undergo a clinical trial for this reason. These tests indicated that malonato complexes were more effective against solid tumours than leukemia screens.

Harrap and his co-workers selected a group of eight complexes largely on the basis of L1210 and ADJ/PC6 screening results (34). These compounds were then further tested against a human bronchogenic carcinoma xenograft and only one compound, $[Pt(1,1-cyclobutanedicarboxylate)(NH_3)_2]$ hereafter called CBDCA, consistently produced cures at non-toxic doses. Other complexes showed activity (Table 25), namely:-

$[Pt(Etmal)(NH_3)_2]$, cisplatin

$[Pt(1,2-dac)(SO_4)(H_2O)]$, cis-$[Pt(i-C_3H_7NH_2)_2(ClAc)_2]$

Studies at the Radiobiological Institute (TNO) in the Netherlands showed that the 1,1-diaminomethylcyclohexane (1,1-damcha) ligand gave rise to a wide range of active complexes (somewhat the same as for

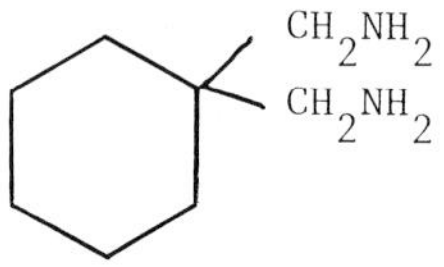

(1-1-damcha)

1,2-dac) with some having good activity against the B16 melanoma as well as L1210 (Tables 7, 13, 17 and 23).

TABLE 22. Tumour Panel testing of promising Pt complexes

COMPLEX	TUMOUR[a]				
	B16 Melanoma (i.p.)	CD8F1 Mammary (s.c.)	Colon 38 (s.c.)	L1210 Leukemia (i.p.)	Lewis Lung (i.v.)
CISPLATIN	++	++	+	++	+
[Pt(en)mal]	++	NT	NT	++	NT
[Pt(1,2-dac)mal]	++	+	+	++	−
CBDCA	++	+	+	+	−
[Pt(1,2-dac)(SO$_4$)(H$_2$O)]	++	+	+	++	−
CHIP	++	+	−	++	−
[Pt(1,2-dac)TMA]	++	+	+	++	−

[a] ++ = significant activity
  + = minimal activity
  − = no activity
 NT = not tested

en = ethylenediamine, mal = malonate, 1,2-dac = 1,2-diaminocyclohexane, TMA = 4-carboxyphthalate, CHIP = [Pt(isopropylamine)(OH)$_2$Cl$_2$].

National Cancer Institute Data (M.K. Wolpert - De Filippes) (14)

TABLE 23. Activity of Complexes [PtAX$_2$] where A = bidentate amine and
X = 2 mono- or 1 bidentate anionic ligand

Tumour = Lewis Lung Carcinoma[a] and B16 Melanoma[b]

A	X	LEWIS LUNG		B16 MELANOMA	
		Optimum Dose (mg/kg/day)[c]	ILS (%)[d]	Optimum Dose (mg/kg/day)[c]	ILS (%)[d]
ethylenediamine	malonate	–	–	25	214[f]
1,2-diamino-cyclohexane	SO$_4$ (H$_2$O)	5	– (9/10)	5	152
1,2-diamino-cyclohexane	malonate	4	141 (7/10)	4	143
1,2-diamino-cyclohexane	hydroxy-malonate	80[e]	112	20	162
1,2-diamino-cyclohexane	oxalate	–	–	3	171
1,2-diamino-cyclohexane	4-carboxy-phthalato	–	–	0.8	168
1,1-diaminomethyl-cyclohexane	SO$_4$ (H$_2$O)	12[e]	117 (1/10)	1.6	154
1,1-diaminomethyl-cyclohexane	4-carboxy-phthalato	–	–	5	141
1,1-diaminomethyl-cyclohexane	Cl	6[e]	127	3.6	173
2,2-diethyl-1,3-diaminopropane	Cl	4[e]	123	2.4	168

[a] 10^6 cells i.p. [b] 0.5ml of 10% tumour brei, i.p.

[c] All treatments q.d1-9 except where indicated otherwise.

[d] Dying mice only. Day 60 survivors in parentheses.

[e] q.d 5, 9, 13. [f] National Cancer Institute data.

Data of Bradner et al (16, 22)

TABLE 24. Activity of complexes $[PtA_2X_2]$ where A = alkyl- or cycloalkylamine and X - 2 mono- or 1 bidentate anionic ligand

Tumour = Lewis Lung Carcinoma[a] and B16 Melanoma[b]

A	X	LEWIS LUNG		B16 MELANOMA	
		Optimum Dose (mg/kg/day)[c]	ILS (%)[d]	Optimum Dose (mg/kg/day)[c]	ILS (%)[d]
i-propylamine	ClAc	8	143	8	163
i-propylamine	NO_3	4	100 (6/10)	8	127
i-propylamine	oxalate	-	-	10	119
n-propylamine	ClAc	4	159 (6/10)	4	175
n-propylamine	SO_4 (H_2O)	-	-	8	144
cyclopentylamine/NH_3	Cl	-	-	1	173

[a] 10^6 cells i.p.   [b] 0.5ml of 10% tumour brei, i.p.
[c] All treatments q.d1-9.   [d] Dying mice only. Day 60 survivors in parentheses.
ClAc = chloroacetate   Data of Bradner et al (16).

TABLE 25. Comparative activity of $[PtA_2X_2]$ complexes against a human
epidermoid carcinoma (P246) xenograph[a]

A_2	X_2	Dose[b] (mg/kg)	$\frac{T}{C}$ x 100	Deaths (week)	% Body Wt. Change
CISPLATIN		6 (2)	1.0	2/6 (3)	-13
		2 (4)	12.0	1/6 (3)	+ 3
$(NH_3)_2$	OHmal	8 (4)	51		+ 2
$(NH_3)_2$	CBDCA	48 (4)	1.0		- 1
		16 (4)	34.0		+ 3
$(NH_3)_2$	Etmal	75 (4)	2.0	1/6 (5) 1/7 (7)	+ 1
i-$PrNH_2$	chloro-acetate	24 (3)	18	1/6 (2)	0
		8 (3)	87		+10
1,2-dac	SO_4 (H_2O)	9 (1)[c]	2.0	2/6 (2,6)	- 6
		3 (3)[c]	27.0		+ 3
CHIP		48 (1)	-	4/6 (1)	
		16 (4)	59		- 7

[a] Grown in immune-deprived mice.   [b] i.p. at twice weekly intervals.
[c] Terminated at 6 weeks.   Number of doses in parentheses.
   Tests completed after 7 weeks
   (except c)
CBDAC = 1,2-cyclobutanedicarboxylate.
1,2-dac = 1,2-diaminocyclohexane.
i-Pr = isopropyl   Data of Harrap et al (34)

4.2. Lack of cross resistance with cisplatin

Burchenal et al derived a line of the L1210 tumour which was approximately 50-fold resistant to cisplatin (in vitro) and this was used to screen a variety of complexes for cross resistance both in vitro and in mice (33). These studies showed that the 1,2-dac structure (and its cycloheptane analogue) conferred a degree of lack of cross resistance with cisplatin and this property was independant of the leaving group (X) which could be malonate, sulphate, chloride or carboxyphthalato (33,36). Using a similar tumour Bradner et al confirmed these results and also demonstrated a lack of cross resistance for 1,1-damcha and related systems including one without a hydrocarbon ring (e.g. 2,2-diethyl-1,3-diaminopropane). They also showed that this applied to Pt(IV) as well as Pt(II) complexes (22) (Tables 26 and 27). The cross resistance of complexes containing 1,2-diaminocyclopentane and orthophenylenediamine, which are closely related to 1,2-dac, suggests that this property cannot be easily related to structure. It is an interesting addition to preclinical screening but a true relationship to the human situation remains to be demonstrated.

TABLE 26. Cross resistance studies for $[Pt(IV)ACl_2X_2]$ species against L1210 leukemia resistant to cisplatin (L1210/cisplatin).

A	X	Optimum Dose (i.p. mg/kg)	L1210[a]	L1210/Cisplatin[a]
CISPLATIN	–	4–8	183	106–121
1,1-diaminomethyl-cyclohexane	Cl	6	183 (1/6)	171 (1/6)
1,1-diaminomethyl-cyclopentane	Cl	4–8	200	138 (3/6)
1,1-diaminomethyl-cyclohexane	OH	12–15	225 (1/6)	229

[a] 10^6 cells i.p. - BDF$_1$ mice

Data of Bradner et al (22)

TABLE 27. Cross resistance studies for $[PtA_2X_2]$ against L1210 leukemia
resistant to cisplatin

A_2	X_2	Optimum Dose (i.p. mg/kg)	L1210[a] (ILS %)	L1210/Cisplatin (ILS %)
CISPLATIN		4-8	183	106-121
$(NH_3)_2$	CBDCA	80-120	146	113
$(NH_3)_2$	Etmal	120-160	183	118
1,2-dac	mal	36-48	169	156
1,2-dac	SO_4 (H_2O)	6-15	217-250	200-371 (2-4/6)
1,2-dac	TMA[b]	10-20	250	176 (2/6)
1,1-damcha	$(Cl)_2$	4-6	217 (1/6)	193 (2/6)
1,1-damcha	SO_4 (H_2O)	9-12	217	171 (1/6)
2,2-diethyl-1,3-diaminopropane	$(Cl)_2$	6-8	175 (2/6)	229 (2/6)

[a] 10^6 cells i.p. - BDF_1 mice. [b] TMA = carboxyphthalato
Data of Bradner et al (22)

4.3. Therapeutic synergism with other agents in animal tumour systems

Cisplatin is active against experimental and human tumours in
combination with other established anti-cancer drugs as well as in single
agent form. Some similar studies have been carried out on analogues,
particularly those containing the 1,2-dac structure (26,42,43). In
general, the effects exhibited by active platinum analogues are broadly
comparable to those shown by cisplatin in the same combination and this
approach does not appear to be a powerful means of identifying clinical
candidates. However, Gale et al have demonstrated strong synergy
against advanced L1210 in mice between 1,2-dac, cyclophosphamide and
ribonucleotide reductase inhibitors such as hydroxy urea (39). Burchenal
and his co-workers have shown synergism against advanced L1210 and P388
for 1,2-dac compounds in combination with VP-16, methotrexate, adriamycin
and arabinosyl cytosine (36).

4.4. Toxicological evaluation

The major toxic limitations of cisplatin have been discussed in Section 2. As nephrotoxicity is the major clinical dose limiting side effect much of the preclinical toxicology has been aimed at an assessment of potential renal damage for active analogues.

The National Cancer Institute used isolated flounder tubules and rat renal tissue slices in vitro to assess renal toxicity potential, and found that six analogues out of the 25 tested had diminished renal toxicity compared to cisplatin (40). This was combined with toxicological evaluation in dogs to identify [Pt(1,2-dac)mal], CBDCA and [Pt(1,2-dac)(4-carboxyphthalato)] (4-carboxyphthallic acid is known as trimellitic acid - compound hereafter called TMA) as potential clinical trial candidates. All six compounds tested were generally less toxic than cisplatin. However, some hepatotoxicity and haematologic toxicity was always observed. CBDCA was particularly interesting as it did not elevate BUN values in dogs at the toxic dose (low) and did not induce emesis even at the lethal dose (Table 28).

TABLE 28. Emetic effect in dogs for $[PtA_2X_2]$

A_2	X_2	BRISTOL LABORATORIES[a] Dose (i.v. mg/kg)	Effect[c]	NATIONAL CANCER INSTITUTE[b] Toxic Dose Low (mg/kg x 5d)	Threshold Emetic Dose (mg/kg x 1d)
CISPLATIN		3	+	0.19	0.75
$(NH_3)_2$	Etmal	12	0		
1,2-dac	$SO_4(H_2O)$	3	+	0.38	1.5
1,2-dac	TMA	3	+	3.5^e	7.0
1,2-dac	mal			3.0	6.0
$(NH_3)_2$	CBDCA			3.0	12.0^d
1,1-damcha	Cl_2	2	+		
CHIP		6	+	0.44	3.5

[a] Data of Schurig et al; 2 Beagles/dose (41).   [b] Data of Guarino et al (40).
[c] + = acute emesis, 0 = no effect.   [d] No emesis even at lethal dose.
[e] Estimated value - some dogs still on test.

1,2-dac = 1,2-diaminocyclohexane
1,1-damcha = 1,1-diaminomethylcyclohexane

Schurig and his colleagues at Bristol Laboratories have evaluated a large number of active platinum analogues for toxic effect in the mouse (41). A large proportion of the compounds studied (Table 29) did not cause significant elevation of BUN levels at optimal doses, with some maintaining this at LD_{50} doses. This confirmed that several platinum compounds were able to combine anti-tumour activity at least comparable to cisplatinum with greatly reduced nephrotoxicity. These analogues, however, did show significant myelosuppression. The following were considered as most promising:- CHIP, $[Pt(NH_3)_2(Etmal)]$, cis-$[Pt(i-C_3H_7NH_2)_2(NO_3)_2]$, $[Pt(1,2-dac)SO_4(H_2O)]$, TMA and $[Pt(1,1-damcha)Cl_2]$. Studies with dogs showed all of the above to cause emesis except $[Pt(NH_3)_2(Etmal)]$ (41) (Table 28).

TABLE 29. Comparative nephro- and myelo- toxicity indicators for active platinum complexes $[PtA_2X_2]$

Acute dosing (Male BDF_1 mice)

A_2	X_2	Test Doses[a] (i.p. mg/kg)	BUN[b] (>30mg%)	Max % Decrease WBC	(day)
CISPLATIN		17.8	8/10	-38	(5)
		13.4	9/10	-53	(3)
$(NH_3)_2$	OHmal	208	1/9	-64	(5)
		156	0/10	-41	(5)
$(NH_3)_2$	Etmal	120	0/10	-44	(3)
		90	0/10	-31	(3)
1,2-dac	$SO_4(H_2O)$	22.5	0/10	-67	(5)
		17	0/10	-64	(5)
1,2-dac	TMA	76.5	0/3	-56	(5)
		57.4	3/7	-33	(5)
		43	0/10	-28	(5)
1,1-damcha	Cl_2	8.7	2/9	-61	(3)
		6.5	0/10	-59	(3)
CHIP		51.5	0/6	-61	(5)
		38.6	1/7	-39	(3)

[a] First dose is LD_{50}. [b] d4 unless indicated.

1,1-damcha = 1,2-diaminomethylcyclohexane
1,2-dac = 1,2-diaminocyclohexane
TMA = 4-carboxyphthalate
Data of Schurig et al (41)

Harrap et al subjected the eight complexes chosen on activity grounds (see earlier) to a toxicological evaluation in the rat in comparison to cisplatin (38). Effects on body weight, blood urea, white blood cell count and selected organ histology were monitored. Overall CBDCA and CHIP were the least toxic derivatives although both were myelosuppressive. CBDCA was selected for Phase 1 study because of its activity against mice carrying the human lung tumour xenograft (Table 25).

5. PHASE 1 CLINICAL TRIALS

The studies outlined in the previous sections have led to the selection of a number of cisplatin analogues for clinical trial. The preclinical studies strongly suggest that new platinum drugs with greatly reduced nephrotoxicity should emerge. However, although there have been suggestions of improved selectivity, activity factors will only emerge in the clinic.

Some complexes have been subjected to limited clinical trials and these are summarised in Table 30. However, it is intended to concentrate here on the present active trials (Table 31) which are the logical extensions of the preclinical studies described in section 4.

TABLE 30. Cisplatin analogues : Past Phase 1 studies

$[Pt(1,2-dac)mal]^a$	Wadley[b] Paris (Mathé)	Some activity Low solubility
$[Pt(1,2-dac)(SO_4)(H_2O)]^a$	Wadley	Stability problems Dose limiting toxicity not reached
$[Pt(1,2-dac)(BrAc)_2]^a$	Wadley	Toxicity (?)
$[Pt(C_5H_{10}NH_2)_2Cl_2]$	Wadley	Low solubility No activity
$[Pt(1,2-daco)(BrAc)_2]^a$	Wadley	Low solubility Toxicity
Pt uracil blue	Wadley	Cardiac arrest Uncertain composition

[a] Trans-1- isomer also tested
[b] Wadley Institutes of Molecular Medicine, Dallas.

1,2-dac = 1,2-diaminocyclohexane   1,2-daco = 1,2-diaminocyclooctane

See reference (43).

TABLE 31. Cisplatin analogues : Active Phase 1 studies

CBDCA (JM-8)	Royal Marsden, Sutton, U.K.	National Cancer Institute, U.S.A.*
CHIP (JM-9)	Roswell Park, Buffalo, U.S.A.	Christie Hospital, Manchester, U.K.*
	M.D. Anderson, Houston, U.S.A.*	Upstate Medical Centre, Syracuse, U.S.A.*
PHIC	Paris	Toulouse
[Pt(1,2-dac)(TMA)] (JM-82)	Sloan Kettering, N. York, U.S.A.	
[Pt(1,1-damcha)(SO$_4$)(H$_2$O)] (TNO-6)	Amsterdam, Netherlands.	
[Pt(en)(mal)] (JM-40)	EORTC*	

* Projected

5.1. Active studies

The only Phase 1 study to be completed has involved CBDCA at the Institute of Cancer Research, Royal Marsden Hospital, Sutton, U.K. (42) (Table 32). Optimum doses vary from 300-520 mg/m^2 (depending on the patients' condition) reflecting the low overall toxicity of the compound. Doses are given as a 1 hour infusion at 4-weekly intervals -- no hydration or diuresis procedures are used. Preclinical work was confirmed in that myelosuppression is the dose limiting toxicity, particularly thrombocytopenia, with the platelet nadir at 21 days post treatment - nephrotoxicity is not apparent at this dose level. Vomiting was seen in all patients at doses above 120 mg/m^2 but was subjectively less severe than with cisplatin. Significant therapeutic activity has been observed for ovarian (8 out of 20) cancer.

TABLE 32. Phase 1 study on CBDCA (JM-8)   (Reference 42)

Location	:	Royal Marsden Hospital, (EORTC) Sutton, U.K.
Schedule	:	Single dose every 4 weeks
Optimum Dose	:	300-520 mg/m^2
No. of Patients	:	47
Toxicities	:	Haematological (Dose limiting) Nausea and vomiting
Responses	:	Ovarian carcinoma - 8/20

Other studies are confirming the lower toxicity, particularly renal, of the new drugs. TMA at Sloan Kettering Memorial Hospital, New York, is being tested at doses around 640 mg/m² with only slight nephrotoxicity. Emesis is apparently less severe than with cisplatin and again haematological effects are dose limiting. The trial is at an early stage but some responses have been observed for solid tumours and a Phase 2 study is envisaged (Table 33) (43). Another 1,2-dac complex with isocitrate as the X group is just commencing Phase 1 trial in Toulouse and Paris. This compound was chosen on activity, toxicity and solubility grounds (Table 34) (18). Its structure is, however, unproven and extensive studies may be required before reproducible large scale production can be achieved.

TABLE 33. Phase 1 study on [Pt(1,2-dac)TMA] (Reference 43)

Location	:	Sloan Kettering Memorial Hospital, New York.
Schedule	:	I.V. infusion over 5 minutes; 3 courses on 3-weekly basis; no diuresis.
No. of Patients	:	29 (19 adenocarcinoma, 9 adenocarcinoma lung)
Maximum Dose	:	800 mg/g²
MTD	:	640 mg/m²
Toxicities	:	Renal (occasional and slight) Emesis (at all levels - less severe than cisplatin) Haematological : Thrombocytopenia > Leucopenia
Responses	:	5

TMA = 4-carboxyphthalate

A platinum(II) compound based on the 1,1-damcha system with aqua sulphate X groups is undergoing Phase 1 evaluation in Amsterdam. Again the trial is at an early stage and dose limiting toxicity has not been reached. However, doses at around 25 mg/m² are much lower than for CBDCA and TMA (43). Haematologic toxicity appears to be dose limiting while nausea and vomiting and nephrotoxicity (slight at 20 mg/m²) have been observed (Table 35). Responses have been noted in ovarian and in one breast cancer. If the latter were to be repeated the drug would be of great interest in terms of an expanded spectrum of activity.

The platinum(IV) complex CHIP has entered Phase 1 at the Roswell Park Memorial Institute (Table 36). Although the dose limiting toxicity has not yet been reached, initial toxicity observations are similar to those for other trials. This compound is expected to go on trial at other institutions in the U.S. (Table 31).

It is anticipated that another malonate analogue, [Pt(en)(mal)], will be undergoing Phase 1 study under the auspices of the EORTC in the near future (Table 31).

TABLE 34. Comparison of Cisplatin and PHIC[a]   (Reference 18)

	PHIC	CISPLATIN
(1) Anti-Tumour Activity		
(a) Therapeutic Index		
L1210	36.3	6.5
S180	21.5	5.2
(b) Surviving Animals		
L1210 (30 days)	YES	NO
S180 (60 days)	YES	NO
(2) Toxicity		
(a) LD_{10} Swiss mice (mg/kg)	135	10
(b) Nephrotoxicity		
Swiss mice (LD_0 level)	NO	YES
(c) Nephrotoxicity 100 mg/kg	NO	YES (LD_0)
Baboon 150 mg/kg	YES	–
(3) Aqueous Solubility	>1500 mg/ml	2 mg/ml
(4) Proven Structure	NO	YES

[a] PHIC = [Pt(1,2-diaminocyclohexane)(iso-citrate)]

TABLE 35. Phase 1 study on TNO6   (Reference 43)

Location	:	University of Amsterdam (EORTC)
Schedule	:	Single dose every 3 weeks
Dose	:	25 mg/m² – MTD not reached
No. of Patients	:	12
Toxicities	:	Haematological (moderate at 20 mg/m²) Renal (slight at 20 mg/m²) Nausea and vomiting
Responses	:	Breast (1 therefore preliminary) Ovarian
Comment	:	MTD expected 25–30 mg/m² Thrombocytopenia to be dose limiting

TABLE 36. Phase 1 study on JM-9

Location	:	Roswell Park Memorial Hospital, Buffalo, U.S.A.
Schedule	:	I.V. infusion over 2 hours - no diuresis
No. of Patients	:	20
Maximum Dose	:	270 mg/m^2
MTD	:	Not reached
Toxicities	:	Renal - not observed Haematological - Thrombocytopenia Emesis - Less severe than cisplatin
Responses	:	No information

5.2. Conclusions to date

These clinical studies are still in progress but some tentative preliminary observations can be made.

Firstly, it is clear that the predictions of greatly reduced nephro-toxicity have been confirmed. Providing that activity is comparable to cisplatin this alone would be sufficient to justify the introduction of a second generation drug.

Other toxicities may not be much affected although nausea and vomiting appears to be somewhat less troublesome. However, again as anticipated from the animal data, myelosuppression remains a major toxicity and it may be necessary to seek an analogue where this effect is reduced (however, preclinical results to date indicate that this may be a difficult task).

There is an indication that side effect toxicity (particularly as reflected by the minimum tolerated dose) is related to the reactivity of the complex. Thus less reactive complexes such as CBDCA, CHIP and TMA (except at high pH) are being used at much higher doses than the more reactive species like cisplatin, TNO6 and, in the past, $[Pt(1,2-dac)SO_4-(H_2O)]$ (43). Toxicities associated with rapidly dividing cells (such as bone marrow) remained essentially unchanged at the optimum doses but side effects such as nephrotoxicity vary from analogue to analogue. One would expect TNO6 to be reactive due to its sulphato group and it is surprising that the drug is not more nephrotoxic than presently reported.

It is too early as yet to assess the extent or spectrum of anti-tumour activity of these second generation drugs. It will be particularly interesting to obtain information on the effect of the 1,2-dac compound (TMA) on cisplatin resistant human tumours. Ultimately the successful candidate will be determined by therapeutic performance in the clinic.

Finally, it is important to note that the classical process of analogue development seems likely, in the case of platinum derivatives, to give results of considerable benefit in clinical practice. It seems appropriate at this stage that the molecular biological mechanisms behind the subtle structure activity variations in activity, toxicity and cross resistance (or lack of) should be studied in detail.

REFERENCES

1. B. Rosenberg, L. Van Camp and T. Krigas, Nature (London), 205, 698 (1965).
2. B. Rosenberg, L. Van Camp, J.E. Trosko and V.H. Mansour, Nature (London), 222, 385 (1969).
3. J.R. Durant in "Cisplatin: Current Status and New Developmets", (Eds. A.W. Prestayko, S.T. Crooke and S.K. Carter), pg.317, Academic Press, 1980.
4. S.D. William and L.H. Einhorn in Reference (3), pg.323.
5. S. Seeber, M.E. Scheulen, R.B. Schilcher, M. Higi, N. Niederle, D. Mouratidou, W.C. Bierbaum and C.G. Schmidt, in Ref. (3), pg.329.
6. J.F. Holland, H.W. Bruckner, C.J. Cohen, R.C. Wallach, S.B. Gusberg, E.M. Greenspan and J. Goldberg, in Reference (3), pg.383.
7. E. Wiltshaw, Personal communication.
8. M.J. Cleare, P.C. Hydes, B.W. Malerbi and D.M. Watkins, Biochemie, 60, 835 (1978).
9. M.J. Cleare, P.C. Hydes, D.R. Hepburn and B.W. Malerbi, in Ref. (3), pg.149.
10. F. Basolo and R.G. Pearson, Mechanisms of Inorganic Reactions, (2nd Ed) Wiley (New York), pg.359, 1967.
11. M.J. Cleare and J.D. Hoeschele, Bioinorg.Chem., 2, 187 (1973).
12. M.J. Cleare and J.D. Hoeschele, Platinum Metals Review, 17, 2 (1973).
13. T.A. Connors, M. Jones, W.C.J. Ross, P.D. Braddock, A.R. Khokhar and M.L. Tobe, Chem-Biol. Interactions, 5, 415 (1972); ibid 11, 145 (1975).
14. M.K. Wolpert-De Filippes in Reference (3), pg.183.
15. G.R. Gale and S.J. Meischen, U.S. Patent Appl. No. 769,888.
16. W.T. Bradner, W.C. Rose and J.B. Huftalen, in Ref. (3), pg.171.
17. J. Berg, E.J. Bulten and F. Verbeek, U.K. Patent Appl. No. 2,024,823 A.
18. J.P. Macquet and J.P. Armand, Proc.Am.Assoc.Cancer Res., 22, 260 (1981); ibid 22, 261 (1981).
19. Y. Kidani, K. Okamato and R. Saito, U.S. Patent No. 4,255,347 (1981).
20. T. Totani and K. Yamaguchi, U.K. Patent Appl. No. 2,074,567 A (1981).
21. C. Yoshikumi, T. Fujii, K. Saito, M. Fujii and K. Niimura, European Patent Appl. No. 41,792 (1981).
22. W.C. Rose, J.E. Schurig, J.B. Huftalen and W.T. Bradner, in press.
23. E.J. Bulton and F. Verbeek, French Patent Appl. No. 2,473,046 (1981).
24. B. Lippert, J.Clin.Haem. and Oncol., 7(1), 26 (1977).
25. J.A. Broomhead, D.P. Fairlie and M.W. Whitehouse, Chem-Biol. Interactions, 31, 113 (1980).
26. G.R. Gale, E.M. Walker, Jr., L.M. Atkins, A.B. Smith and S.J. Meischen, Res.Commun.Chem.Pathol.Pharmacol., 7, 529 (1974).
27. S.J. Meischen, G.R. Gale, L.M. Lake, C.J. Frangakis, M.G. Rosenblum, E.M. Walker, Jr., L.M. Atkins and A.B. Smith, J.Natl.Cancer Inst. 57, 841 (1976).

28. H.J. Ridgway, R.J. Speer, L.M. Hall, D.P. Stewart, A.D. Newman and J.M. Hill, J.Clin.Haematol.Oncol., 7, 220 (1977).

29. P. Schwartz, S.J. Meischen, G.R. Gale, L.M. Atkins, A.B. Smith and E.M. Walker, Jr., Cancer Treat. Rep., 61, 1519 (1977).

30. C.G. von Kralingen and J. Reedijk, Ciênc Biol (Portugal), 5, 159 (1980).

31. F. Basolo, H.B. Gray and R.G. Pearson, J.Amer.Chem.Soc., 82, 4200 (1960).

32. Y. Kidani, M. Noji and T. Tashiro, Gann., 71, 637 (1980).

33. J.H. Burchenal, L. Lokys, J. Turkevich, G. Irani and K. Kern, Recent Results Cancer Res., 74, 146 (1980).

34. K.R. Harrap, M. Jones, C.R. Wilkinson, H. McD. Clink, S. Sparrow, B.C.V. Mitchley, S. Clark and A. Veasey, in Ref. (3), pg.193.

35. P. Lelieveld and L.M. Van Putten, Proc. 12th Int. Congr. Chemother. Abs., 21 (1981).

36. J.H. Burchenal, L. Lokys, J. Turkevich and C. Ramachandran, in Ref. (3), pg.113.

37. E.M. Walker, Jr. and G.R. Gale, Res.Commun.Chem.Pathol.Pharmacol., 6, 419 (1973).

38. R.J. Speer, H. Ridgway, D.P. Stewart, L.M. Hall, A. Zapata and J.M. Hill, J.Clin.Haematol.Oncol., 7, 210 (1977).

39. G.R. Gale, L.M. Atkins, S.J. Meischen and P. Schwartz, Cancer, 41, 1230 (1978).

40. A.M. Guarino, D.S. Miller, S.T. Arnold, M.A. Urbanek, M.K. Wolpert-De Filippes and M.P. Hacker, in Reference (3), pg.237.

41. J.E. Schurig, W.T. Bradner, J.B. Huftalen, G.J. Doyle and J.A. Gylys, in Reference (3), pg.227.

42. H. Calvert, personal communication.

43. K.R. Harrap, Platinum Analogues: Criteria for Selection, Series on Chemotherapy, Volume 1, (Ed. F.M. Muggia), Martinus Nijhoff, in press.

BIOREDUCTIVE ALKYLATION – NATURALLY OCCURRING QUINONES AS POTENTIAL CANDIDATES

H.W. MOORE, K.F. WEST, K. SRINIVASACHER AND R. CZERNIAK

INTRODUCTION

Bioreductive alkylation is the term used to describe the effect of those compounds which express their mode of biological action as alkylating agents, but do so subsequent to their in vivo reduction.[1] That is, they are pro-drugs which are activated by a bioreduction. A class of compounds ideally suited to function as the reducible moiety of bioreductive alkylating agents is the quinones since their facile in vivo and in vitro reduction to the corresponding hydroquinones is a well known and extensively studied reaction.[2] If the quinone is further substituted with a side-chain bearing a leaving group (X) at the 2-position of the substituent, then quinone methide formation can result by an elimination of HX from the hydroquinone.[3] The reactive quinone methide is suggested as the discrete alkylating agent and functions as such by a Michael addition of a biologically important nucleophile (Nu$^-$: DNA, protein, carbohydrate, etc.) to the enone of the methide. This postulate is represented by the sequence of reactions outlined in Scheme 1, i.e., $1 \to 2 \to 3 \to 4$. Further comments concerning the details of this proposed mechanism of action follow. 1) Although a two-electron reduction is represented, a one-electron process can also be envisaged. That is, rather than the hydroquinone 2, a semiquinone radical-anion could be formed initially. This could then proceed to the radical form of 3 and subsequently to a radical anion of 4. 2) The facility of quinone methide formation, and thus biological activity, may be enhanced as the half-wave reduction potential $(E_{1/2})$ of the quinone decreases. That is, electron-releasing substituents attached to the quinone nucleus will retard the reduction step, i.e.,

D.N. Reinhoudt, T.A. Connors, H.M. Pinedo & K.W. van de Poll (eds.), Structure-Activity Relationships of Anti-Tumour Agents.
© 1983, Martinus Nijhoff Publishers, The Hague/Boston/London. ISBN 90-247-2783-9.

Scheme I

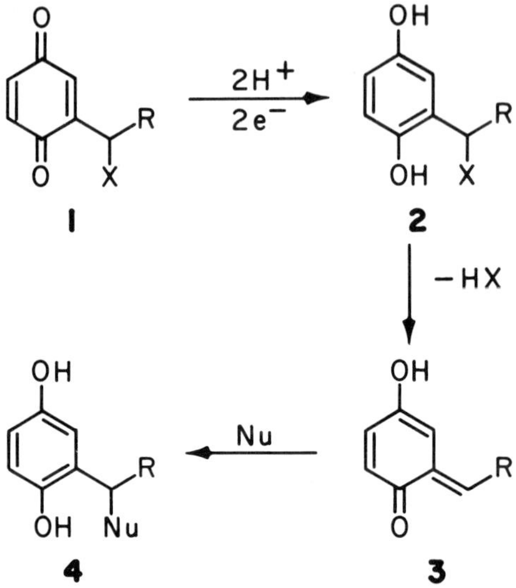

lower the half-wave potential. However, once reduced, the electron-rich hydroquinone will be activated towards HX elimination and thus quinone methide formation. This would be particularly true if the electron-releasing substituents are ortho- and/or para to the side-chain bearing the leaving group. In such cases, the electron-releasing substituents would facilitate loss of the leaving group X and thus enhance quinone methide formation. 3) The ease of quinone methide formation should also be affected by the character of the leaving group, X. Specifically, good leaving groups (weak bases) in the sense of the SN_1 or SN_2 reaction would also enhance quinone methide formation from the hydroquinone, 2. 4) It is also noted that the generalized structure 1 is an oversimplification since the quinone nucleus need not be limited to the benzoquinones. Indeed, quinone methides can be envisaged as arising by a reductive elimination from appropriately substituted benzoquinones, naphthoquinones, anthraquinones, anthracyclines, and many other quinone and related systems. Additionally, the leaving group need not be located only at the position adjacent to the quinone nucleus. Rather, it could be bonded to a number of possible vinylogous sites in compounds more complex than 1 and still give rise to quinone methides or related reactive intermediates.

Not all of the above proposed structural requirements have been probed experimentally. However, Sartorelli and his co-workers at Yale have elegantly shown that a number of benzoquinones, naphthoquinones, and anthraquinones, meeting the general structure 1, do express antineoplastic activity.[1,4] Furthermore, the biological activity is generally enhanced as the half-wave reduction potential of the quinones decreases and as the leaving group ability increases. These workers have further suggested that quinones of structure 1 might be logical chemotherapeutic agents to attack hypoxic tumor cells, i.e., those cells remote from blood vessels such as are found at the core of solid tumors.[5] The oxygen deficiency of hypoxic cells suggests them to be potentially good candidates for selective cancer chemotherapy by bioreductive alkylating agents since they are believed to provide a more efficient reducing environment than do oxygen-rich tumor or normal cells. Thus, their ability to reduce the quinone 1 to the "activated" hydroquinone 2 may be enhanced. Indeed, some progress in this direction has been reported.[6] For example, mitomycin C, as well as some 9,10-anthraquinones which are substituted so as to allow quinone-methide formation, have recently been shown to possess significantly enhanced toxicity towards hypoxic tumor cells as compared to analogous oxygen-rich cells.

NATURALLY OCCURRING QUINONES AS POTENTIAL BIOREDUCTIVE ALKYLATING AGENTS

The term, bioreductive alkylation, was coined by Lin, Cosby, Shansky, and Sartorelli in 1972[1] to explain the antineoplastic activity of some synthetic quinones of general structure 1. However, the genesis of the concept stems from the earlier report of Iyer and Szybalski[7] who suggested that the natural product, Mitomycin C, expressed its antineoplastic activity as a cross-linking agent for DNA, and that this alkylation occurred only subsequent to an in vivo reduction. Indeed, they demonstrated the in vitro cross-linking of calf thymus DNA by Mitomycin C, and this occurred only in the presence of a reducing agent. A possible molecular mechanism of action of mitomycin C (5) which falls within the framework of bioreductive alkylation is outlined in Scheme 2. The salient features of this proposed mechanism follow: 1) Mitomycin C is reduced to the hydroquinone which then eliminates CH_3OH to give the indole, 6; 2) opening of the aziridine ring by an elimination reaction would give the quinone methide, 7; 3) nucleophilic

Scheme 2

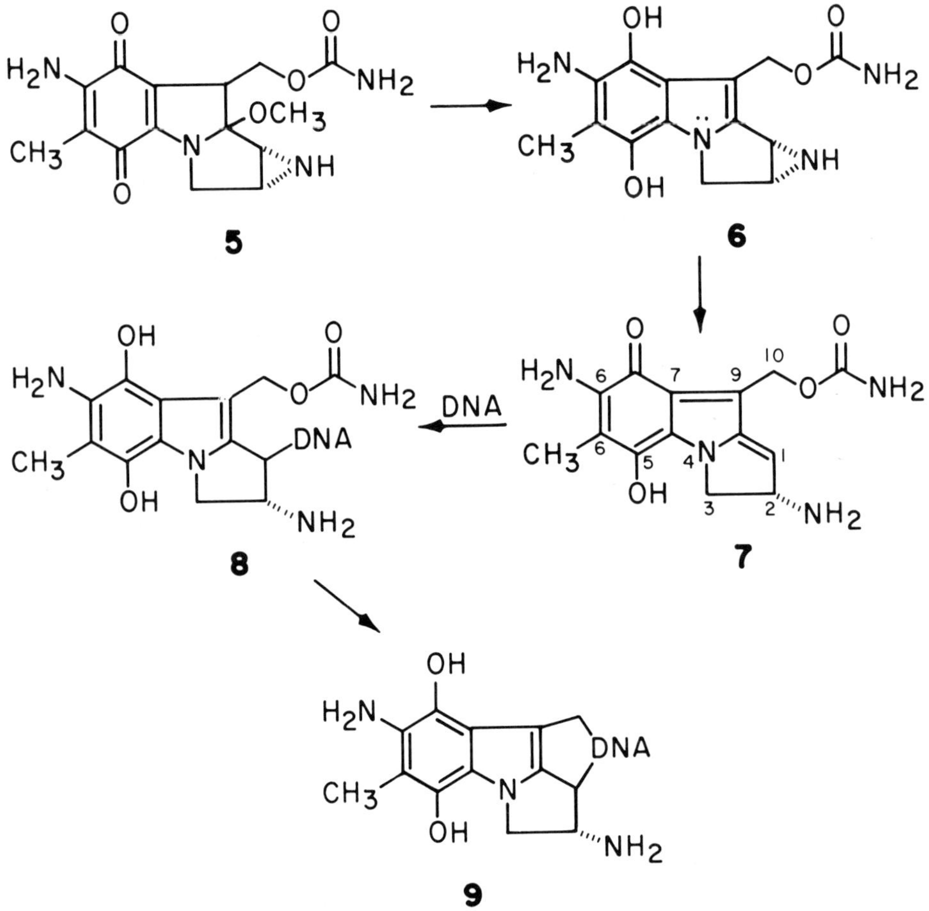

addition of DNA to the quinone methide would give the monoalkylated adduct, 8; 4) intramolecular SN_2 displacement of the carbamate would result in the cross-linked adduct 9. Two interesting model experiments which lend support for this proposed mechanism have recently been reported. Hornemann, Keller, and Kozlowski have observed the first 1-substituted mitocene to be generated from Mitomycin C under reductive conditions.[8] Specifically, an adduct analogous to 8 was obtained when a mixture of Mitomycin C and potassium ethylxanthate was treated with the reducing agent sodium dithionite. This product most likely arises from nucleophilic attack of the xanthate ion at position -1 of the quinone methide 7. A related result was reported by Hashimoto, Shudo, and Okamoto who generated the quinone methide by reduction of Mitomycin C with H_2/Pd/C and trapped it in situ with 5'-guanylic acid.[9] Interestingly, only the cis-adduct 10 was reported. Such a stereochemical consequence

10

is clearly counter to that expected for a mechanism involving an SN_2 opening of the aziridine ring. However, the quinone methide 7 could account for this result. For example, interaction of the phosphoric acid moiety of 5'-guanylic acid with the C-2 amino group of the quinone methide, 7, could result in delivery of the nucleophile from the α-face and thus give the observed adduct, 10. In any regard, the critical point is that adducts such as 10 have now been observed, and are formed only under reductive reaction conditions.

The work of Sartorelli which now spans a period of 10 years as well as the earlier report that Mitomycin C cross-links DNA, but only in the presence of a reducing agent, stimulated our interest in this area. These results caused us to ask the following simple question: If nature has provided one quinone, i.e., Mitomycin C, which needs a reductive activation to express its biological activity, is it possible that many other natural quinones exist which could behave analogously? The answer is clearly affirmative. At least it is with respect to the availability of a large number of naturally occurring quinones which possess the appropriate structural features to allow them to function as precursors to quinone methides subsequent to an in vivo reduction. A detailed survey of naturally occurring quinones was accomplished;[10] the prime objective of the search was to catalogue those natural products which could function as potential bioreductive alkylating agents. The desirable detailed structural features sought will not be elaborated here. However, in their simplest form, those outlined in Scheme 1 constitute the foundation. This survey has now been published and thus only selected examples will be represented in this manuscript. Suffice it to say that nearly 200 naturally occurring quinones can be so catalogued, and a complete listing of these appear in our review.[10] The majority of these compounds have not been tested for anticancer activity. However, a large fraction of them have been reported to show some form of biological activity, e.g., antibiotic, antifeedants, antifungal agents, wilting agents, and indeed some are anticancer agents. A selected few of these compounds are represented here, along with some examples which were not previously known at the time of our review, e.g., U 58,431[11] and P 1894B[12].

A few general comments suggesting potentially important structure-activity relationships are in order with regard to the examples given here. Many other relationships can be seen after inspection of the entire listing. For example, C-glycosides of quinones are very rare, e.g., Aquayamycin, P 1894B, Carminic Acid, and Kidamycin. However, those which are known all appear to show biological activity. Other examples are Hedamycin, Neopluramycin, and Pluramycin A, all of which are closely related to Kidamycin. In addition, it is noteworthy that the leaving group in these C-glycosides would be the ether linkage of the sugar; this is located in a position strictly analogous to the O-glycosidic linkage of most of the anthracyclines, e.g., Adriamycin.

I. Benzoquinones

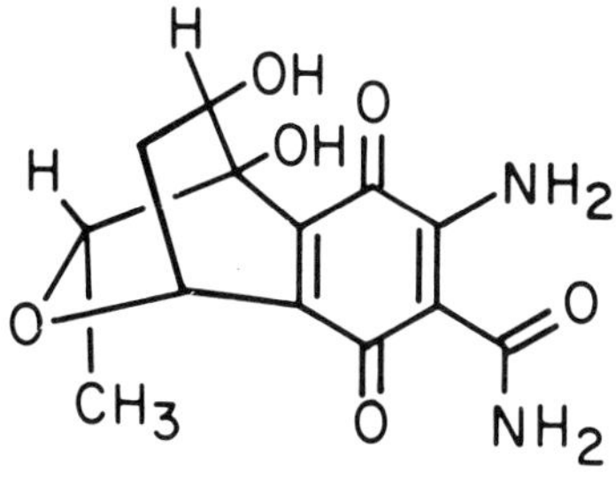

u 58,431

Antibiotic

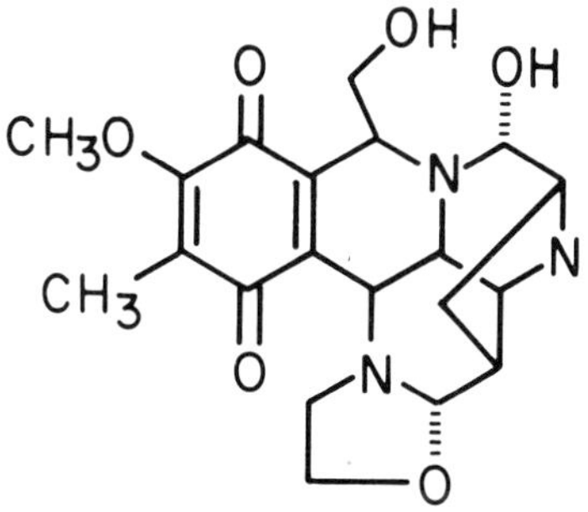

Naphthyridinomycin

Antibiotic

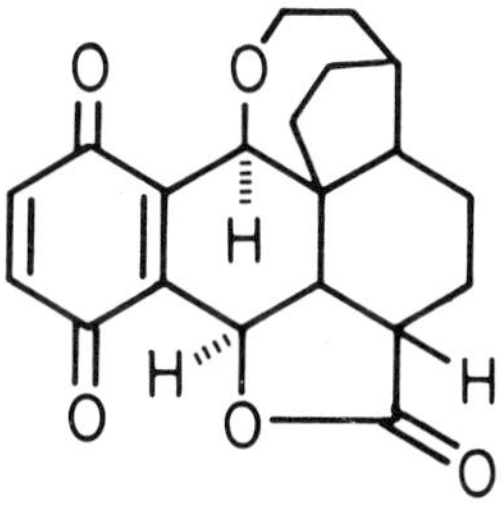

Pleurotin

Antibiotic

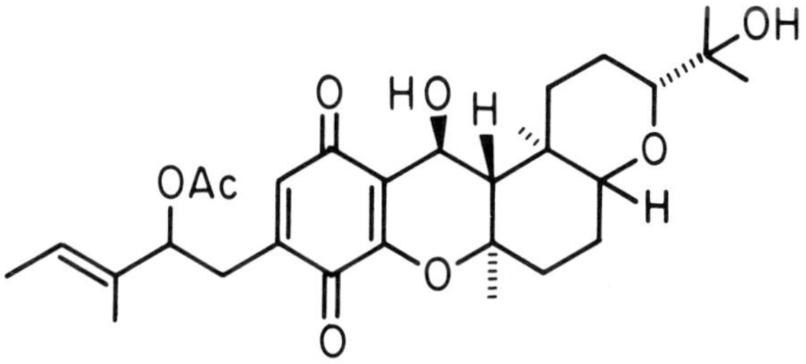

Stemphone

Antibiotic

Furthermore, a reaction of note is the observation that reduction of Adriamycin (sodium dithionite) gives a quantitative yield of the 7-desoxy aglycone, and this transformation most likely proceeds via a quinone methide intermediate.[13] Thus, an analogous reductive elimination of the C-glycosidic quinones would be a most reasonable possibility. However, unlike the anthracyclines, this should be a favorable reversible reaction since it would be intramolecular in character. As a result, the C-glycosides could provide greater selectivity as an alkylating agent. No

2. Naphthoquinones

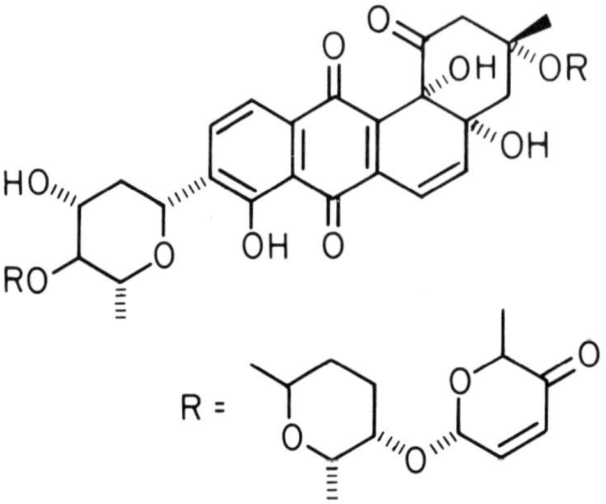

Aquayamycin

Antibiotic

R = H

R =

P 1894B

Proline Hydrase Inhibitor

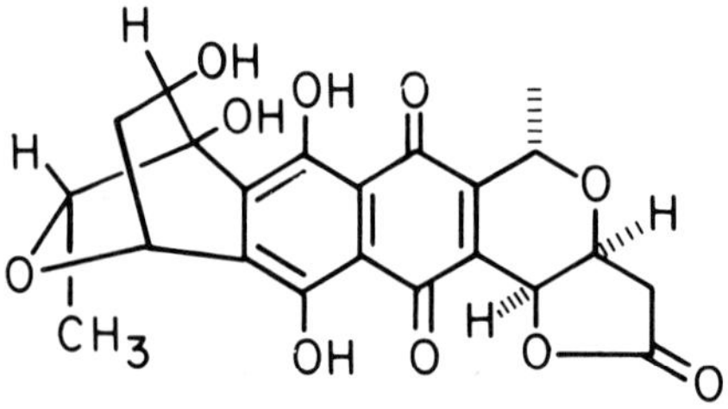

Granaticin

Antitumor – Antibiotic

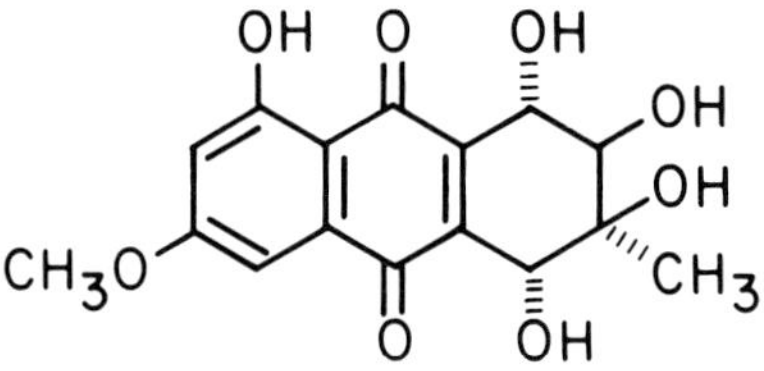

Altersalanol A

Phytotoxin

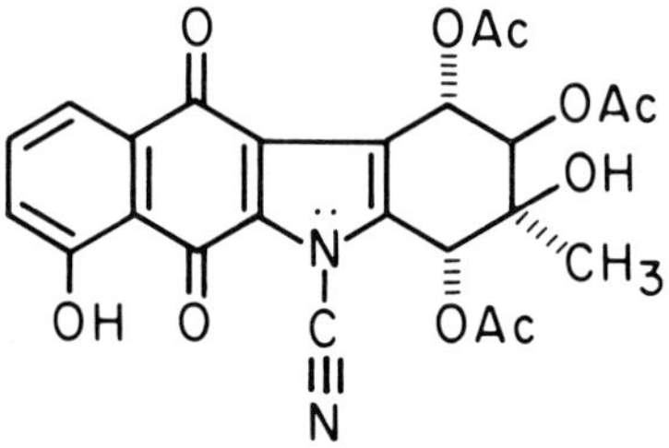

Kinamycin C

Antibiotic

study has appeared whose objectives are the synthesis and biological evaluation of C-glycosidic quinones. This could be a worthwhile endeavor.

3. Anthaquinones

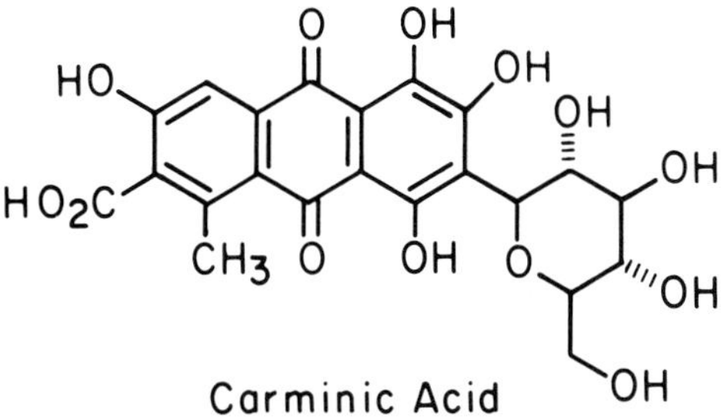

Carminic Acid
Antitumor

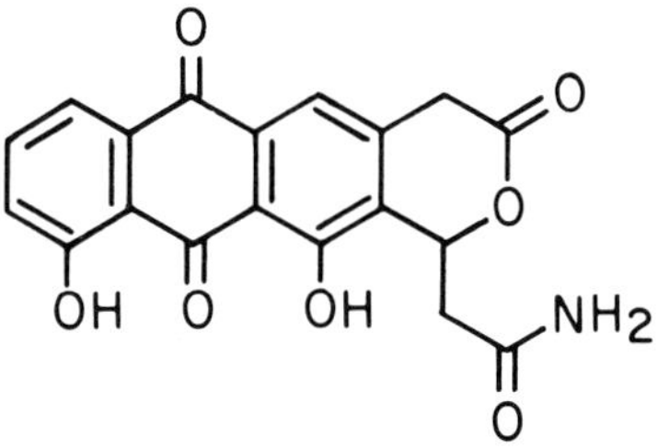

Ekatetrone
Antitumor – Antibiotic

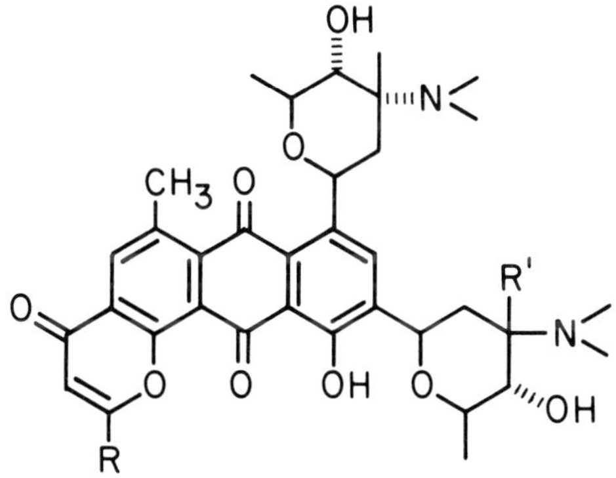

R = (structure) R' = H

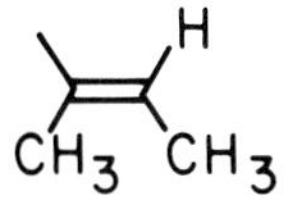

Kidamycin
Antitumor – Antibiotic

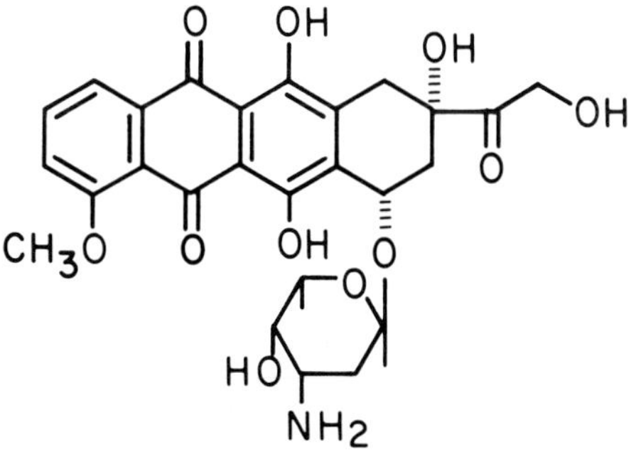

Adriamycin
Antitumor – Antibiotic

Antibiotic U58,431 is one of only four known naturally occurring primary amino-1,4-quinones. The others are Mitomycin C, Streptonigrin, and Rhodoquinone. The amino group in U58,431 is ideally located to facilitate quinone methide formation at the hydroquinone stage by assisting in the cleavage of the ether linkage of the bicyclic ring situated in the para-position. A Mitomycin C derivative having the amino and methyl groups on the quinone ring interchanged would provide an analogous situation; this would be a most interesting compound to compare with the Mitomycin C/DNA cross-linking ability and biological action. Also note that the bicyclic ring of U58,431 is identical to that found in Granaticin, a compound showing both antibiotic and anticancer properties. Antibiotic U58,431, like Mitomycin C, can also be viewed as a possible bis-alkylating agent; that is, a bis-quinone methide can be viewed as arising from the above-mentioned ether cleavage followed by dehydration. Other potential bis-alkylating agents listed here would be Naphthyridinomycin, Pleurotin, Aquayamycin, P1894B , Altersalanol A, Kinamycin C, and Kidamycin. Granaticin is unique in that it has at least four possible alkylating sites, i.e., the two associated with the bicyclo-[2.2.2] ring as well as an additional two associated with the γ-lactone and pyrone rings. Thus, conceivably it could give the equivalent of a tetraquinone methide under reductive conditions. It is also interesting to note that Granaticin is one of approximately 25 natural quinones having the pyrone-γ-lactone ring system fused to a quinone nucleus, and all of these show activity as antibiotics and/or antifungal agents.

The Kinamycins and Mitomycins appear to be the only examples - of naturally occurring indolequinones. They both meet the structural requirements for bioreductive alkylating agents, and upon close inspection, their similarity is rather remarkable. For example, comparison of the hydroquinone of Kinamycin C with the mitocene hydroquinone, 6, reveal the potential leaving groups in both compounds to be in strictly analogous positions with respect to the indole nucleus. A closer inspection of these natural products suggest an even more interesting structural similarity. That is, Mitomycin C would appear to be "activated" towards alkylation by reduction and loss of CH_3OH to give 6 which functions as the penultimate precursor to the quinone methide 7. The driving force for methide formation would be enhanced by the release of the strain energy of the aziridine ring. This elimination would be further assisted by the C-7 hydroxy group as well as the availability of the non-bonding electron pair on the indole nitrogen. Note that this electron pair would not assist bond cleavage of the aziridine ring at any quinoid stage since it would be vinylogously conjugated to the quinone carbonyl group. The pyrrole nitrogen electron pair in Kinamycin would be even less available for assisted ionization than that of Mitomycin since it is in conjugation with both the quinone carbonyl and the cyano substituent. Thus, both natural products would be expected to be reasonably stable in their quinone forms. However, Kinamycin, like Mitomycin, may unleash its alkylating sites by a sequence of reduction and elimination steps. For example, reduction to the hydroquinone followed by loss of HCN and proton transfer would result in the decyanated quinone form of Kinamycin. A second reduction step would then provide an indole having the electron pair on the indole nitrogen as well as that on one of the hydroquinone hydroxy groups appropriately situated to assist ionization. This sequence of reactions would result in 11 which would function as a potent alkylating agent. A less esoteric possibility worth considering is that Kinamycin's activity is simply due to HCN which is released upon bioreduction.

11

Finally, it is noted that both KinamycinC and Altersalanol A contain an identical polyoxygenated cyclohexenyl ring which bears the potential leaving groups for quinone methide formation. An analogous structural feature is also found in Bostrycin, Altersalanol B, and Kinamycin

A, B, and D.

ALKYNYLQUINONES AS POTENTIAL PRECURSORS TO BIOREDUCTIVE ALKYLATING AGENTS

Our interests in the concepts of bioreductive alkylating agents are multifaceted. However, at this time, the prime objective is to develop viable synthetic routes to functionalized quinones which could be employed as versatile precursors to both synthetic and natural bioreductive alkylating agents. Such a class of quinones would be alkynylquinones having the general structure 12 since they could be converted by standard methods to potential bioreductive alkylating agents of general structure 13.

The synthetic utility of alkynylquinones seemed obvious; their availability, however, was not. In fact, to our knowledge, quinones of this type had not previously been described. This problem has now been at least partially resolved by the synthetic methodology outlined below.

A variety of possible synthetic routes to alkylated quinones can be envisaged from the reactions of quinones with organometallic reagents. Unfortunately, such reactions are often fraught with complexities due to electron transfer processes. An exception to this is the ability of alkyne lithium reagents to undergo synthetically useful 1,2-additions to the quinone carbonyl groups.[14] We have taken advantage of this to develop a potentially general route to alkynylquinones.[15] Specifically, alkynylation of alkoxyquinones followed by acid hydrolysis of the resulting β-hydroxy enol ether linkages of the quinols regenerates a quinone which now bears the alkyne group. For example, alkynylation of 2,5-diethoxy-1,4-benzoquinone followed by treatment with an alkyl, aryl, or alkynyl lithium reagent and finally acid hydrolysis give good overall yields of 2,5-dialkylated-1,4-benzoquinones. Selected examples are given in Scheme 3. A more complex utilization of this methodology is the synthesis of 7-chloro-6-methyl-1,2,5,8-tetrahydro-3H-pyrrolo-[1,2a]indole-5,8-dione, an indolequinone having the basic mitomycin

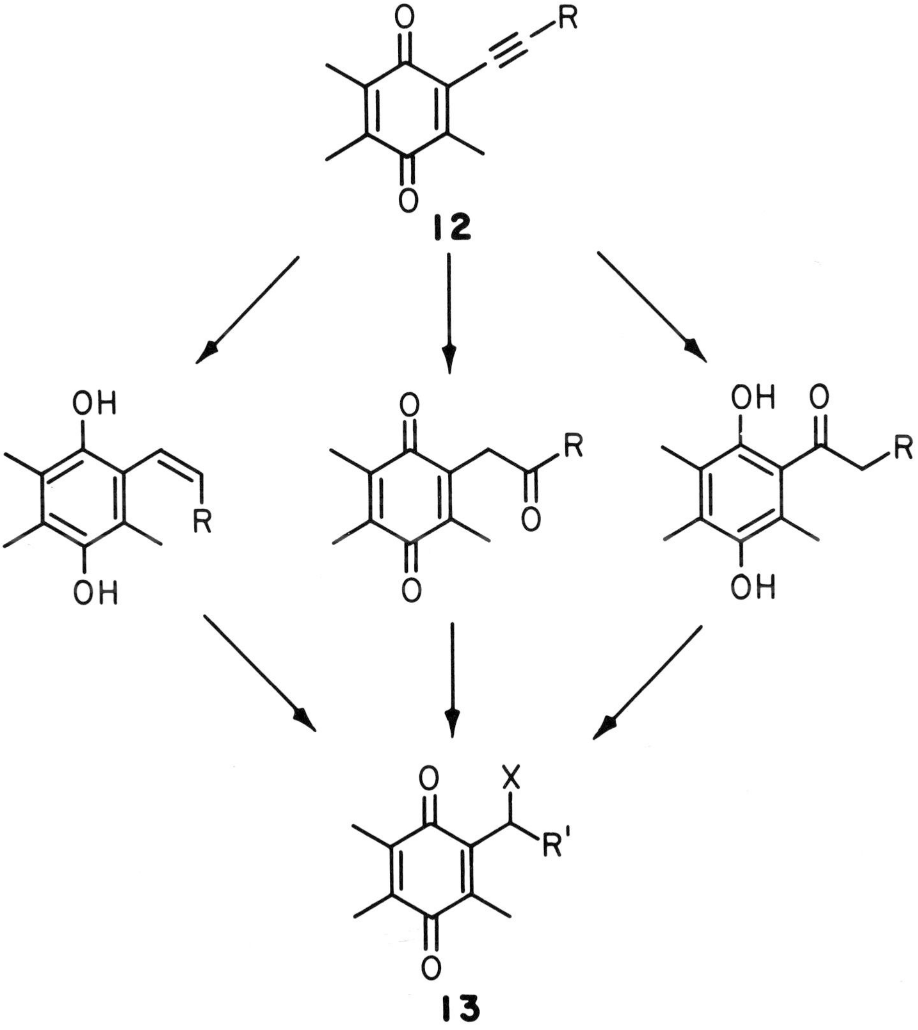
12
13

ring system (Scheme 4).

Scheme 3

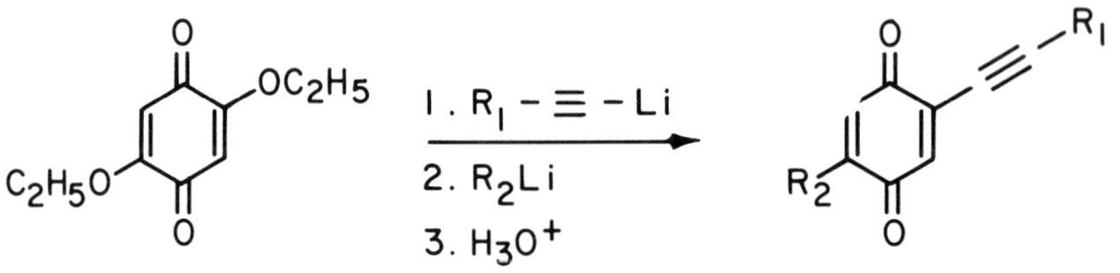

R_1	R_2	Yield
$-CH_2-O-CH_2C_6H_5$	$-CH_2-O-CH_2-C_6H_5$	56
$-CH_2-O-CH_2-C_6H_5$	$-C_6H_5$	60

A particular desire was to employ this quinone-alkynylation methodology to prepare 2-alkynyl-5-methoxy-1,4-benzoquinones. Such a substitution pattern would provide an ideal situation for subsequent conversion to bioreductive alkylating agents. For example, the alkyne group
could be modified to incorporate the appropriate side-chain as generally
outlined above.   This would then provide a series of bioreductive
alkylating agents having the electron-releasing methoxyl group para to
the side-chain bearing the leaving group. This structural pattern speaks
directly to those features deemed necessary for enhanced biological
activity. Specifically, the methoxy group will lower the half-wave reduction potential and, in addition, it is located in conjugation with the site
of methide formation. Thus, it should facilitate loss of the leaving group
at the hydroquinone stage. These desired 2-alkynyl-5-methoxy-1,4-
benzoquinones have now been prepared in good yields as outlined in
Scheme 5.[16]

The synthetic methodology outlined here shows the potential of developing into a general route to alkynylquinones. Depending upon the specific
structure of the starting alkoxy-substituted quinone, one can envisage
synthetic routes to a large variety of mono- and dialkynylated 1,4- and
1,2-benzoquinones. These, in turn, are viewed as ideal precursors

Scheme 4

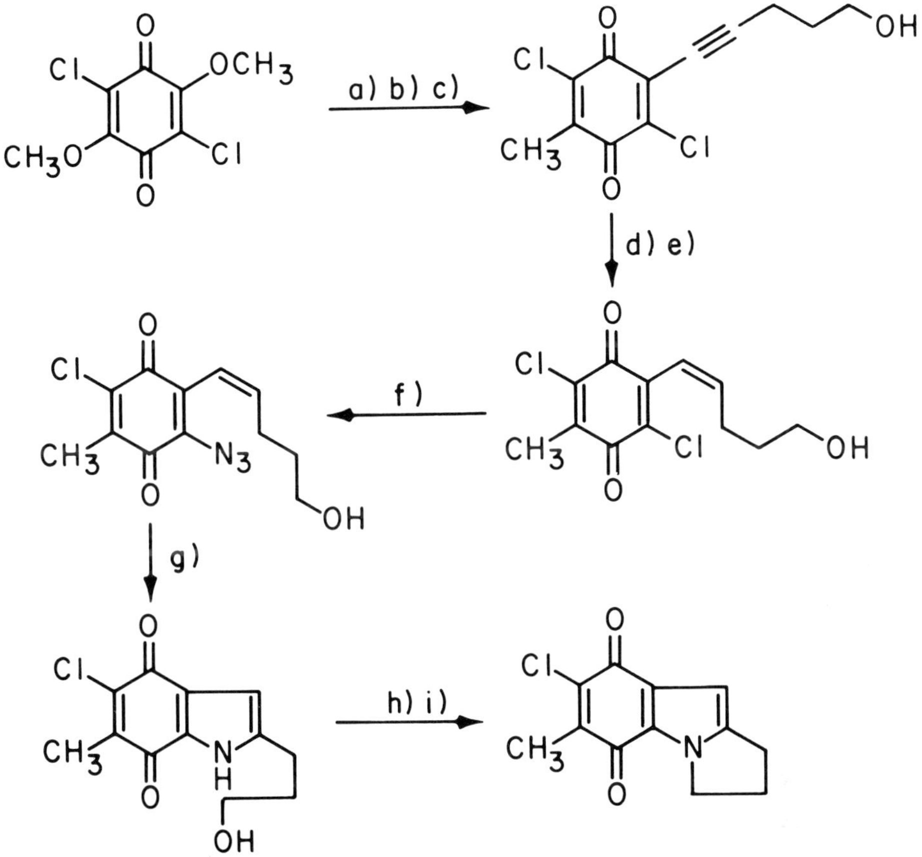

a) Li$-\equiv$ $\{$CH$_2\}_3$ OTHP   b) CH$_3$Li   c) H$_3$O$^+$

d) H$_2$/Pd/ BaSO$_4$ e) FeCl$_3$ f) KN$_3$ g) Δ, C$_6$H$_6$

h) MSCl   i) tBuOK

Scheme 5

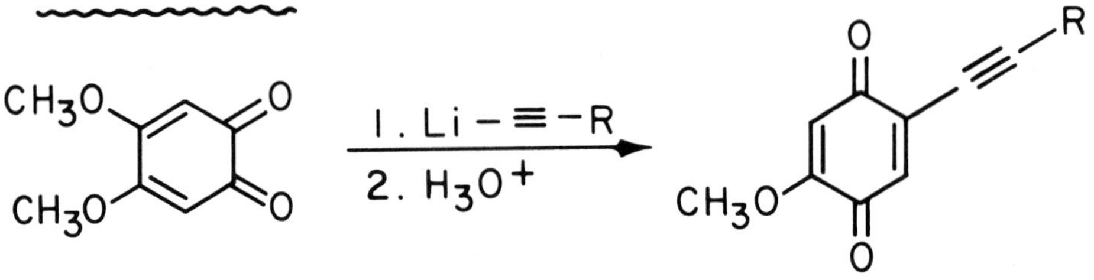

R	Yield
— C_6H_5	92
— $CH_2-O-CH_2C_6H_5$	87
— $C=CH_2$ $\quad$ CH_3	84
— $CO_2C_2H_5$	86
— $(CH_2)_4 C \equiv CH$	60
— H	65

to potential bioreductive alkylating agents.

CONCLUSION

The concept of bioactivation of quinones to give reactive quinone methides which function as alkylating agents is a powerful predictive model. The credence of this idea finds experimental support in the work of Sartorelli. Its implications in the field of natural products remains speculative, but it does suggest a number of important research areas. For example, nearly 200 natural quinones can be catalogued as potential bioreductive alkylating agents. Certain of these pose challenging synthetic problems to the synthetic organic chemist. In addition, a variety of synthetic problems concerning structure-activity relationships can be considered. The toxicology of these natural products should be investigated. Since they are potential alkylating agents, their mutagenicity and carcenogenicity would be of interest. Their ability to covalently bind to DNA in the presence of a reducing agent would be a worthwhile study. Finally, a systematic study of their possible anti-neoplastic activity would be most instructive.

ACKNOWLEDGEMENT

The authors wish to thank the National Cancer Institute for financial support of this work (CA 11890).

REFERENCES

1. A. J. Lin, L. A. Cosby, C. W. Shansky, and A. C. Sartorelli, J. Med. Chem., 15, 1247 (1972).
2. See for example, S. Patai, Ed., "The Chemistry of the Quinoid Compounds," Parts 1,2, J. Wiley and Sons, Inc., 1974; R. A. Morton, "Biochemistry of Quinones", Academic Press, 1965.
3. For reviews of quinone methide chemistry see, for example, a) ref. 2; b) A. B. Turner, Quart. Rev., (London), 18, 347 (1964).
4. A. J. Lin, R. S. Pardini, L. A. Cosby, B. J. Lillis, C. W. Shansky, and A. C. Sartorelli, J. Med. Chem., 16, 1268 (1973); A. J. Lin, C. W. Shansky, and A. C. Sartorelli, J. Med. Chem., 17, 558 (1974); A. J. Lin, B. J. Lillis and A. C. Sartorelli, J. Med. Chem., 18, 917 (1975); A. J. Lin and A. C. Sartorelli, ibid., 19, 1336 (1976); A. J. Lin and A. C. Sartorelli, J. Org. Chem., 38, 813 (1973).
5. K. A. Kennedy, B. A. Teicher, S. Rockwell, and A. C. Sartorelli, Biochem. Pharmacol., 29, 1 (1980).
6. K. A. Kennedy, S. Rockwell, and A. C. Sartorelli, Cancer Res., 40, 2356 (1980).
7. V. N. Iyer and W. Szybalski, Science, 145, 55 (1964).
8. P. J. Keller, J. F. Kozlowski, and U. Hornemann, J. Am. Chem. Soc., 101, 7121 (1979).

110

9. Y. Hashimoto, K. Shudo, and T. Okamoto, Chem. Pharm. Bull, 28, 1961 (1980).

10. H. W. Moore and R. Czerniak, Med. Res. Rev., 1, 249 (1981).

11. L. Slechla, C. G. Chidester, and F. Reusser, J. Antibiotics, 33, 919 (1980).

12. K. Ohta, and K. Kamiya, Chem. Comm., 154 (1981).

13. T. H. Smith, A. N. Fujiwara, D. W. Henry, and W. W. Lee, J. Am. Chem. Soc., 98, 1969 (1976).

14. W. Reed, Angew. Chem., 23, 933 (1964).

15. H. W. Moore, Y. L. Sing, and R. S. Sidhu, J. Org. Chem., 45, 5057 (1980).

16. H. W. Moore and K. West, unpublished results.

STRUCTURE–ACTIVITY RELATIONSHIPS IN DOXORUBICIN RELATED COMPOUNDS

F. ARCAMONE

1. INTRODUCTION

Doxorubicin (*Ia*) belongs to the anthracycline family of antibiotics, not rarely encountered as pigmented products of the
metabolism in cultures of different species of the genus *Streptomyces*. The classical anthracyclines such as the rhodomycins, the
pyrromycins and the cinerubins, although displaying cytotoxic
activity, are not clinically useful compounds because of their
low therapeutic index. On the other hand, daunorubicin (*Ib*) and
especially doxorubicin have received considerable attention because of their efficacy in the chemotherapic treatment of different human cancers. The use of doxorubicin in the clinical
practice is however not devoid of undesirable side effects (1).

Ia : R = OH
Ib : R = H

D.N. Reinhoudt, T.A. Connors, H.M. Pinedo & K.W. van de Poll (eds.), *Structure-Activity Relationships of Anti-Tumour Agents.*
© 1983, Martinus Nijhoff Publishers, The Hague/Boston/London. ISBN 90-247-2783-9.

The molecular behaviour of doxorubicin is clearly determined by its chemical structure and by the shape of the molecule itself in space. The presence of the amino and phenolic functionalities determines the existence, in aqueous media, of different charged species (the chromophore is red in acid and blue-violet in alkaline solution) whose relative concentrations at equilibrium are dictated by the values of the dissociation constants. The chromophoric quinone system is responsible for the oxido-reduction behaviour and for the tendency of the drug molecules to aggregate forming dimeric species whose importance becomes negligible only at concentrations below 10^{-5}M. As deduced from nuclear magnetic resonance and X-ray diffraction studies, cyclohexene ring A is in the half-chair conformation and the sugar moiety lays almost perpendicularly to the planar chromophoric system (1,2).

According to a generally accepted view, the cytotoxicity of antitumour anthracyclines is related with an impairment of nuclear DNA structure and function in sensitive cells. Other important mechanisms operating in living systems are the active drug extrusion process demonstrated in resistant cells and the metabolic transformations due mainly to two reactions, namely (a) the reduction of the side-chain ketone to a secondary alcohol, and (b) the reductive splitting of the glycosidic bond to give the 7-deoxy aglycone (1).

In the last ten years several daunorubicin and doxorubicin related glycosides have been obtained in our laboratory by semi-synthesis, partial or total synthesis and biosynthesis, with the aim of discovering new anticancer agents endowed with higher antitumour efficacy, wider spectrum of activity and lower toxicity in respect to the parent compounds. Different lines of investigation were therefore carried out, namely (a) the simple chemical derivatization of the parent drugs, (b) the synthesis of amino-sugar derivatives related to daunosamine and the coupling of the same with the biosynthetic aglycones, (c) the total synthesis of new aglycones and their glycosidation, (d) the chemical modification of the biosynthetic glycosides, (e) the partial synthesis starting from the biosynthetic aglycones, and (f) the isolation of anthracycline-type compounds from cultures of mutants of *S. peucetiu.* the original daunorubicin and doxorubicin producing microorganism. The analogues resulting from these different approaches can be clas sified as (a) compounds showing modifications on ring A (including the C-9 side-chain), (b) configurational and/or structural analogues modified in the carbohydrate moiety, and (c) compounds showing a different substitution on the anthraquinone chromophore (rings B and D) (1).

The study of structure-activity relationships is an essential part of the above mentioned programme and is aimed to rationalize chemical modifications for the optimization of pharmacological behaviour. Drug activity results from the combination of two properties, namely potency and selectivity of action (efficacy). According to Albert (3) intrinsic biological activity (potency) is a function of tridimensional shape of the molecule, of electric charge distribution and of lipophilicity (it is clear that these parameters dictate the affinity for the ultimate biological receptor(s)), whereas selectivity is a function of tissue distribution, metabolism and pharmacokinetics of drug and its metabolites.

2. THE DNA COMPLEX

There is little doubt that cell DNA be the major site of action of antitumour anthracyclines. This conclusion is derived from results of investigations carried out in cell cultures, in experimental animals and in clinical patients indicating, *inter alia,* the nuclear localization of the drug, the depression of nucleic acid synthesis in cells and tissues, chromosomal damage, and DNA fragmentation as consequences of doxorubicin (or daunorubicin) treatment (for reviews see ref. 1, 4-6). Current views accept the conclusion that the main type of anthracycline-DNA interaction corresponds to the formation of an intercalation complex (1,4,7). Equilibrium studies performed by different investigators, using a variety of physico-chemical techniques, have given values of the apparent stability constant, K_{app}, of the doxorubicin intercalation complex with double-stranded calf thymus DNA in the range 0.37 to 11.6 $l \cdot mol^{-1} \cdot 10^6$, and of the apparent number of binding sites per nucleotide, n_{app}, in the range 0.09 to 0.25 (reviews 7,8).

Similar ranges of K_{app} values have been reported for daunorubicin, the deviations being attributed to differences in experimental con ditions, DNA preparations, buffers and treatment of results (reviews: 7,8). The ability of anthracyclines to intercalate is clearly related with the molecular shape of these compounds, which are characterized by the presence of an electron deficient planar chromophore (rings B, C and D) and a sugar moiety oriented almost perpendicularly to the plane of the chromophore and linked to the a-licyclic ring A, the latter being in the half-chair conformation (1,7). The results of X-ray diffraction and nuclear magnetic resonance investigations of the DNA complex of daunorubicin and its derivatives (reviews: 7,8) indicate the planar aglycone oriented at right angle to the long dimension of the base pairs, ring B being located in the shielding region of base pairs, whereas the aminosugar moiety would be,in contrast with previous deductions (9,10), in the narrow groove displaying no electrostatic interaction with the charged phosphate groups (11). However, the size of the binding site, also because of the bulky sugar moiety, was sug gested to correspond to three base pairs, in agreement with most of the mentioned, and more recent (8, 12), equilibrium studies. In the cited paper (8), reporting the results of investigations recently carried out in our laboratory, data concerning the dimerization of the antitumour anthracyclines and equilibrium dialysis experiments using $[^{14}C]$-doxorubicin and different concentrations of native calf thymus DNA are given. In particular, when account is taken of the dimerization and binding data are treated according to a model corresponding to two classes of indipendent binding sites, the following values for K_{app} and n_{app} were found:

$K_1 = 1.0 \times 10^7$, $n_1 = 0.084$; $K_2 = 2.0 \times 10^5$, $n_2 = 0.109$.

The classification of 36 daunorubicin and doxorubicin analogue on the basis of the values of the apparent binding constant of the corresponding DNA complex in *high*, *intermediate*, and *low* relative affinity groups has been attempted (13,8). Viscometric dat were also used as a measure of binding,according to the known enhancement of DNA viscosity upon intercalation (14-16), as such determinations were also available for the said analogues (17,18, 8). A substantial qualitative agreement has been found between the two different techniques (8). A general relationship was found between the ability of the compounds to bind to DNA and cytotoxicity on *in vitro* cultured HeLa cells or toxicity in the animal tests. An exception was represented by the 4'-O-methyl analogues and by the 14-esters of doxorubicin, the latter probably because of their hydrolysis to the parent compounds. On the other hand antitumour efficacy at optimal doses appeared to be dependent on other factors related with the structure of the C-9 side chain (doxorubicin derivatives exhibit higher selectivity than daunorubicin ones) and on other properties such as distribution and rate of metabolization *in vivo* (19).

3. MOLECULAR REQUIREMENTS FOR BIOACTIVITY

3.1. Analogues modified on ring A

Chemical variations of the non aromatic portion of the anthraclinone moiety can be divided in (a) modifications of the C-9 side chain and (b) modifications at the carbon atoms of the alicyclic ring itself. As regards to the former, it should be pointed out that the anthracyclines of the daunorubicin-doxorubicin type are the only members of this family of antibiotics in which the side chain is in oxidized form, whereas in the other biosynthetic compounds the same appears in the form of an ethyl group. On the other hand the importance of positions 9 and 10 is indicated by the fact of being the first the site of ring closure in the original biogenetic polyketide intermediate and of appearing the second a site of substitution in the other anthracyclines such as for instance in rhodomycin (the C-10 hydroxyl can also be in glycosylated form in some congeners) and in aclacinomycin (1).

Doxorubicin analogues modified at the C-9 side chain considered in this section are daunorubicin (*Ib*), doxorubicin octanoate (*IIa*), 9-deacetyl-9-hydroxymethyldaunorubicin (*IIb*), and 9-deacetyl daunorubicin (*IIc*). As it is shown in Table 1, the ester IIa, althoug showing a low relative affinity for DNA ($K_{anal}/K_{dox} < 0.5$) retains the full activity of the parent, in agreement with the observed metabolic conversion to doxorubicin and doxorubicin derived metabolites (21) and with the behaviour

Table 1. Binding to calf thymus DNA (17,18,20) and antitumour
activity in the P 388 murine system of doxorubicin
and related compounds bearing modifications at the
C-9 side chain

Compound	$\dfrac{K_{anal}}{K_{dox}}$ [a]	$\dfrac{\eta'_{sp}}{\eta_{sp}}$ [b]	O.D. [c]	T/C [c]
Ia	1.00	2.03	7.5	168
Ib	1.22	2.16	13.3	134
IIa	0.27	–	10	176
IIb	0.84	–	10.5	136
IIc	0.59	1.51	75	156

(a) Ratio of K_{app} of the compound over K_{app} of doxorubicin
determined by equilibrium dialysis. (b) Ratio of specific
viscosities of native calf-thymus DNA ($5.2 \cdot 10^{-4}$M as DNA-P)
treated (η'_{sp}) and untreated (η_{sp}) with the drug ($5.2 \cdot 10^{-5}$M)
(c) Optimal dose, mg/Kg and survival time of animals bear-
ing experimental leukemia treated on days 5,9,13 expressed
as per cent of untreated controls (NCI data). Average values
of experiments n. 4832, 4961, 5186, 5214, 5391, 5391, 5392,
5620, 5765.

IIa: R = $COCH_2OCO(CH_2)_6CH_3$
IIb: R = CH_2OH
IIc: R = H

IIIa: R = H
IIIb: R = OH

of doxorubicin-14-glycolate (19). Compound *IIb* shows the same values of optimal doses as daunorubicin and doxorubicin but is less effective than the latter, thus confirming the importance of the ketol side chain of doxorubicin for pharmacological selectivity. Compound *IIc*, lacking the C-9 side chain, shows a reduced ability of DNA binding and concomitantly a higher dose is necessary to obtain the antitumour effect. Additional evidence concerning the importance of the C-14 hydroxyl can be deduced from the lower antitumour efficacy in the P 388 system of different derivatives substituted at C-14, including thioesters, ethers, aminoderivatives and 14-alkyl analogues (1).

The higher selectivity of doxorubicin when compared with the analogues possessing different side chains at C-9 is in agreement with the generally observed superiority of doxorubicin over daunorubicin derivatives (19). The reasons for this behaviour are still unknown, although the different efficacy of the two parents be possibly related with differences in the selectivity factors as defined above, namely distribution, metabolism and pharmacokinetics (19).

Structures *III-V* indicate compounds modified at positions 9 and 10 of alicyclic ring A, namely 9-deoxydaunorubicin (*IIIa*), 9-deoxydoxorubicin (*IIIb*), 10(R)-methoxydaunorubicin (*IVa*), 10(R)--methoxydoxorubicin (*IVb*), 10(S)-methoxydaunorubicin (*IVc*), 9,10--anhydrodaunorubicin (*Va*).

IVa: $R^1 = R^3 = H$, $R^2 = OMe$
IVb: $R^1 = OH$, $R^2 = OMe$, $R^3 = H$
IVc: $R^1 = R^2 = H$, $R^3 = OMe$

Va: R = H
Vb: R = Me

Table 2 shows the binding data and antitumour activity of the said analogues. Compounds *IIIa*, *b* and *IVa*, *b*, clearly able to bind to DNA, show marginal activity, as does daunorubicin, in the Q4D 5,9,13 P 388 system, in which however doxorubicin affords approximately 70% increase of life span of treated animals. The behaviour of *IIIb* and *IVb*, possessing the same side chain as doxorubicin, suggests that the presence of the ketol side chain is by itself a necessary but not sufficient requirement for optimal response in this particular test system, the substitution at nearby positions 9 and 10 being critical in this respect. On the other hand compounds *IVc* and *Va*, poor complexing agents, do not show antitumour activity, in agreement with the relationships between affinity for DNA and bioactivity already established (19). It could be pointed out that in both *IVc* and *V* the conformation of ring A is completely different than that of the DNA intercalating anthracyclines (22,23). These conclusions are confirmed by the lack of activity shown by totally synthetic derivative *VI* (24) on one hand and by compounds *Vb*, *VIIa*, *VIIb and VIII* (23) in the Q4D 5,9,13 P 388 test at maximum dosages tested, the latter being in the range 50 to 200 mg/kg.

VI

VIIa : R = CHOHMe
VIIb : R = OMe

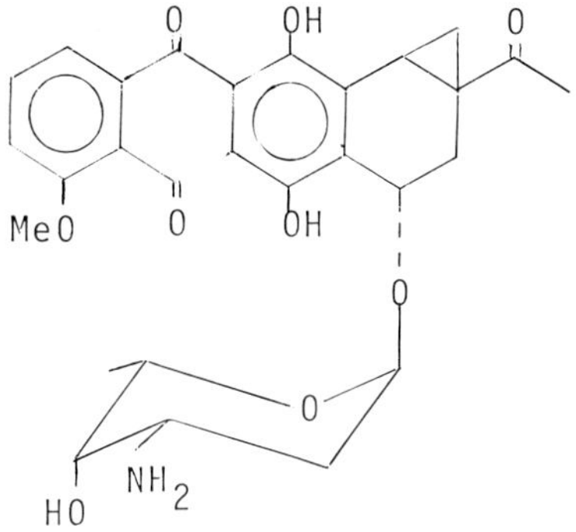

VIII

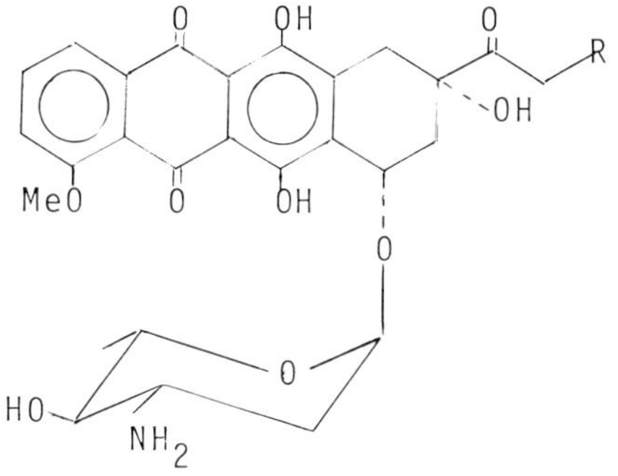

IXa : R = H

IXb : R = OH

Table 2. Binding to calf thymus DNA (8,17,18) and antitumour
activity in the P 388 murine system of daunorubicin
and doxorubicin analogues modified at C-9 and/or C-10

Compound	$\dfrac{K\ anal^a}{K\ dox}$	$\dfrac{\eta'sp^b}{\eta\ sp}$	O.D.^{c}	T/C^c
IIIa	0.70	2.01	18.8	128
IIIb	0.62	2.01	37.5	128
IVa	0.87	2.47	12.5	128
IVb	–	2.84	10.4	132
IVc	–	1.24	50.0	115
Va	0.55	1.20	–	(d)

(a) - (c) See footnotes to Table 1. (d) No antitumour activity in L 1210 leukemia (19). Activity data are median values
obtained in experiments 6280, 6452, 6505, 6696, 6794, 6795,
6947, 7007, 7810. Doxorubicin (Ia) : O.D.=7.3, T/C% = 168;
Daunorubicin (Ib) : O.D.=3.5, T/C% = 129.

3.2. Analogues modified in the sugar moiety

Special consideration has been given in our laboratory to
the synthesis of daunorubicin and doxorubicin analogues showing modifications in the daunosamine residue. The reasons for
this, as well as synthetic procedures used and products ob-

tained have been reviewed (1). Data concerning configurational analogues *IXa*, *IXb*, *Xa*, *Xb*, *XI* are presented in Table 3.
The 4'-epimers (L-arabino configuration) *IXa* and *IXb* are

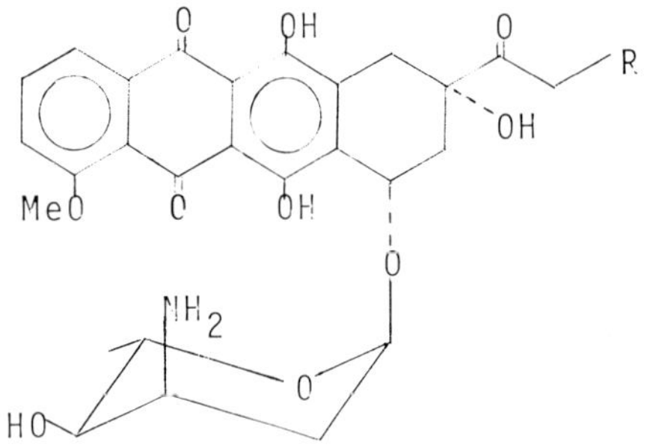

Xa : *R = H*

Xb : *R = OH*

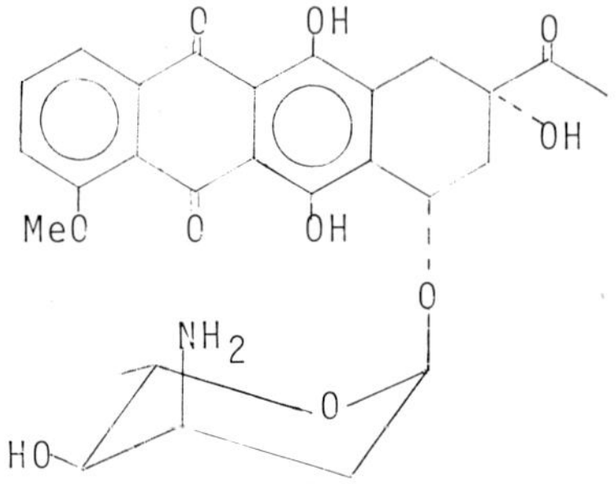

XI

Table 3. Binding to calf thymus DNA (8,17,18) and antitumour
activity in the L 1210 murine system (1) of configurational analogues

Compound	$\frac{K\_anal}{K\ dox}$ [a]	$\frac{\eta'\ sp}{\eta\ sp}$ [b]	O.D. [c]	T/C [c]
Ib	1.22	2.16	4	150
IXa	–	–	4	143
Xa	0.70	1.88	50	137
XI	0.35	1.60	50^d	no activity
Ia	1.00	2.03	5	166
IXb	0.97	1.90	5	150
Xb	0.92	1.83	60	161

(a) - (c) See Table 1 but treatment ip on day 1. (d) Max.dose
tested.

equivalent to the parent compounds (L-lyxo configuration) both
in terms of binding affinity for DNA and antitumour activity

in the L 1210 test (24). On the other hand the 3',4'-diepi a
nalogues *Xa* and *Xb* (L-ribo configuration) are 12 fold less
toxic than the parents, the varied response being not fully
explainable with the moderate decrease in affinity for native DNA. Other factors (e.g. intracellular concentrations)
may be important as shown by the markedly lower cytotoxicity
in cultured cells of *Xa* in respect to *Ib* (19). The same considerations should apply to the 3'-epimer (L-xylo configuration) *XI*.

A detailed comparison of doxorubicin and 4'-epidoxorubicin
in different experimental mouse systems has been reported
(25). The analogue displayed the same antitumour activity as
the parent drug in L 1210 and P 388 leukemies, but showed a
reduced toxicity, and therefore a superior therapeutic ratio.
In an experimental mammary carcinoma, in MSV induced sarcoma,
in metastatic diseases such as Lewis lung carcinoma and MS-2
sarcoma, the 4'-epi compound was as active as doxorubicin at
the same dose levels in different treatment schedules but the
lower toxicity allowed higher dosages with consequent improved results. The analogue appeared to be less cardiotoxic than
the parent drug in the rabbit, and also in a mouse system (26).
In agreement with the observed similarity of the affinity for
DNA, 4'-epidoxorubicin did not differ from doxorubicin in cytotoxicity in cultured cells and in the inhibition of DNA dependent polymerases (25), the more favourable pharmacological
properties of the analogue being attributed to differences in
distribution, rate of metabolism and pharmacokinetic behaviour
(19).

Owing to the favourable properties of 4'-epidoxorubicin, we
gave particular attention to other modifications at C-4' such
as those exemplified in 4'-deoxy and 4'-O-methyl analogues
XIIa, *XIIb*, *XIIIa*, *XIIIb*, *XIVa*, *XIVb*. Table 4 shows the DNA
binding properties and the antitumour properties in the P 388
system of these analogues. 4'-Deoxydoxorubicin displays bind
ing properties and antitumour efficacy similar to those of do
xorubicin, in agreement with the behaviour of 4'-epidoxorubi-

cin, albeit at a three fold lower dose.

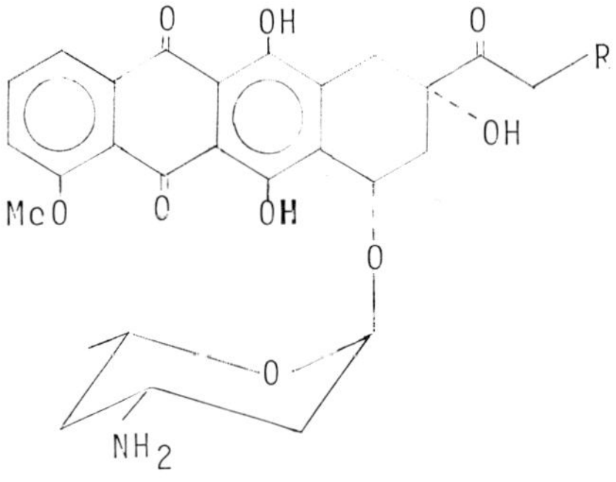

XIIa : R = H
XIIb : R = OH

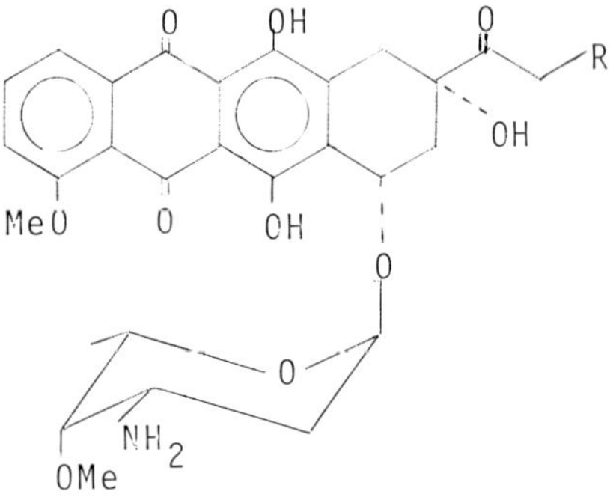

XIIIa : R = H
XIIIb : R = OH

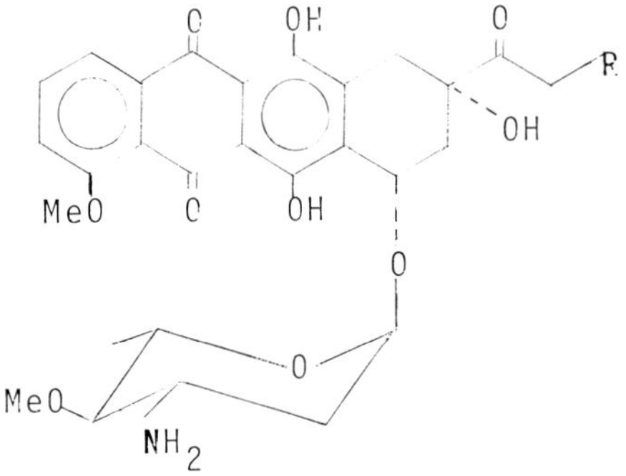

XIVa : R = H
XIVb : R = OH

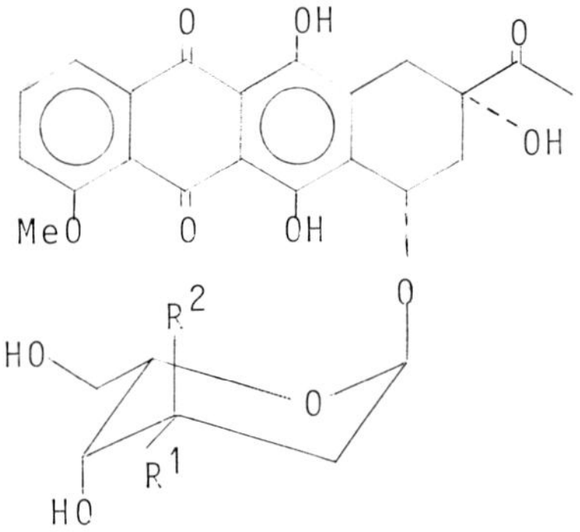

XVa : R^1 = NH_2, R^2 = H
XVb : R^1 = H, R^2 = NH_2

Table 4. Binding to calf thymus DNA (17,18,19) and antitumour
activity in the P 388 murine test of 4'-deoxy and 4'-
-O-methyl analogues.

Compound	$\dfrac{K\ anal^{a}}{K\ dox}$	$\dfrac{\eta'\ sp^{b}}{\eta\ sp}$	MTD^{c}	T/C^{c}
XIIa	0.84	--	4.0^{d}	162,187
XIIb	1.19	2.03	2.0	204
XIIIa	0.68	2.01	4.4	156
XIIIb	0.48	1.88	4.4	200
XIVa	0.27	1.80	20.0	174,180
XIVb	–	–	10.0^{d}	187^{d}

(a), (b) see Table 1. (c) Maximum tolerated dose ($\geq$ optimal
non toxic dose) in mg/kg and T/c as already defined (treatment
ip   on day 1 after tumour inoculation). Daunorubicin (Ib),
MTD = 4.3, T/C% = 179; Doxorubicin (Ia), MTD = 7.0, T/C% = 228.
(d) Experimental L 1210 leukemia (doxorubicin, MTD = 10.0,
T/C% = 187).

4'-C-Methyl derivatives XIIIa and XIIIb, on the other hand, although displaying a somewhat lower value of K_{app}, exhibit the
same toxicity as the parent compounds. Aside from the possibil
ity that approximations accepted for K_{app} evaluation be not
valid in the case of the said derivatives, it could be that
other molecular properties, such as for instance the increased
lipophilicity of the sugar moiety, play a role in this case.
The particularly higher efficacy of XIIIb in L 1210 leukemia
of the mouse (27) may also be related with this behaviour and
still unknown aspects of distribution, metabolism and pharmaco
kinetics may also be involved. In XIVa, the presence of an
equatorial methoxyl at C-4' reduces the affinity for DNA and
consequently the toxicity in biological systems (19).

4'-Deoxydoxorubicin has been selected for further development owing to the outstanding antitumour effects in different
mouse tumours and of the absence of cardiac damage at non lethal
doses in the animal models (28). Fluorescence based data concerning the tissue distribution and elimination of the compound

in laboratory mice have been reported (29). It appears that
further investigation of the "selectivity parameters" as defin
ed above will provide explanation of the favourable properties
of 4'-deoxydoxorubicin, a very promising analogue.

Seven out of the eight 3-amino-2,3-dideoxy-L-hexopyranosyl
possible derivatives of daunomycinone or adriamycinone have also
been prepared. According to the studies performed in Author's
Laboratory, the presence of the 6'-hydroxyl reduces the affin
ity for DNA (Table 5). Within this series, 6'-hydroxy-3',4'-
-diepi analogues *XVIa* and *b* have been demonstrated to possess
good antitumour properties in the P 388 system at optimal dosages (30). Data reported by Di Marco et al. (31) indicate that
the L-arabino compounds *XVIIa* and *b* display a DNA association
constant whose value is 0.58 times that of daunorubicin and
doxorubicin respectively and this may explain, at least in part,
the lower toxicity and the higher values of active doses.

XVIa : *R = H*
XVIb : *R = OH*

XVIIa : *R = H*
XVIIb : *R = OH*

Table 5. DNA binding properties and antitumour properties in
the L 1210 system of 6'-hydroxylated analogues (17,18).

Compound	$\dfrac{K\ anal}{K\ dox}$ [a]	$\dfrac{\eta'\ sp}{\eta\ sp}$ [b]	O.D. [c]	T/C [c]
XVa	0.76	–	–	–
XVb	–	1.86 [d]	>75	100
XVIa	0.68	1.70	$\geq$17.2	150
XVIb	0.32	1.55	–	–

(a)-(c) See Table 3. (d) Unpublished result.

N - Acyl derivatives of daunorubicin or doxorubicin have
been obtained and studied by different investigators (1).
Claims concerning the favourable pharmacological properties of
N-trifluoroacetyldoxorubicin-14-O-valerate (AD 32) and of ami-
noacyl derivatives (32, 33) make a discussion on this class of
analogues of interest.

N-acetyldaunorubicin and N-acetyldoxorubicin are rather in-
efficient DNA intercalators (8). However, the latter shows dis
cernible antitumour activity in experimental mouse leukemias,
albeit lower than the parent doxorubicin and at a much higher
dosage (19). N-trifluoroacetyldoxorubicin and its derivative
AD 32 are endowed with antitumour properties comparable to that
of doxorubicin at approximately 10 to 20 higher doses (1). For
AD 32 a different, albeit unknown, mechanism of action has been
suggested (34). However, recent reports indicate the presence
of the parent drug as a product of metabolism of AD 32 and of
N-leucyldaunomycin in vivo (32, 35). A quantitative study using
$\underline{/}^{-14}\underline{C}\underline{/}$AD 32 in rats in order to evaluate the excretion, the
distribution, and the metabolism of the compound has been per
formed in our laboratory (unpublished studies). At 24 hours
after the administration about 80% of the i.v. dose of radioactivity was excreted, mainly in the faeces (doxorubicin 37.5%)
tissue levels of carbon-14 being lower (with the exception of
blood and liver) than after a 10 times lower dose of $\underline{/}^{-14}\underline{C}\underline{/}$
doxorubicin. In liver, kidney, spleen and lung tissues the

main radioactive species present were AD 32 itself and doxorubicin, N-trifluoroacetyl doxorubicin and its 13-dihydro derivative accounting for most of urinary radioactivity. It can
be deduced, therefore, that deacylation to give the parent
drug is certainly an important activation process explaining,
at least in part if not completely, the antitumour effects of
the N-acyl derivatives known so far.

3.3. Analogues modified in the anthraquinone moiety

Modifications of the chromophoric moiety in antitumour anthracyclines have been carried out by either total synthesis
or semisynthesis starting from the biosynthetic aglycones,
mainly daunomycinone. The first approach has allowed the prep
aration of different analogues showing variations in the sub
stitution on ring D (XVIIIa-g, XIX), whereas the second one has
been used for the synthesis of O-methyl derivatives (XXa-d,
XXI a and b). Also the 7(R), 9(P) and 1'(S) (β-glycoside)
configurational isomers of XVIIIa were obtained (1).

XVIII   XIX

	R	R¹	R²
a	H	H	H
b	OH	H	H
c	H	H	Me
d	OH	H	Me
e	H	Me	H
f	H	Cl	H
g	H	H	Cl

	R	R^1	R^2
a	H	H	H (carminomycin)
b	H	Me	H
c	H	H	Me
d	OH	Me	H

XXIa : $R^1 = H$, $R^2 = Me$
XXIb : $R^1 = Me$, $R^2 = H$

The remarkable antitumour activity of 4-demethoxy analogues
XVIIIa, b, c, d and some related compounds, such as the 4'-
-epi analogue of XVIIIb, is an established knowledge (1). With
the exception of the 7(R), 9(R) stereoisomer, all compounds of
types XVIII and XIX were bioactive, indicating the loose requirements of ring D substitution at this regard (in agreement
with the peripheral condition of this position of the anthracycline molecule within the structure of DNA intercalation complex).
Of particular interest is the activity displayed by compound
XVIIIa, 4-demethoxydaunorubicin, when administered by the oral
route (36). 4-Demethoxydaunorubicin has also been proved to be
less cardiotoxic in laboratory animals (see below) and therefore
proposed for clinical trials.

The substitution of the 4-methoxy group in daunorubicin with
an hydrogen atom has probably no effect on the affinity towards
DNA (Table 6), this property not accounting for the markedly
higher toxicity of XVIIIa when compared with Ib (19). An im-

portant feature of the demethoxy analogue is however its high
er (up to 4 times after two hours exposure) intracellular con
centration when compared to daunorubicin in cultured cells
treated with the drugs (39). Additional studies of the *in vitro*
and *in vivo* behaviour of the new drug are clearly necessary
for understanding the said pharmacological differences.

Table 6. Comparison of DNA binding properties of 4-demethoxy-
-daunorubicin *(XVIIIa)* with those of daunorubicin
(Ib) according to different studies.

Method	*XVIIIa*		*Ib*	
	K_{app}	η	K_{app}	η
Equilibrium dialysis[a]	5.9×10^5	0.17	4.9×10^5	0.17
Fluorometry[b]	2.4×10^6	0.20	3.3×10^6	0.16
Spectrophotometry[c]	9.4×10^5	0.21	13.3×10^5	0.20

(a) Arlandini et al. (17, 18). (b) Zunino et al. (37).
(c) Plumbridge & Brown (38).

The antitumour activity of daunorubicin analogues differing in the methylation of the phenolic groups is presented in
Table 7. The biosynthetic derivative *XXa* (carminomycin) is
clearly more effective than daunorubicin *(Ib)* and its isomers
XXb and *XXc*, the latter showing a distinctly lower activity.
The 6-O-methyl analogue *XXb* appears to behave similarly to
daunorubicin in the P 388 leukemia system. On the other hand
compounds with two methyl groups such as *XXIa* and *XXIb* are
even less effective, the optimal doses being ten times or more
greater than the optimal dose of the parent *Ib*.

Because of the appreciable activity of *XXb*, the corresponding doxorubicin analogue *XXd* was prepared (41).
Interestingly, the new compound displayed antitumour activity
similar to that of the isomeric doxorubicin together with the
exhibition of a marked toxocity (unpublished work from
Author's Laboratory). Notwithstanding the presence of the
bulky methoxy group at C-6 on ring B, that is thought to be

(together with ring C) the portion of the molecule that is in-
tercalated between the base pairs inside the double DNA-helix.

Table 7. Antitumour activity in the P 388 murine system of ana
logues differing in the methylation of phenolic group.

Compound	Schedule of Treatment (ip)	O.D. (mg/kg)	T/C (%)	Number of Experiments
XXa[a]	Q4D 5,9,13[b]	2.35[c]	156[c]	3
XXb	"	12.50	129	1
XXc	"	50.00[c]	125	1
Ib	"	11.00	134	4
Ia	"	7.2	190	5
XXIa	Day 1	50.00	127	(d)
XXIb	"	200.00[c]	122	"
Ib	"	4.40	148	"

(a) Carminomycin. (b) NCI data. (c) Max. dose tested. (d) Ref.40

4. CONCLUSIONS AND ADDENDA

The analysis of a selected group of structural variations of
the daunorubicin and doxorubicin molecules confirms previous de
ductions (19) and allows drawing some relationships that are
summarized below. It is clear, however, that additional investigations are needed, both at molecular and biological level,
in order to reach a full understanding of the complex picture
represented by the different parameters of anthracycline action
on tumour proliferation and of the molecular requirements for
optimal bioactivity.

Available experimental evidence supports the current view
indicating nuclear DNA as the main receptor of antitumour anthracyclines in biological systems. In fact those chemical modi
fications of the anthracycline molecule that reduce the affinity for DNA also reduce the toxicity and optimal antitumour effects are obtained with higher dosages as compared with the par
ent drugs. Results of C-9 side chain modifications indicate that
doxorubicin-type hydroxyacetyl structure at C-13 and C-14 is
related with the highest selectivity, i.e. greater antitumour
efficacy at optimal doses. Ring A conformation is a strict re-

quirement for bioactivity suggesting that a given orientation
in space of the sugar moiety relative to the aglycone is requir
ed for intercalation. As regards the sugar moiety, doxorubicin
derivatives modified at C-4' appear to maintain the DNA complex
ing properties of the parent and may exhibit enhanced selectivity (probably related with variations in pharmacokinetics and
metabolism) in some important biological system. Metabolic conversion to the parent drug is also responsible for bioactivity
in vivo of derivatives, such as esters or amides, that show low
affinity for DNA. Finally, modification of the substitution on
the anthraquinone chromophore may have profound consequences on bioactivity because of the importance of the moiety in the intercalation process.

An important pharmacological property that is dependent on
structural changes is the already mentioned cardiotoxicity in
laboratory animals. For instance, the optimal dose shown by doxorubicin in the P 388, Q4D, 5,9,13 ip schedule is of the same
order of magnitude as the minimal cumulative cardiotoxic dose in
a rat model (42), whereas the latter is twice the optimal anti-
tumour dose for doxorubicin 14-octanoate, -nicotinate, and
-stearoylglycolate and for 4'-epidoxorubicin, the same ratio
being three for 4-demethoxydoxorubicin and five for 4'-deoxy-
doxorubicin!

Notes concerning recent develoments of compounds reported
here may be added. 4'-Epidoxorubicin has already entered phase
2 clinical trials in different centres. It appears to have
(a) the same activity as doxorubicin on doxorubicin responsive
tumours, (b) a somewhat lower incidence of undesirable side effects and (c) activity on malignant melanomas, a tumour naturally resistant to doxorubicin (43-51). 4'-Deoxydoxorubicin
has been demonstrated (52) to be active in inhibiting the proliferation of human colorectal tumours transplanted in nude
mice, an observation that has aroused much interest on this
compound. 4-Demethoxydaunorubicin has been submitted to phase
1 clinical trials, both by the iv and oral route, the results
being in full agreement with the animal data (53, 54).

REFERENCES

1. Arcamone F. 1981. "Doxorubicin", Medicinal Chemistry Series, 17, Academic Press, New York.
2. Arcamone F. 1978. Topics in Antibiotics Chemistry , 2, 100, P.G. Sammes Ed., Ellis Horwood Ltd, Chichester.
3. Alberts A. 1981. 182nd ACS Nat. Meeting, New York, Aug.23-28, Abstracts MEDI 56.
4. Di Marco A, Arcamone F, Zunino F. 1974. Antibiotics, 3, 101, Springer Verlag, Berlin (Corcoran JW & Hahn FE Eds.).
5. Di Marco A. 1975. Cancer Chemother. Rep., 6, 91.
6. Di Marco A, Arcamone F. 1975. Adriamycin Review, 11, European Press Medikon, Ghent, Belgium (Staquet M et al. Eds.)
7. Neidle S. 1978. Topics in Antibiotic Chemistry, part D, 2, 240, Ellis Horwood Ltd, Chichester.
8. Arcamone F, Arlandini E, Menozzi M, Valentini L, Vannini E. 1981. Symposium on Anthracycline Antibiotics in Cancer Therapy, New York, Semptember 16-18.
9. Pigram WJ, Fuller W, Hamilton L.D. 1972. Nature New Biol., 235, 17.
10. Di Marco A, Arcamone F. 1975. Arzneim. Forsch., 25, 368.
11. Quigley GJ, Wang A H J, Ughetto G, Van Der Marel G, Van Boom JH, Rich A. 1980. Proc. Natl. Acad. Sci. USA, 77, 7204.
12. Bauer E, Förster W, Gollmick FA, Schütz H, Stutter E, Walter A, Berg H. to be published.
13. Arcamone F. 1981. Paper presented at the Symposium on Anthracyclines, Paris, June 24 - 25.
14. Zunino F, Gambetta R, Di Marco A, Zaccara A. 1972. Biochim. Biophys. Acta, 277, 489.
15. Saucier JM, Festy B, Le Pecq JB. 1971. Biochimie, 53, 973.
16. Gabbay EJ. 1976. Internat. Quantum Chem. No. 3, 217, J.Wiley & Sons Inc.
17. Arlandini E, Vigevani A, Arcamone F. 1977. Il Farmaco, 32, 315, Ed. Sci.
18. Arlandini E, Vigevani A, Arcamone F. 1980. Il Farmaco, 35, 65, Ed. Sci.
19. Arcamone F, Casazza A, Cassinelli G, Di Marco A, Penco S. 1981. Paper presented at the Symposium on Anthracycline Antibiotics in Cancer Therapy, New York, September 16-18.
20. Penco S, Angelucci F, Vigevani A, Arlandini E. 1977. J.Antib., 30, 764.
21. Arcamone F, Franceschi G, Minghetti A, Penco S, Redaelli S, Di Marco A, Casazza AM, Dasdia T, Di Fronzo G, Giuliani F, Lenaz L, Necco A, Soranzo C. 1974. J. Med. Chem., 17, 335.
22. Penco S, Gozzi F, Vigevani A, Ballabio M, Arcamone F. 1979. Heterocycles, 13, 281.
23. Penco S, Angelucci F, Gozzi F, Franchi G, Gioia B, Arcamone F. 1980. C.A., 92, 42256. Paper presented at the 11th International Symposium on Chemistry of Natural Products, Golden Sands, Bulgaria, September 17-23, 1978.
24. Di Marco A, Casazza AM., Gambetta R, Supino R, Zunino F. 1976. Cancer Res., 36, 1962.
25. Arcamone F, Di Marco A, Casazza AM. 1978. Advances in Cancer Chemotherapy, p.297, Japan Sci. Soc. Press, Tokyo/Univ. Park Press, Baltimore.

26. Casazza AM, Di Marco A, Bonadonna G, Bonfante V, Bertazzoli C, Bellini O, Pratesi G, Sala L, Ballerini L. 1980. Anthracyclines (Proc.Workshop), p. 403. Academic Press, New York.
27. Cassinelli G, Ruggieri D, Arcamone F. 1979. J. Med. Chem., 22, 121.
28. Casazza AM. 1981. Paper presented at the Symposium on Anthracyclines, Paris, June 24-25.
29. Formelli F, Pollini C, Casazza AM, Di Marco A, Mariani A. 1981. Cancer Chemother. Pharmacol. 5, 139.
30. Arcamone F, Bargiotti A, Di Marco A, Penco S. 1976. Germ. Offen. 2,618,822, C.A. 86, 140416, (1977).
31. Di Marco A, Casazza AM, Dasdia T, Necco A, Pratesi G, Rivolta P, Velcich A, Zaccara A, Zunino F. 1977. Chem. Biol. Interactions, 19, 291.
32. Masquelier M, Baurain R, Trouet A. 1980. J. Med. Chem., 23, 1166.
33. Sela Ben-Ami, Levin Yehuda. 1981. Cancer Treatment Reports, 65, 277.
34. Krishan A, Israel M, Modest EJ, Frei III E. 1976. Cancer Res., 26, 2114.
35. Israel M. 1981. Papre presented at Symposium on Anthracycline Antibiotics in Cancer Theraphy, New York Univ. Med.Center, September 16-18.
36. Di Marco A, Casazza AM, Pratesi G. 1977. Cancer Treat. Rep. 61, 893.
37. Zunino F, Gambetta R, Di Marco A, Luoni G, Zaccara A. 1976. Bioch. Biophys. Res. Comm., 69, 744.
38. Plumbridge TW, Brown JR. 1978. Biochem. Pharmacol., 27, 1881.
39. Formelli F, Casazza AM, Di Marco A, Mariani A, Pollini C. 1979. Cancer Chemother. Pharm., 3, 261.
40. Zunino F, Casazza AM, Pratesi G, Formelli F, Di Marco A. 1981. Biochemical Pharmacology, 30, 1856.
41. Arcamone F, Cassinelli G, Penco S. to be published in ACS Symposium Series:"Anthracycline Antibiotics", H.S. El Khadem Ed.
42. Arcamone F. 1979. Advances in Medical Oncology, Research and Education. Basis for Cancer Therapy I, 5, 21, Pergamon Press Oxford and New York.
43. Bonfante V, Bonadonna G, Villani F, Di Fronzo G, Martini A, Casazza AM. 1979. Cancer Treat. Rep. 63, 915.
44. Bonfante V, Bonadonna G, Villani F, Martini A. 1980. Recent Results in Cancer Research, 74, 202, Springer Verlag.
45. Schauer PK, Wittes RE, Gralla RJ, Casper E.S, Young C.W. 1981. Cancer Clinical Trials (in press).
46. Bonfante V, Villani F, Bonadonna G. 1981. Cancer Chemotherapy and Pharmacology (in press).
47. Hurteloup P, Mathé G, Hayat M, & the EORTC Clinical Screening Group. 1981. Paper presented at the 12th Int. Congress of Chemotherapy, Florence (Italy), July 19-24 and at the UICC Conference on Clinical Oncology, Lausanne (Switzerland) October 28-31.
48. Robustelli della Cuna G, Pavesi L, Cuzzoni Q, Ganzina F, Tramarin R. 1981. Paper presented at the 12th Int. Congress

of Chemotherapy, Florence (Italy), July 19-24.
49. Robustelli della Cuna G, Ganzina F, Tramarin R, Pavesi L. 1981. Paper presented at the UICC Conference on Clinical Oncology, Lausanne (Switzerland), October 28-31.
50. EORTC Clinical Screening Group, De Jager R. 1981. Paper presented at the Symposium on Anthracyclines, Paris, June 24-25.
51. Campora E, Sertoli M.R, Vinci P, Nobile MT, Boccardo F, Rosso R. 1981. Paper presented at the 12th Int. Congress of Chemotherapy, Florence (Italy), July 19-24.
52. Giuliani F, Zirvi K.A, Kaplan N.O, Goldin A. Int. J. Cancer, in press
53. Varini M, Kaplan S, Togni P, Cavalli F. 1981. Abstracts 57, Third NCI-EORTC Symposium on New Drugs in Cancer Therapy, Brussels (Belgium), October 15-17.
54. Bonfante V, Villani F, Bonadonna G. 1981. Abstracts 61, Third NCI-EORTC Symposium on New Drugs in Cancer Therapy, Brussels (Belgium), October 15-17.

STRUCTURE—ACTIVITY RELATIONSHIPS AMONG ANTITUMOUR QUINONES

J.S. DRISCOLL

1. INTRODUCTION

The quinone function appears with considerable frequency among compounds which demonstrate clinical and pre-clinical antitumor activity. Sources of these compounds include fermentation products, synthetic materials and plant products. Familiar names among antitumor quinones include daunorubicin, adriamycin, mitomycin C, streptonigrin, lapachol, trenimon and carbazilquinone. New quinoid compounds currently under investigation by the National Cancer Institute (NCI) in the United States are AZQ, dihydroxyanthracenedione, aclacinomycin A and 7-OMEN.

The quinone ring has a unique combination of structural features which allows a degree of both stability and reactivity. The ability of a quinone to participate in redox reactions and to activate ring substituents make this function a very versatile nucleus on which to build antitumor properties.

Since several other presentations will emphasize certain quinone containing drugs, I will limit my discussion to representatives of two quinone classes which the NCI currently has in Phase II clinical trial (AZQ and anthracene-dione) and two hydroquinone classes (catechols and hydroxypyridones) which are presently under investigation in our laboratories at the NCI.

2. AZIRIDINYLBENZOQUINONES

An analysis of the structure-activity relationships among the more than 2,000 quinones which the NCI had tested for antitumor activity by 1970 revealed that the aziridinyl-p-benzoquinones were the only members of this family which possessed very good activity against murine leukemia L1210 (1). These non-ionic, lipophylic molecules appeared to possess the physical and chemical properties required for penetration of the blood-brain barrier (2). Once we established that some of the molecules already available possessed intracerebral (IC) as well as intraperitoneal (IP) L1210 activity, a series of diaziridinylquinones was designed taking into account the lipophilic,

D.N. Reinhoudt, T.A. Connors, H.M. Pinedo & K.W. van de Poll (eds.), Structure-Activity Relationships of Anti-Tumour Agents.
© 1983, Martinus Nijhoff Publishers, The Hague/Boston/London. ISBN 90-247-2783-9.

electronic and steric effects of the other two ring substituents (Table 1). Emphasis was placed on diamino derivatives, since few of these compounds

TABLE 1. Aziridinylquinone design considerations.

> Water solubility
>   log P (-2 to +2)
>   non-ionic functional groups for
>   blood-brain-barrier penetration
> Electronic and steric effects
>   redox potential
>   aziridine reactivity

were known and amino groups should make the quinoid ring difficult to reduce, a property suspected to be important in the reactivity of aziridinylquinones (3). An additional objective was the preparation of a compound with water solubility adequate for formulation purpose. About 20 compounds were synthesized and evaluated against both IC and IP murine tumor models (4,5). Representative structures are shown in Fig. 1.

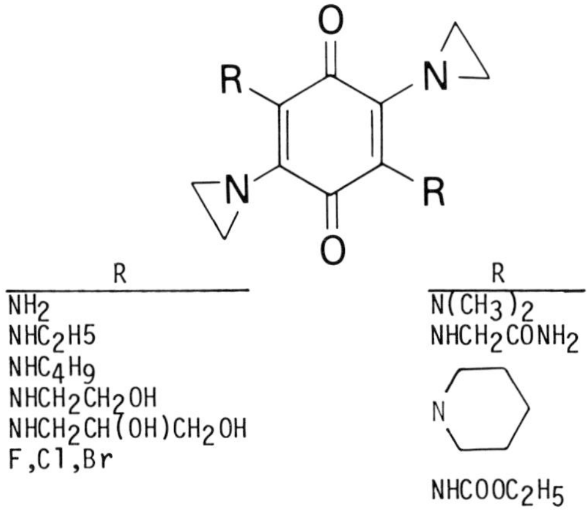

R	R
NH$_2$	N(CH$_3$)$_2$
NHC$_2$H5	NHCH$_2$CONH$_2$
NHC$_4$H$_9$	
NHCH$_2$CH$_2$OH	
NHCH$_2$CH(OH)CH$_2$OH	
F,Cl,Br	
	NHCOOC$_2$H5

FIGURE 1. Representative structures of synthesized aziridinylquinones.

The compounds synthesized at the NCI, as well as analogs previously prepared by other organizations and submitted to the NCI for evaluation, were compared using IP drug treatment against five murine tumor models (Table 2).

TABLE 2. Tumor models utilized.

> IC ependymoblastoma
> IP L1210 leukemia
> IC L1210 leukemia
> IP P388 leukemia
> IP B16 melanoma

Among the 31 compounds fully evaluated in this manner (6), the carbamate, subsequently named AZQ, was determined to have the best overall activity, especially if emphasis was placed on brain tumor activity. This compound produced multiple 60 day survivors in the IC ependymoblastoma (EM) tumor system and was active in numerous tumor models (Table 3).

TABLE 3. AZQ antitumor activity.

$$H_5C_2OOCHN \quad \overset{O}{\underset{O}{\bigcirc}} \quad N\triangle$$

$$\triangle N \qquad NHCOOC_2H_5$$

Tumor Model	Treatment Route	%ILS or (%TWI)*
IC ependymoblastoma	IP	349
IC P388 leukemia	IP	60
IC L1210 leukemia	IP	84
IP L1210 leukemia	IP	169
IP L1210 leukemia	Oral	88
IP B16 melanoma	IP	70
IP P388 leukemia	IP	138
IP P388 leukemia	IV	71
IP colon 26	IP	225
SC CD8F$_1$ mouse mammary	IP	(89)
SC colon 38	IP	(83)
RC MX-1 breast xenograft	SC	(100)

*ILS - increase in life span
 TWI - tumor weight inhibition

AZQ is presently undergoing Phase II clinical trials in the United States. Clinical pharmacology studies show that AZQ readily enters cerebrospinal fluid and this compound has demonstrated activity against human brain tumors.

Several structure-activity relationships became apparent upon evaluation of the 31 aziridinylquinone analogs. The polar, water soluble derivatives were more active in IP ascites tumor systems than the lipophilic analogs. However, the reverse was true against the intracerebral tumors. A parabolic relationship was observed against IP tumors in the series methyl-, ethyl-, propyl- and butylamino. Replacing alkylamino groups with halogen (F, Cl, Br) abolished antitumor activity. Increasing the number of alkyl groups on the amino function actually increased the water solubility of the derivatives, probably through reduction of internal crystal forces by disruption of hydrogen bonding. Addition of one or two methyl groups to the aziridine rings in carbamate derivatives reduced antitumor activity, probably through steric effects.

While AZQ was judged to have the best overall activity in the series, a second analog, called BZQ, was found to possess an interesting and somewhat different spectrum of activity. It had less IC but greater IP leukemia activity (Table 4). In addition, BZQ has a significantly higher ratio of water solubility to optimum dose than AZQ. This parameter is of importance relative to how easily a parenteral formulation can be prepared.

TABLE 4. Comparison of AZQ and BZQ antitumor activity.

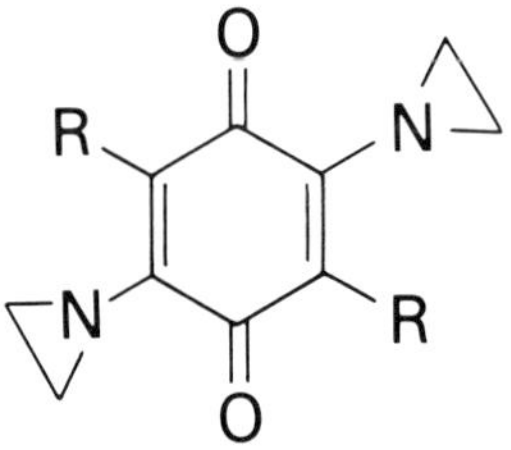

AZQ, R = $NHCOOC_2H_5$
BZQ, R = $NHCH_2CH_2OH$

Compound	IC		Activity % ILS, (cures/6)		IP	
	EM	L1210	P388	B16		L1210
AZQ	170(6)	79	112(1)	62		113
BZQ	83	48	160(2)	61		175(5)

The EORTC, in cooperation with the NCI, is presently evaluating the feasibility of a clinical trial for BZQ in Great Britain and Europe.

3. ANTHRACENEDIONES

In 1973, the anthraquinone (I) was obtained during a random collection of compounds offered by the Allied Chemical Company.

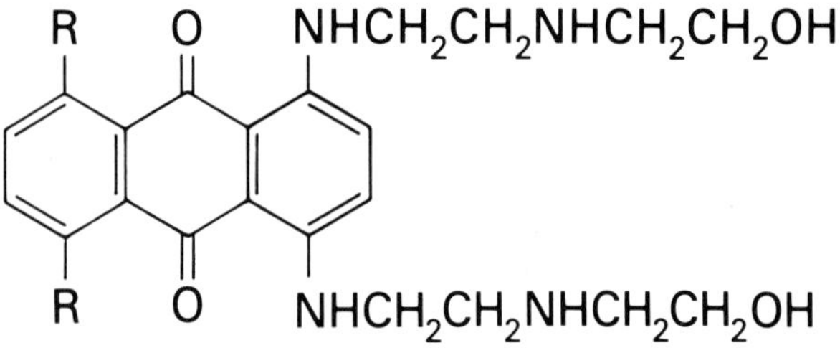

I, R=H
II, R=OH

The initial tests against L1210 and P388 leukemia showed a remarkable degree of activity. Subsequent tests showed activity in other tumor systems including B16 melanoma where I produces more than 50% long-term survivors. With the permission of the supplier of compound I, the NCI sponsored a structure-activity study by Dr. C.C. Cheng (Midwest Research Institute) in an attempt to optimize the antitumor properties in this series. These results (7,8), as well as those from Lederle Laboratories (9), show that certain structural features found in the parent molecule, I, are critical. Much of the synthetic effort in the Midwest study was directed towards a study of the effect of changes in the ethanolamino side chain (7). Table 5 shows some of these results. All alterations shown reduced activity relative to the parent, I. The aliphatic nitrogen atom is very important. Replacement with sulfur or carbon abolished activity entirely. P388 leukemia activity appears to correlate with hydrophilic character.

TABLE 5. Anthracenediones. Side chain effects.

R	P388 activity (% ILS)
$NHCH_2CH_2OH$ (I)	176
$NHCH_2CH_2CH_3$	25
$NHCH_2CH_3$	68
$NHCH_3$	100
NH_2	115
N⬡	28
SCH_2CH_2OH	N*
$CH_2CH_2CH_2OH$	N
$CH_2NHCH_2CH_2OH$	33
$NH(CH_2)_2NH(CH_2)_2OH$	20

*N = not active

Although only a few examples were reported involving alterations in the aromatic nucleus (7,9), one of these compounds, the 5,8-dihydroxy analog (II), was found to possess excellent activity and to be more water soluble and more than ten times as potent as I (Table 6).

Compound I has undergone early clinical trials at the Jules Bordet
Institute. Phase II trials are anticipated under EORTC sponsorship.
Compound II is currently in Phase II clinical trial in the United States.

TABLE 6. Antitumor activity of anthracenedione analogs.

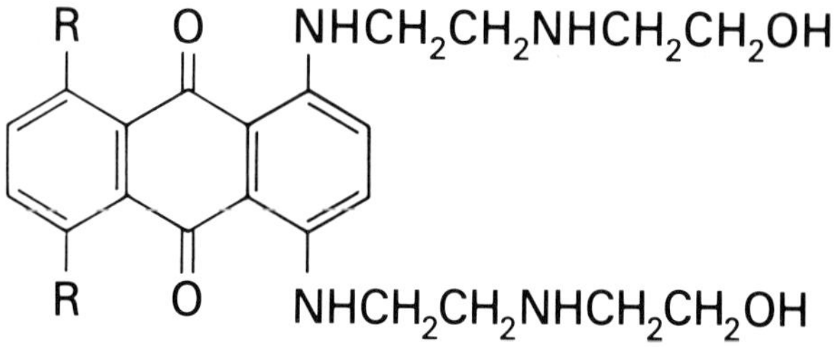

In Vivo antitumor activity

R	P388		B16	
	O.D.*	% ILS (cures)	O.D.	% ILS (cures)
H	8	176(4/6)	8	162(7/10)
OH	0.5	199(4/6)	0.5	162(8/10)

*O.D. - optimum dose (mg/kg/day, QD 1-9)

4. CATECHOL DERIVATIVES

During a study of the antitumor properties of psychotropic drugs (10),
dopamine (III) was found to possess reproducible activity against L1210
and P388 leukemia. Dopamine, a catecholamine, has long been recognized
as an important neurotransmitter substance. L-DOPA (IV), the biochemical
precursor of III, was inactive against these tumors.

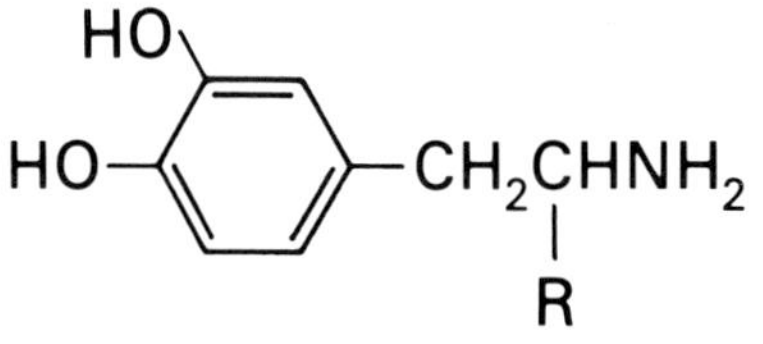

III,R=H
IV,R=COOH

A study was designed to identify the structural fractures critical for
antitumor activity and to establish whether antitumor activity was somehow
related to neurotransmitter activity (11).

Dopamine is a catechol, and as such, is the reduced form of an orthoquinone. o-Quinones are, in general, reactive molecules and our initial
hypothesis was that III might be oxidized at a tumor target site to produce
an o-quinoid form which could react with a nucleophilic group on a
physiologically important molecule (Figure 2).

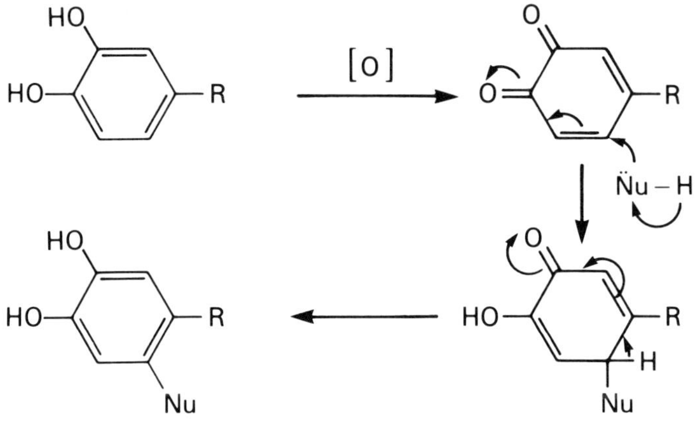

FIGURE 2. Possible mechanism of action for antitumor active catechols.

An evaluation of over 30 analogs of dopamine was made against P388 leukemia (11). The compounds studied fell into several sub-structural groups.

4.1. Aminoethylcatechols

Table 7 shows structures representative of those compounds evaluated in this group.

TABLE 7. Aminoethylcatechols evaluated.

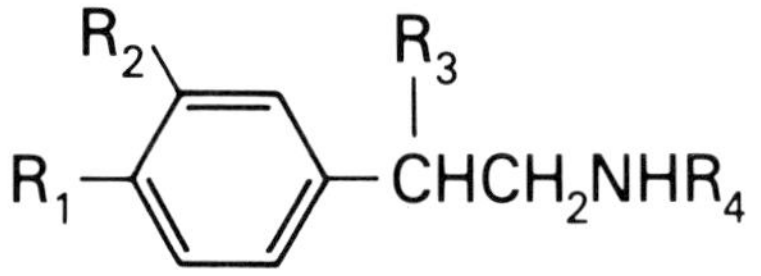

Aminoethylcatechol	R₁	R₂	R₃	R₄
III	OH	OH	H	H
V	OH	OH	H	CH₃
VI	OH	OCH₃	H	H
VII	OH	H	H	H
VIII	NH₂	H	H	H
IX	NO₂	H	H	H
X	H	H	H	H
XI	OH	OH	OH	H
XII	OH	H	OH	H
XIII	H	OH	OH	H
XIV	OH	OH	OH	isopropyl

Only N-methyldopamine (V) and isoproterenol (XIV) were active in this series with P388 ILS values of 56% and 31%, respectively. Dopamine (III) gave ILS values of 50-70% in multiple tests.

4.2. Aminomethylcatechols (benzylamines)

Five benzylamines (Table 8) were tested. Compound XV (dopamine minus a methylene group) gave a P388 ILS of 58%. This indicated that the neurotransmitter properties of III are probably unrelated to the observed antitumor activity of this molecule.

TABLE 8. Aminomethylcatechols evaluated.

Benzylamine analog	R_1	R_2
XV	OH	OH
XVI	OH	OCH_3
XVII	OCH_3	OCH_3
XVIII	Cl	Cl
XIX	H	H

This series, therefore, became of interest for structural optimization since dopaminergic side effects should not pose a problem in the aminomethyl series.

4.3. Nonamino catechols

Table 9 shows some of the compounds evaluated in an attempt to determine whether the amino group in III and XV was was critical to the P388 leukemia activity observed.

TABLE 9. Nonamino catechols tested.

Catechol analog	R_1	R_2	R_3
XX	OH	OH	H
XXI	OH	OH	CH_3
XXII	OH	OH	CHO
XXIII	OH	OH	COOH
XXIV	OH	OH	CH_2COOH
XXV	OH	OH	CH_2CH_2COOH
XXVI	OH	OH	$CH=CHCOOH$

With the finding that both XXI and XXII were active (ILS 30%), it became clear that an amino group was not necessary for activity.

4.4. Trihydroxyphenethylamines

Comparison of the P388 activity of 5-hydroxydopamine (XXVII) and
6-hydroxydopamine (XXVIII) revealed the 5-hydroxy isomer to have significant
activity (ILS 68%) while XXVIII was inactive. This finding suggested that
the positioning of the potentially oxidizable hydroxyl groups was important
and that compounds which are potential p-quinones may not be optimum for
antitumor activity.

Based on the benzylamine and trihydroxybenzene data, a new series was
designed and a number of compounds synthesized (12). Among the 15 compounds
tested, XXIX, XXX, and XXXI were active with ILS values of 57%, 37% and
49%, respectively. In addition, a comparison of three dihydroxybenzaldehydes

| XXIX | XXX | XXXI |

showed that only the one capable of being oxidized to an o-quinone (XXII)
was active.

| XXII | XXXII | XXXIII |

The following conclusions can be reached regarding structure-activity
relationships among catechol analogs evaluated here. Ortho-hydroxy groups
are required. N-methylation does not abolish activity but O-methylation
does by making the aromatic ring non-oxidizable. Neither the aminoethyl
side chain nor the amino group are critical to activity in this series.
Polyhydroxybenzenes which cannot be oxidized to an o-quinone or which can
be oxidized to a p-quinone are not active.

5. HYDROXYPYRIDONES

Pyridine derivatives containing more than one hydroxyl group are heteroaromatic counterparts of catechol (XXXIV) and other dihydroxybenzene isomers (Figure 3).

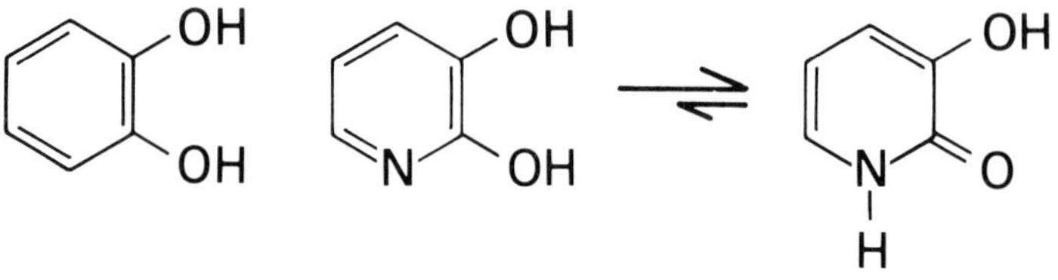

XXXIV	XXXVa	XXXVb

FIGURE 3. Relationship of pyridones to catechols.

While pyridine derivatives with hydroxyl groups in the 2- or 4- position prefer to exist in the lactam form (XXXVb) and are called pyridones, they are oxidizable to quinoid forms analogous to those of catechols.

The discovery in the NCI screening program a number of years ago that XXXV and its 3-acetoxy derivative (XXXVI) possessed P388 leukemia activity; as well as the structural similarities of these compounds to the catechols, led to the design of a series of pyridones for the study of structure-antitumor activity relationships. The activity of the lead compounds is shown in Figure 4.

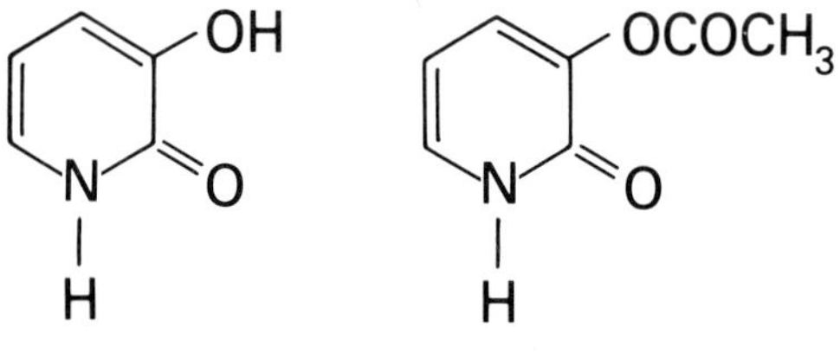

XXXVb
P388 (ILS 34%)

XXXVI
P388 (ILS 65%)
L1210 (ILS 53%)

FIGURE 4. Initial pyridones found to be active.

Approximately 20 2-pyridones were synthesized and a total of 32 evaluated for their effects against P388 leukemia during our initial study (13). These results then were used to expand the investigation to bioisosteres and 4-pyridones (14). The compounds studied fell into several sub-classes and addressed different structure-activity questions.

5.1. Monohydroxylated pyridines

Four compounds, 2-, 3- and 4-hydroxypyridine as well as 3-acetoxy-pyridine were found to be devoid of activity. This indicated that at least two hydroxyl groups were required for activity.

5.2. Hydroxy-2-pyridone isomers

The positional relationships between the two hyroxyl groups were studied in a series of six compounds (Figure 5).

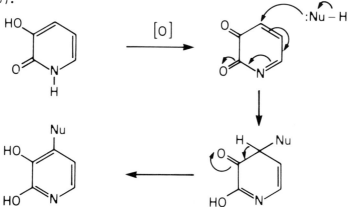

R (P388 active)
3-OH
3-OCOCH$_3$
5-OH
(5-OCOCH$_3$)

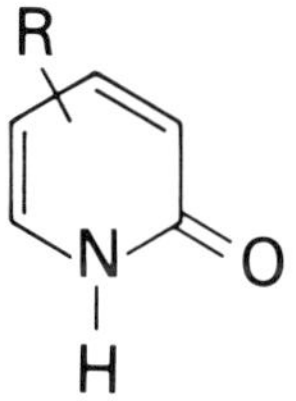

R (P388 inactive)
4-OH
6-OH

FIGURE 5. Dihydroxypyridone isomers and derivatives.

The 4- and 6-hydroxy isomers, which are not capable of being oxidized to a quinoid form were inactive. The 5-hydroxy isomer, which has the possibility of oxidation to a p-quinoid form, was active (ILS 28%), but somewhat less so than its 3-substituted position isomer. The 5-acetoxy analog had variable activity in three P388 tests with ILS values of 32, 21, and 19%. It should be noted that 4-hydroxy-2-pyridone, the aglycon of the very active nucleoside 3-deazauridine, was inactive. These results indicated that vicinal hydroxyl groups were optimum. This finding was consistent with the data from the catechol series and leads to a similar hypothesis for the mechanism of action (Figure 6).

FIGURE 6. Possible mechanism of action for hydroxypyridones.

5.3. 3-Substituted-2-pyridones

From the above described results, it was apparent that the 3-substituted-2-pyridone series was the one to optimize. The significantly better 2-pyridone activity for the 3-acetoxy (XXXVI) vs the 3-hydroxy (XXXV) analog led to the speculation that the acyl group might be affording some degree of protection against premature oxidation of 2,3-dihydroxypyridine during biological transport to the target tumor site. Hydrolyzable protecting groups appeared necessary, however, since it was established early in the study that ether groups in the 3-position (e.g. 3-methoxy-2-pyridone) abolished activity. If the protection hypothesis were correct, groups other than acetyl might prove better by providing an optimized hydrolysis rate. Twenty 3-acyloxy derivatives of 2-pyridone were synthesized and tested. Some representative structures are shown in Figure 7.

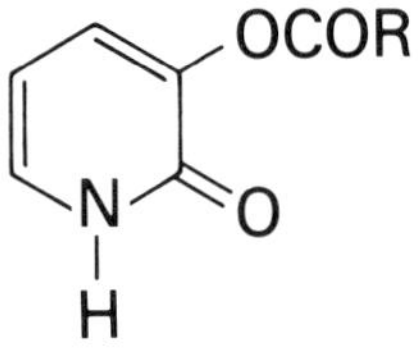

R (active, % ILS)		R (inactive)
CH_3	(65)	cyclopropyl
C_2H_5	(40)	t-butyl
$NHCH_3$	(44)	C_6H_5
NHC_6H_4F	(32)	OC_2H_5

FIGURE 7. Activity of 3-substituted-2-pyridones.

Although eight new P388 active compounds were discovered in this 2-pyridone study, none had any advantage over XXXVI, the initial lead compound. For this reason, we turned our attention to bioisosteres of the 2-pyridones and to the 4-pyridones (14).

5.4. Bioisosteres of 2-pyridone

The compounds shown in Figure 8 were prepared and evaluated to determine the necessity for hydroxyl groups in the 2- and 3-positions. Active compounds are designated with %ILS values.

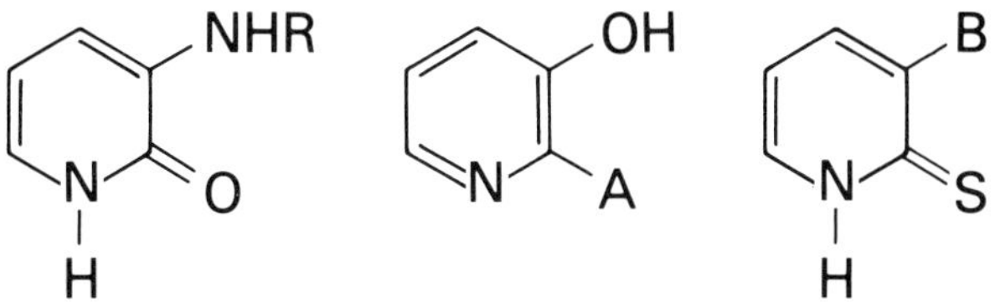

XXXVII,R=H (33%)   XXXVIII,A=NH₂   XXXIX,B=OH (39%)
R=COCH₃   A=Cl   B=OCOCH₃
R=CONHCH₃

FIGURE 8. Bioisosteres evaluated.

Activity was retained when an amino group was substituted for hydroxyl in the 3-position (XXXVII), but not the 2-position (XXXVIII). Sulfur was a successful substitution for oxygen in the 2-position. Acyl protecting groups, contrary to results with XXVb, reduced activity.

5.5. 4-Pyridones

The natural product maltol (XL) was used to prepare several compounds in the 4-pyridone series (Figure 9).

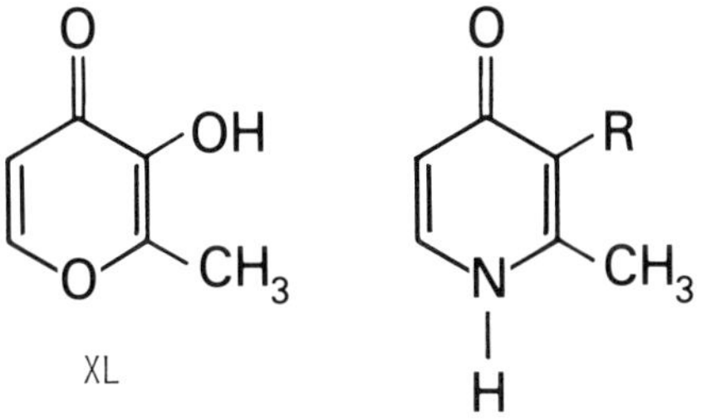

XLI,R=OCH₃
XLII,R=OH   (53%)
XLIII,R=OCOCH₃ (79%)

FIGURE 9. 4-Pyridones evaluated for P388 activity.

Neither maltol nor the XLI were active. These compounds are not oxidizable to quinoid forms. The 4-pyridone analogs of our 2-pyridone lead compounds, however, possessed substancial P388 activity. Compound XLIII, with a P388 ILS of 79%, is the most active compound prepared in the pyridone series.

Work is continuing on both the 2- and 4-pyridones and the study has been broadened to include the synthesis and evaluation of nucleosides of these aglycons.

REFERENCES

1. Driscoll JS, Hazard GF, Wood HB, Goldin A. 1974. Cancer Chemother. Rep. Part 2, 4 (no. 2), 1.

2. Rall DP, Zubrod CG. 1962. Ann. Rev. Pharmacol., 2, 109.

3. Ross WCJ. 1962. "Biological Alkylating Agents," Butterworths, London.

4. Khan AH, Driscoll JS. 1976. J. Med. Chem., 19, 313.

5. Chou FT, Khan AH, Driscoll JS. 1976. J. Med. Chem., 19, 1302.

6. Driscoll JS, Dudeck L, Congleton G, Geran RI. 1979. J. Pharm. Sci., 68, 185.

7. Zee-Cheng RKY, Cheng CC. 1978. J. Med. Chem., 21, 291.

8. Cheng CC, Zee-Cheng RKY, Narayanan VL, Ing RB, Paull KD. 1981. Trends Pharmacol. Sci., 2, 1.

9. Murdock KC, Child RG, Fabio PF, Angier RB, Wallace RE, Durr FE, Citarella RV. 1979. J. Med. Chem., 22, 1024.

10. Driscoll JS, Melnick NR, Quinn FR, Ing R, Abbott BJ, Congleton G, Dudeck L. 1978. Cancer Treat. Rep., 62, 45.

11. Driscoll JS. 1979. J. Pharm. Sci., 68, 1519.

12. Lin AJ, Driscoll JS. 1981. J. Pharm. Sci., 70, 806.

13. Hwang DR, Driscoll JS. 1979. J. Pharm. Sci., 68, 816.

14. Hwang DR, Proctor GR, Driscoll JS. 1980. J. Pharm. Sci., 69, 1074.

IN VITRO OXIDATIVE ACTIVATION: A MODEL FOR THE CYTOTOXIC ACTION OF 9—HYDROXY ELLIPTICINE DERIVATIVES

B. MEUNIER, C. AUCLAIR, J. BERNADOU, G. MEUNIER, M. MAFTOUH, S. CROS, B. MONSARRAT AND C. PAOLETTI ∗

I N T R O D U C T I O N

Ellipticines derivatives have been first described as natural antitumor alcaloïds (1). It has been later shown that hydroxylation in position 9 increases the antitumor activity of ellipticine itself (2). Furthermore, it was established that the quaternarization of the pyridine nitrogen of 9-hydroxy ellipticine (9-OH-E) leads to a compound, N2-methyl 9-hydroxy ellipticinium (NSC 264137) (9-OH-NME+) which is one of the most efficient anti-cancer drug in these series (3) and has been retained for clinical use in humans (4).

The actual mode of antitumor action of these compounds is still unknown. They all are strong cytotoxic compounds when tested on in vitro grown cells (5). They all bind to double stranded DNA with an affinity coefficient of about 10^5-$10^6 M^{-1}$ in usual experimental conditions(2). They intercalate between DNA base-pairs (6, 7). It has been assumed that a relatively high affinity for DNA is a necessary condition for anticancer potency but not a sufficient one (2). Moreover, they induce protein associated DNA strands breaks when put in contact of mouse leukemia L1210 cells (8, 9). They are highly mutagenic (10, 11) ; 9-OH-E is also recombinogenic in the mouse (12).

A clue for elucidating their mode of action might be to consider the 9 hydroxylated ellipticine derivatives as stable reduced forms of p-quinone-imine structures. Nitrogen analogues of

∗ To whom correspondence should be sent.

D.N. Reinhoudt, T.A. Connors, H.M. Pinedo & K.W. van de Poll (eds.), Structure-Activity Relationships of Anti-Tumour Agents.
© *1983, Martinus Nijhoff Publishers, The Hague/Boston/London. ISBN 90-247-2783-9.*

the quinones share many of their chemical properties with the quinones and about 200 of these have recently been screened by the National Cancer Institute for antitumor action and seven have proved activities against mouse and rat cancers (13). The quinone chemicals comprise approximatively 15 % of the compounds which show some activity against experimental tumors (14). Among them, some derivatives have been used in humans, such as streptonigrin, lapachol, mitomycin C or are presently largely retained in cancer therapy such as the anthracyclines Adriamycin and Daunorubicine.

Two main hypothesis have been put forward to explain the mode of cytotoxic action of these quinones. The first one proposes that electrophilic intermediates generated through a two electron reduction of the quinones are good alkylators of the pharmacological target, probably nucleic acids or proteins. This process has been named bioreductive alkylation (15, 16). It has recently received some tentative experimental support in the case of strepto-nigrin (17), anthracyclines (18) and mitomycin C (19, 20) and has been thoroughly described, documented and reviewed by Moore (16, 21). The second hypothesis (oxidation stress) assumes that activated species of oxygen, mostly superoxide ion $O_2^{\cdot-}$ are generated in situ by the reductive activation of molecular oxygen. The quinones would serve as electron carriers between one of the following enzymatic complexes : cytoplasmic aldo-ceto reductase, mitochondrial NADH-succinate flavodehydrogenase and microsomal NADPH-cytochrome P450 reductase and oxygen. During the electron transport process, the quinones would be transiently reduced to the corresponding unstable radical semi-quinones (for anthracyclines, see (22) and (23)). The cellular damages are generally considered as the consequence of the formation of hydroxyl radical, $OH^{\cdot}$, although this mechanism is still considered as not completely established. It has also been claimed (18) that the semi-quinone radicals of anthracyclines were able to covalently bind DNA and proteins.

In this paper, we review and summarize our _in vitro_ experimental data which suggest that both hypothesis could be extended to 9-hydroxy ellipticine (9-OH-E) and 2-N-methyl-9-hydroxyellipticinium (9-OH-NME$^+$) viewed as reduced derivatives of quinone imine compounds and might give clues for understanding their cytotoxic properties.

Its first part will document the capability of 9-hydroxylated ellipticine derivatives (oxoellipticines) to form reactive electrophilic species after a two-electron oxidation. These species are formally analogous to the quinone methide intermediate described by Moore (16) in his bioreductive alkylation model. The oxoellipticines are strong alkylating agents which lead _in vitro_ to new ellipticine adducts in presence of molecules carrying nucleophilic centers such as pyridine, amino-acids, sulfhydryl derivatives and nucleosides. Their occurence _in vivo_ has been inferred from the appearance of a 10S- glutathione conjugate, as a bile excretion metabolite of rats treated with N_2-methyl 9-hydroxyellipticinium. Its second part will be devoted to the generation of O_2^- and phenoxy radicals from these drugs submitted to one electron oxidation either by molecular oxygen of by H_2O_2 in presence of myeloperoxidase.

A major difference between the original model and the model applied to the 9-hydroxy ellipticine derivatives lies in the mode of generation of the electrophilic species which is an oxydative one in the present case : such as biooxydative alkylation, viewed as a potential mechanism of metabolic activation of some chemicals, leading to their cytotoxicity, has already been proposed for other drugs submitted to an oxidative metabolism such as acetanilides, hydrazines, aromatic benzenoids, thiol derivatives, chloramphenicol, alkenes and alkynes (see General Review by S.D. Nelson (24)), and the anticancer agent dacarbazine (25). Numbering and structure of ellipticinium derivatives quoted in this paper are found on Figure 1.

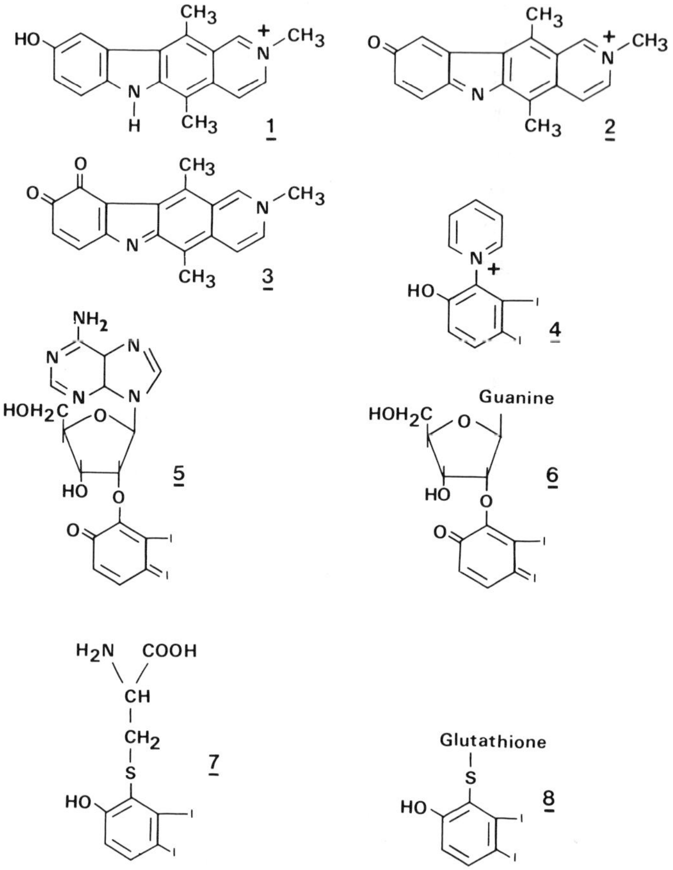

Fig. 1 : Ellipticinium derivatives

I. TWO ELECTRON OXIDATION OF 9-HYDROXY-ELLIPTICINE DERIVATIVES GENERATES STRONG ELECTROPHILIC QUINONE-IMINE SPECIES.

As previously stated, the oxidation of 9-OH ellipticine derivatives yield 9-oxo-derivatives, either in presence of H_2O_2 and peroxidase or in presence of molecular oxygen (26) (27). Up to now, the oxo-derivative 2 of 9-OH-NME$^+$ could not be purified and isolated as a defined stable product and fully characterized due to its high reactivity in solution. However we have obtained compelling evidence of the occurrence of this quinone-imine in solution. It is possible to obtain a solution of the hexafluorophosphate salt of 2 by extraction of the aqueous phase with methylene chloride in presence of NH_4PF_6. This solution is stable at low temperature (below - 20°C) but a slow transformation, probably into polymers, can be surveyed at room temperature. Unfortunately, the solution of 2 in deuterated methylene chloride are too diluted to allow ^1H NMR records with well defined peaks. However, the electron impact mass spectra of this organic solution of 2 displays the expected molecular peak M^+ at 275 whereas in identical conditions, the molecular peak of the drug 1 appears at 277. The UV-visible spectrum of solution of 2 (Figure 2) correlates well with the existence of a quinonoid structure according to the three maxima at λ = 255, 310 and 470 nm. This spectrum is nearly the same of the one observed for the stable quinone-imine prepared by chemical or biochemical oxidation from the non-quaternarized 9-hydroxy ellipticine (26).

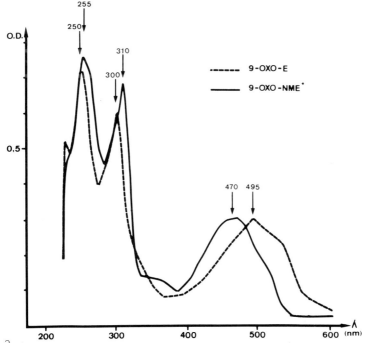

Fig. 2 :
UV visible spectrum of 9-oxo-ellipticine and 9-oxo-NME$^+$ in CH_2Cl_2
Experimental conditions : phosphate buffer, pH 5, $5 \times 10^{-2}M$, [9-OHE] = [9-OH-NME$^+$ 1] = $2.5. 10^5M$, [HRP] = $10^{-8}M$, [H_2O_2] = $5.10^{-5}M$; Extraction with CH_2Cl_2 at t = 2 mn in presence of NH_4PF_6 ($2.5.10^{-4}M$).

Moreover, the quinone-imine 2 is not the only product of the peroxidase oxidation of 1 ; it is itself rather unstable and yields a second product of oxidation of 1, an ortho-quinone derivative 3, 9, 10-dioxo- 2 NME. As shown on Fig. 3, the stability of 2 is highly pH dependent and is optimal at pH 5.0.

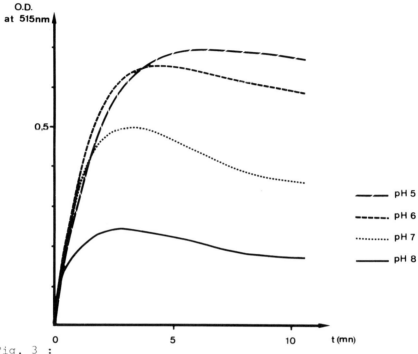

Fig. 3 :
pH dependent formation and stability of 9-oxo-NME$^+$ 2 followed by light absorbance at 515 nm : phosphate buffer 5 x 10^{-2}M, [1] = 10^{-4}M, [H$_2$O$_2$] = 2 x 10^{-4}M, [HRP] = 5 x 10^{-9}M ; t = 20°C.

We shortly suspected that the difficulties we met to characterize the quinone-imine 9-oxo-NME$^+$ arose from the high reactivity of compound 2. This hypothesis was confirmed and led to demonstrate the strong electrophilic properties of the quinone-imine 2, 9-oxo-NME$^+$ and to use it for preparing new adducts.

The subsequent presentation describes this preparation, the nature and properties of these adduct in the case of the following nucleophiles (a) H$_2$O and H$_2$O$_2$ (b) ribonucleosides (c) N-donors such as pyridine and amino-acids (d) SH-donors such as cysteine and glutathione.

(1) FORMATION OF 2-N-METHYL 9, 10 - DIOXOELLIPTICINE (9, 10-DIOXO NME) FROM 9-OH-NME[+] BY H_2O AT ACIDIC PH AND BY H_2O_2.

Figure 4 summarizes the assumed mechanisms of the nucleophilic attack of the compound 2, 9-oxo-NME[+], which lead to the formation of compound 3, the unchanged 9, 10-dioxo-NME. Full account of this work will be found in a recent paper (42).

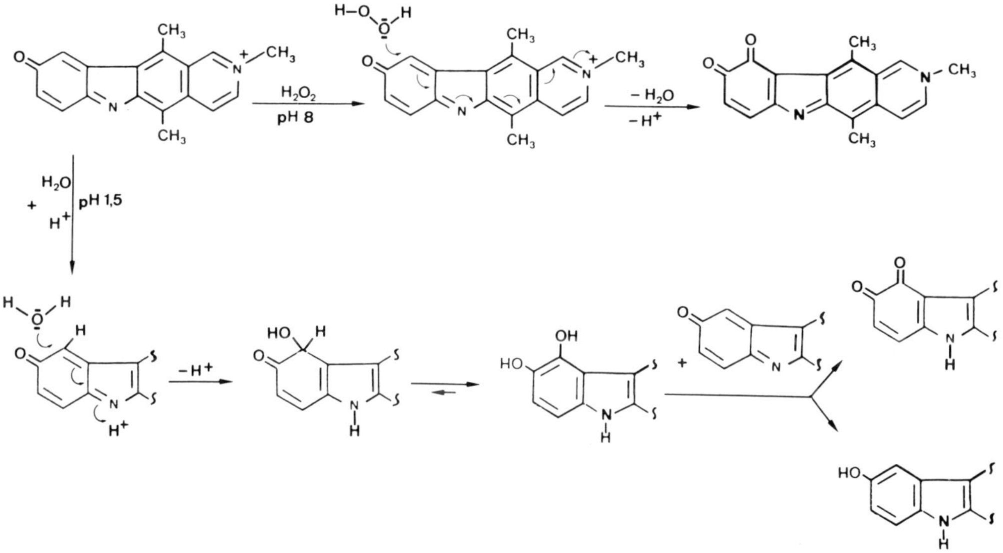

Fig. 4 : Proposed mechanisms of formation of the orthoquinone 9.10-dioxo-NME.

To obtain some informations on the stability of the qui-none-imine compound 2, we undertook experiments in which its con-centration was monitored during its formation through the peroxi-dase oxidation of 1 by visible spectroscopy at 515 nm at which the absorbance of 1 is low. Above pH 5.0, the quinone-imine absorption rapidly decreased. The UV-visible spectra in the range 200-600 nm (Fig. 5a and b) were recorded during the formation of the quinone-imine 2 accompanied by its pH- dependent conversion to a new compound 3 (λ max = 230 and 307 nm at pH 8.0 ; 220 and 288 nm at pH 5.0) (Fig. 5c). This interconversion of products in the HRP-H_2O_2 oxidation of 1 could also be monitered by HPLC (Fig. 6). At pH 5.0, the rapid formation of 2 and the slow apparition of the

156

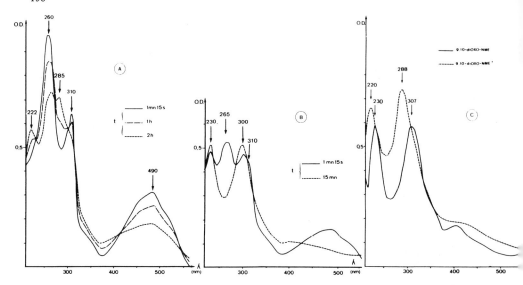

Fig. 5 : Spectroscopy studies during the peroxidative formation
of 9-oxo-NME.

(A) pH 5 : phosphate buffer, pH 5.5 x 10^{-2}M, [1] =
2.5.10^{-5}M, [H_2O_2] = 5 x 10^{-5}M, [HRP] = 10^{-8}M

(B) pH 8 : phosphate buffer, pH 8.5 x 10^{-2}M, [1] = 2.5
10^{-5}M, [H_2O_2] = 5 x 10^{-5}M, [HRP] = 10^{-8}M ;

(C) - UV-visible spectrum of 9,10-dioxo-NME 3 (26.8 x
10^{-6}M in CH_3OH) ; (30.9 x 10^{-6}M in H_2O).

new dioxo compound 3 were observed within 3-4 hours. As we
increased the pH of the solution, the formation of 3 is
accelerated : at pH 8.0, 2 is rapidly converted to 3 in 15-20 min.
This new orthoquinone derivative was isolated and characterized by
usual spectroscopic methods : it is stable at room temperature in
methanol over 5-6 hours. Its degradation occurs beyond this
period. In boiling methanol a substitution product with a methoxy
group in position 7 was obtained after two hours.

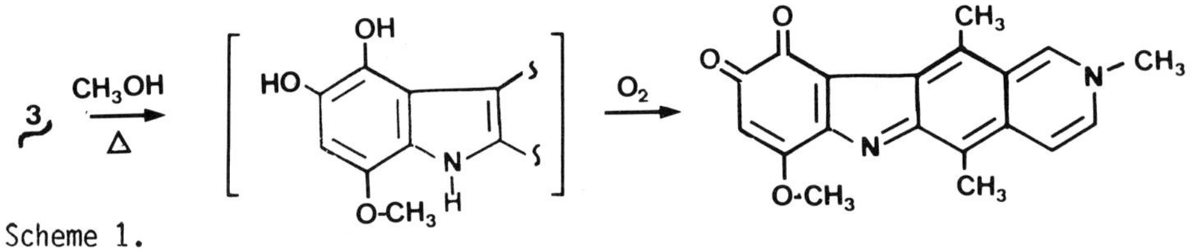

Scheme 1.

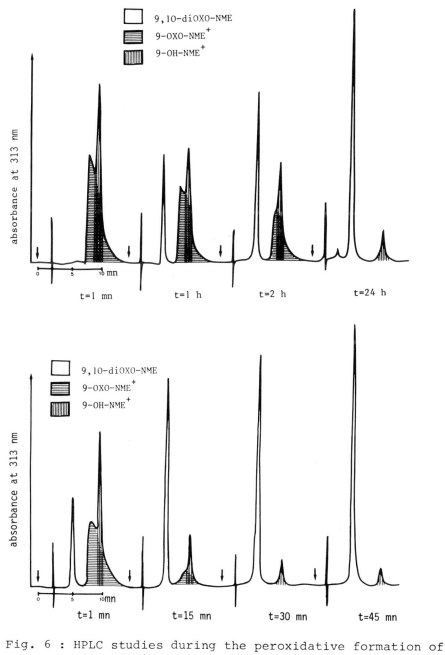

Fig. 6 : HPLC studies during the peroxidative formation of
9-oxo-NME[+]

(A) at pH 5 ; (B) at pH 8

Conditions : phosphate buffer 5×10^{-2}M [4] = 10^{-4}M,
$[H_2O_2]$ = 2×10^{-4}M, [HRP] = 5×10^{-8}M OD at = 313 nm.

The reaction between 3 and cysteine in methanol yielded only cystine ; original the starting orthoquinone was probably regenerated through the aerial autoxidation of the corresponding bisphenol. It should be noted that the orthoquinone 3 could not be reduced under aerobic conditions to the bisphenol with ammonium sulfide or sodium borohydride ; the starting material was again recovered due to the extremely rapid oxidation by oxygen of the corresponding bisphenol to the orthoquinone. Therefore, we consider that this orthoquinone 3 is a poor electrophile. In contrast, it is an active electron carrier.

It increased the flow of electrons from NADPH to molecular oxygen as measured by enhanced oxygen consumption in presence of rat liver microsomes as described by BACHUR et al. for quinone-containing anticancer drugs (28, 29). The stimulation of oxygen consumption has also been established in presence of the xanthine oxidase/NADH system (Fig. 7).

The cytotoxicity of the hydroxy derivative 9-OH-NME[+] has been tested in vitro on experimental tumors such as murine leukemia L1210. This molecule is close to the most cytotoxic antitumoral drugs (5). Its ID_{50} is 0.05 μM. In identical conditions, the ID_{50} of the orthoquinone 3 and its protonated form obtained by protonation with acetic acid of the indolic nitrogen are respectively 9.6 μM and 5.8 μM. So the cytotoxicity of this orthoquinone is lower than that of 9-OH-NME[+] by about a 200-fold/factor.

(2) FORMATION OF NUCLEOSIDES ADDUCTS FROM 9-OXO-NME[+].

The above described work shows that 9-oxo-NME[+] is a strong electrophilic agent which can regiospecifically react at position 10 with O donors such as H_2O and H_2O_2. Obvious extension of this work was a search for reactions of this compound with other donors.

The results of experiments involving a peroxidase oxidation of the 9-OH-NME[+] in presence of various nucleosides and nucleotides are summarized in Table 2. The structure of two adducts prepared from adenosine 5 and from guanosine 6 has been elucidated by determining their mass spectra and NMR studies. Se-

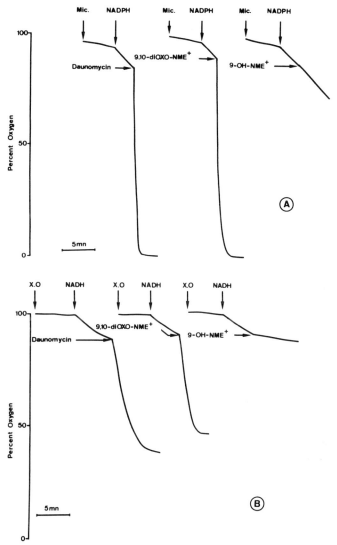

Fig. 7 :

Stimulation of oxygen consumption by 9,10-dioxo-NME
in presence of rat liver microsomes or xanthine oxydase.
Experimental conditions :

(A) rat liver microsomes/NADPH system : phosphate buffer
5×10^{-2}M, pH 8, [$\underline{1}$] = 0.5 mM, [NADPH] = 6 mM,
[microsomes]= 2 mg/ml

(B) xanthine oxydase/NADH system : phosphate buffer
5×10^{-2} M, pH 8, [$\underline{1}$] = 0.5 mM, [NADH] = 0.2 mM
[xanthine oxydase] = 0.240 mg/ml.

TABLE 1 :

Structure of ellipticine derivatives.

R_1	R_2	R_3	R_4	name	abbreviations
H	H		H	ellipticine	E
H	H	CH_3	H	ellipticinium	NME^+
OH	H		H	9-hydroxyellipticine	9-OH-E
OH	H	CH_3	H	9-hydroxyellipticinium	$9-OH-NME^+$
0			H	9-oxoellipticine	9-Oxo-E
0		CH_3	H	9-oxoellipticinium	$9-Oxo-NME^+$

TABLE 2 :

Formation of adducts between 9-oxo-NME$^+$ and various nucleosides and nucleotides detected on HPLC.

	RUNS	Guanine derivatives	Adenine derivatives
1	Free Purine	n.a.d.*	n.a.d.
2	R.Nucleoside	R_t=0.85**(98-0)	1.30 (98-2)
3	dR. "	n.a.d.	n.a.d.
4	R. 5'P nucleotide	0.65 (98-2)	0.90 (92-8)
5	dR. 5'P "	n.a.d.	n.a.d.
6	5'P-N^2-benzoylguanosine	3.30 (72-28)	
7	N^6-benzyladenosine		8.0 (95-5)
8	adenine-9-β-arabino-furanoside		n.a.d.

* n.a.d. :

no adduct detected, the only product observed is the orthoquinone derivative.

** :
A Rt value is associated to each product and defined as the ratio of the retention time of the product to the retention time of the 9-OH-NME$^+$, product 1 with the injection used as 0. The R_t value of orthoquinone 3 is 0.58.
(   ) Ratio of area peak of adduct to orthoquinone 3.
R = Ribose   dR = deoxyribose.

*** :
In presence of 1 equivalent of H$_2$O$_2$ with respect to the 9-OH-NME$^+$, it is possible to isolate an adduct with deoxyribonucleotides, the structures of which are currently under investigations (C. Auclair, unpublished results).

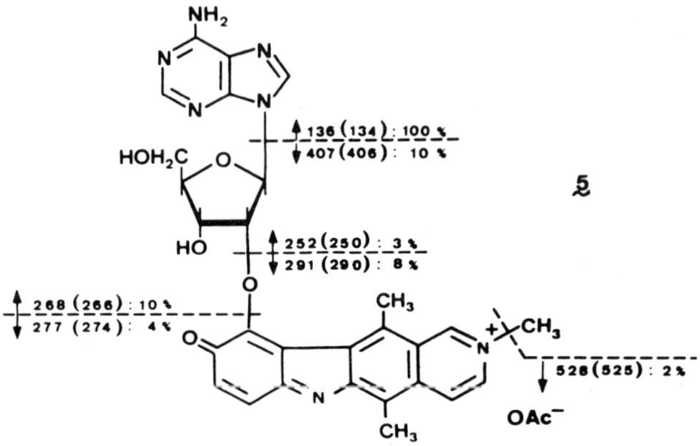

Fig. 8 :

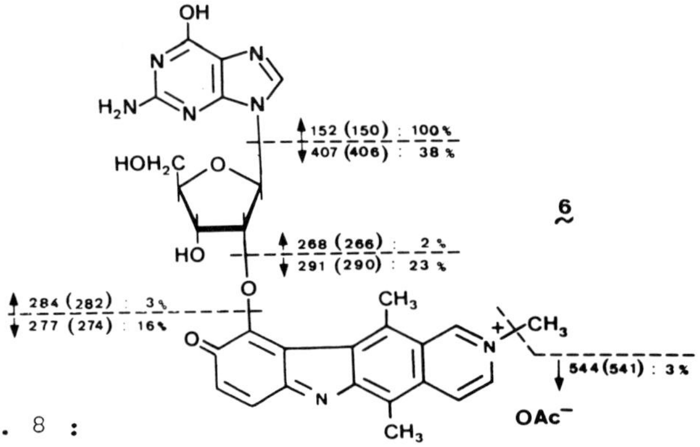

Mass spectra of the adducts between 9-oxo-NME$^+$ and adenonine or guanosine. The adducts were obtained by CI(NH$_3$). For each fragment the calculated mass is indicated in parentheses and followed by the relative percentage.

Molecular peaks (540 for 5 and 556 for 6) are observed in FD spectra

veral observations support the conclusion that the ribose ring of the nucleosides was specifically alkylated (i) the same ellipticinium-ribose fragment was observed in mass spectra at 407 for both compounds 5 and 6 (see figure 8) and (ii) the ribose was the only moiety to be disturbed in the ^{1}H NMR spectra. The quasi-absence of a coupling constant (less than 1.0 Hz) between H$_1^1$ and H$_2^1$ strongly suggested that the hydroxy group in 2' was the alkylated site. Furthermore no adduct were detected with free purines, deoxyribo-

nucleosides, deoxyribonucleotides or with the adenine-9-β-
arabinofuranoside which carries the hydroxy group on carbone 2'
in β configuration. Therefore, formula 5 and 6 account for the
structure of the adducts derived from adenosine and guanosine ;
they involve the formation of a regiospecific covalent bond
between the oxygen 2' of the ribonucleoside and the carbon 10 of
the ellipticinium ring.

The regiospecificity of the alkylations reaction at ribose 2-C site was an unexpected result. It allows substituted
nucleosides the NH_2 group of which was blocked, to still yield 2'-C
ribose adducts (Table 2-runs 6 and 7)

It should be noted also that neither 5-phosphate ribose
or deoxyribose or β -methyl riboside reacted in the same conditions. This observation points out the importance of the anomeric
link to the base for enhancing the reactivity of the 2' (or 3')
position in the alkylation reaction. The alkylation rate of 9-
oxo-NME[+] generated in the presence of different substrats depends
on the nature of the nucleosides ; the pyrimidine nucleosides are
less reactive that the purine ones.

However, the alkylation reaction competed with the formation of the orthoquinone 3 (pathway b).

$$9\text{-OH-NME}^+ \xrightarrow[\text{H}_2\text{O}_2]{\text{HRP}} 9\text{-oxo-NME}^+ \begin{array}{l} \nearrow \text{ adduct} \\ \quad \textit{pathway a} \\ \\ \searrow \textit{pathway b} \\ \quad 9, 10\text{-dioxo-NME} \end{array}$$

These alternative pathways are illustrated in Table 2
which displays ratios between adduct versus orthoquinone peaks.

The absence of adduct formation might not express a complete lack of reactivity of the purine derivatives ; it could result from a too slow addition reaction rate when compared to that
of the orthoquinone formation.

(3) FORMATION OF ADDITION ADDUCTS FROM 9-OXO NME$^+$ AND N DONORS.

(a) PYRIDINE ADDUCT.

When the biochemical oxidation of the drug 9-OH-NME$^+$ by the HRP/H$_2$O$_2$ system was carried out in presence of pyridine it was possible to isolate an adduct bearing a pyridine at position 10 on the ellipticine skeleton. Its structure was elucidated by mass spectra and ^{1}H NMR data (30) (adduct 4, Fig. 1)

(b) AMINO-ACIDS ADDUCTS.

Carbon-nitrogen bond formation was also observed with the primary amines of various amino-acids. When 9-oxo-NME$^+$ was generated in presence of amino-acid in excess, adducts formed by a covalent bond between the carbon 10 of the ellipticinium and the nitrogen of the amino-acid were isolated with a satisfactory yield (40-60 %).

It is assumed (Figure 9) that the nucleophilic addition of the nitrogen of the amino-acid led to an intermediate which was oxidized in a second undefined step to produce an orthoquinoneimine. This product should have been transformed in the final adduct by removal of the proton linked to the Carbon of the amino-acid . This absence of the Cα -H is clearly indicated in ^{1}H NMR studies by the presence of a singlet at S = 2.41 in the case of the methyl resonance of the alanine adduct (30).

This fact has been confirmed for the valine or leucine derivatives by homonuclear decoupling experiments for Cβ and Cγ protons. In these compounds, the Cβ proton(s) appear(s) as a singlet when the Cγ protons are irradiated.

These results point out the high affinity of 9-oxo NME$^+$ for the -NH$_2$ function of amino-acids.

Amino-acid adducts tested for their cytotoxicity on L1210 cells in vitro are less active than 9-OH-NME$^+$.

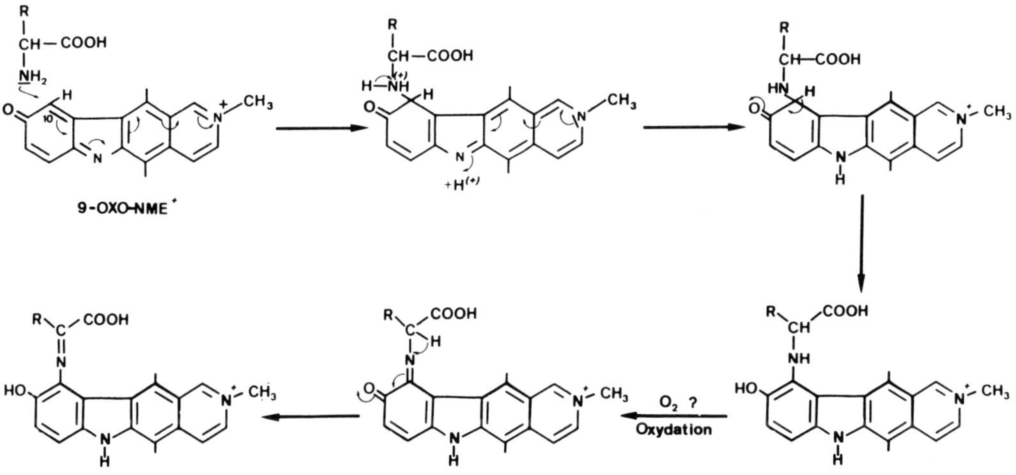

Fig. 9 : Proposed mechanisms of formation of some amino-acids
adducts from HRP-H$_2$O$_2$ oxidation of 9-OH-NME$^+$.

However, they still are highly cytotoxic drugs whose ID 50 lies in
the 0.2 - 0.5 μM range. Glycine and alanine adduct are not active
against mice L1210 leukemia in vivo ; more hydrophobic amino-acid
adducts (valine and leucine) are moderately efficient against this
leukemia (ILS ranging between 30 and 40 % at 1/2 LDo).
These adducts display two remarkable properties.

a) They have a marked affinity for DNA (ranging between
0.5 10^5 M^{-1} and 5 10^5 M^{-1}. b) in spite of the fact that the p-
hydroxy-imino structure is an oxidation-prone one, they resisted
any attempt to oxidize them in mild or moderatly strong conditions.

(4) FORMATION OF ADDITION ADDUCTS BETWEEN 9-OXO-NME$^+$
AND-SH MOLECULES.

The above described alkylation at -NH$_2$ sites of amino-
acids is not observed at the same site in the case of -SH
containing amino-acids or derivatives. Cysteine derivatives or
glutathione (GSH) were only alkylated on the sulfur atom. To avoid
the direct contact between the -SH containing molecules and the
oxidant mixture, the coupling reaction was performed after the
extraction of 9-oxo-NME$^+$ 2 by CH$_2$ Cl$_2$ in presence of ammonium

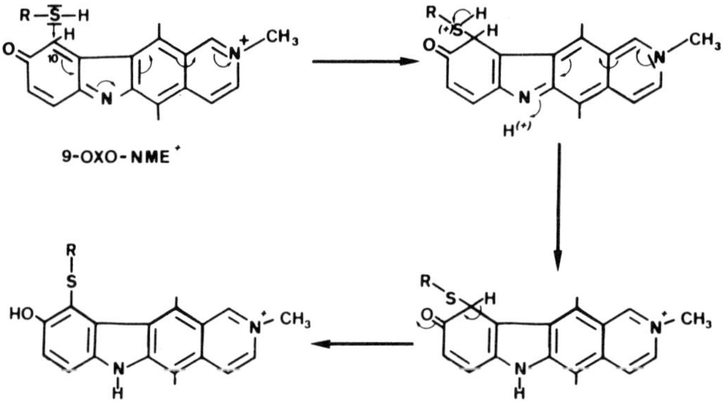

166

Fig. 10 :

Proposed mechanism of formation of cysteine and glutathione adducts from HRP-H$_2$O$_2$ oxidation of 9-OH-NME$^+$.

hexafluorophosphate. The spectroscopic data are compatible with
the adduct structure presented on Fig. 10 characterized by a C-S
bond at the C-10 position. These adducts 7, 8 resulting of a
Michael condensation of the -SH nucleophile with the quinone-imine
are likely candidates as metabolites of the drug 1 if the quinone-
imine is generated from it in vivo by enzymatic oxidative
processes as those carried out by peroxidases, oxidases and
microsomal mixed function oxidases ; this later reaction has been
actually observed in the case of acetaminophene or thiophene (35).
Our hypothesis was recently confirmed by studies on the metabolism
of the drug after its administration in rats (I.V. route) and a
direct analysis of biliary excretion by HPLC. Beside two excreted
compounds, the unchanged drug in minor proportion and its O-
glucuronide derivative, we have been able to detect and isolate a
minor metabolite (4 %) which present the chromatographic behaviour
of the authentic GSH-conjugate prepared in vitro by biochemical
oxidation, as well as an identical UV absorbance spectrum.

ONE ELECTRON TRANSFER FROM 9-HYDROXY-ELLIPTICINE DERIVATIVES GENERATES FREE RADICALS SPECIES AND O_2

We have shown in the first part of this paper that the oxidation of 9-hydroxy-ellipticine derivatives might occur along two different pathways, an autooxidative one, involving oxygen as electron acceptor and an enzymatic peroxidative one involving H_2O_2 as electron acceptor. The second part of this work summarizes some of our experiments which establish that in each case free radical species are generated.

(a) INVOLVEMENT OF ONE ELECTRON TRANSFER IN 9-OH-E AND 9-OH-NME$^+$ AUTOXIDATION.

During 9-OH-E autoxidation in presence of molecular oxygen, electrons are transferred from the drug to oxygen. This reaction may occur either through a two-electron transfer generating directly H_2O_2 and the quinone 9-oxo-E (26) or through one-electron transfer, generating superoxide anion ($O_2^{\cdot-}$) and the free radical of the drug as intermediates according to eq. 1.

$$9\text{-}O^-\text{-E} + O_2 \longrightarrow 9\text{-}O^\cdot\text{-E} + O_2^{\cdot-} \quad (1)$$

where $9\text{-}O^-\text{-E}$ is the phenolate form of the drug considered as the efficient electron donor. A possible approach to test the ability of 9 hydroxy ellipticines to transfer one electron on molecular oxygen is to perform experiments in strong alkaline solutions such as NaOH 1N or alkaline DMSO. This allows the formation of a great amount of the phenolate form of the drugs and in the presence of oxygen the reaction indicated in eq.1 may occur. In proton deficient solutions, the free radicals possibly generated remain stable in solution and can be easily detected by E.P.R. spectroscopy. Accordingly, free radicals of 9-OH-E and 9-OH-NME$^+$ can be detected at room temperature.

The figure 11A shows the EPR spectrum of 9-OH-E in 1N NaOH. The poor resolution obtained do not permit the determination of the hyperfine splitting constants.

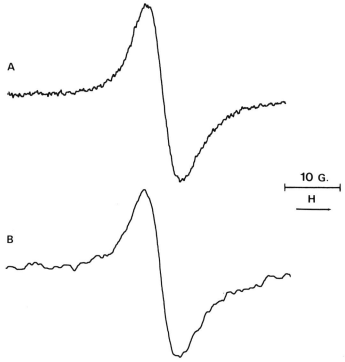

Fig. 11 :
EPR spectra of 9-OH-E in 1N NaOH. Spectra were recorded at room temperature. Microwave frequency was 9.770 GH_z with 1 Gauss modulation and 200 mW microwave power. The concentration of 9-OH-E in 1N NaOH was 10^{-4} M. Spectrum A was recorded 2 min. after the addition of 9-OH-E in NaOH and spectrum B Was recorded 28 min. later.

Moreover, secondary radicals are likely formed since, as shown in Fig. 11B the EPR spectrum becomes asymetric and may be representative of polymer formation. In 1N NaOH no signal was detected in the presence of 9-OH-NME[+] indicating that the free radical is not stable under these conditions. The use of alkaline DMSO allows to obtain a better stability of the radicals.

Fig. 12A shows the EPR spectrum of 9-OH-E and Fig. 12B the spectrum of 9-OH-NME[+] in DMSO containing 0.1 N NaOH and 1 % water. As well as in 1N NaOH the spectra obtained are not resolved,

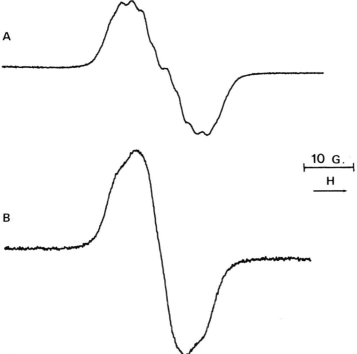

Fig. 12 :
EPR spectra of 9-OH-E (A) and 9-OH-NME[+] (B) in
alkaline DMSO. Spectra were recorded at room temperature using a microwave frequency of 9.770 GH_z,
1 Gauss modulation and 200 mW microwave power. The
mixtures was composed of DMSO, 0.55 M water,
5×10^{-3}M NaOH and 10^{-4}M drugs.

however the radicals remain stable in solution for several hours.
From these results, the structure of the free radicals cannot be
determined but it may be concluded that 9-OH-E and 9-OH-NME[+] can
transfer one electron on molecular oxygen according to eq. (1).
$O_2^{\bar{}}$ can be effectively identified at low temperature from the
appearance of a spectrum which exhibits a gauss near 2.09 GAUSS
(Fig. 13), the absorbance being superimposed to the signal of the
free radical of this drug. $O_2^{\bar{}}$ is detected with both 9-OH-E and 9-
OH-NME[+] in alkaline DMSO at 110°K.

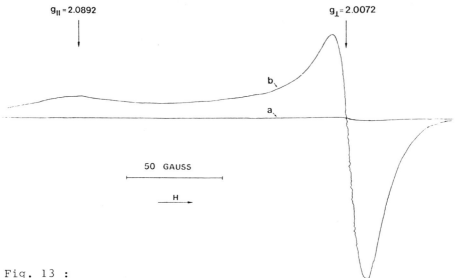

$g_{\text{II}} = 2.0892$ $g_{\perp} = 2.0072$

50 GAUSS

H

Fig. 13 :
EPR spectrum of 9-OH-E in alkaline DMSO at low
temperature. Spectra were recorded at 110°K in
similar conditions as those indicated in Fig. 11
and 12. The concentration of 9-OH-E was 10^{-4}M. A
indicates the spectrum recorded with alkaline
DMSO in the absence of 0-OH-E.

        In aqueous buffer near neutral pH, the free radicals of
the drug and O_2^{-} readily dismutate according to the following
reactions :

$$9\text{-}O\text{-}E + 9\text{-}O\text{-}E \xrightarrow{\text{H+}} 9\text{-}OH\text{-}E \quad + 9\text{-}oxo\text{-}E \qquad (2)$$

$$O_2^{-} + O_2^{-} \xrightarrow{2H^{+}} H_2O_2 + O_2 \qquad (3)$$

        At physiological pH, the amount of the phenolate form of
the drug is very low whereas the dismutation rate constants are
expected to be very high. Consequently, the concentration of the
radicals remains very low at the steady state, and cannot be observed directly by EPR spectroscopy. However, O_2^{-} can be detected
using the spin trap DMPO which react with O_2^{-} to generate a stable
free radical. The incubation of 9-OH-E in phosphate buffer

(ph 7.40) in the presence of 50 mM DMPO resulted in the spectra of Fig. 14A. The 1 : 2 : 2 : 1 quartet (g : 2.0060, $a^N = a^H$ = 15.0G) is comparable to the spectrum attributed to the hydroxyl free radical (OH°) spin adduct of DMPO. However, when superoxide dismutase (SOD) was added to the reaction mixture the signal was suppressed (Fig. 14B) indicating that O_2^- is initially involved in the generation of the DMPO adduct. It may be concluded that at physiological pH, 9-OH-E and 9-OH-NME$^+$ may transfer one electron on molecular oxygen and thus undergo a spontaneous oxidation generating free radicals as intermediates.

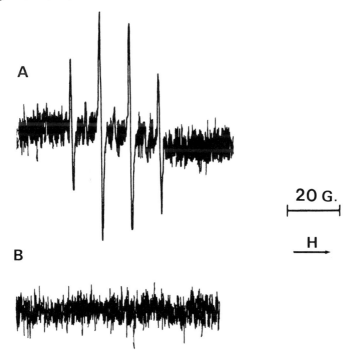

Fig. 14 :

EPR spectra of DMPO spin adducts. Spectra were recorded at room temperature using a microwave frequency of 9.750 GH$_z$, 1.25 Gauss modulation and 250 mW microwave power. Spectrum A is obtained with a mixture composed of 0.05 M phosphate buffer (pH 7.40), 10^{-4}M EDTA, 50 mM DMPO and 10^{-4}M 9-OH-E. In B 10 μg SOD was added to the mixture.

(b) GENERATION OF FREE RADICALS DURING THE PEROXIDASE CATALYZED OXIDATION OF 9-OH-E and 9-OH-NME$^+$.

Peroxidases are enzymes known to catalyze the oxidation of various organic compounds such as aryl-amines and phenols in the presence of H_2O_2 as electron acceptors.

Free radicals of the electron donor molecules are initially formed according to the following reactions :

$$peroxidase + H_2O_2 \longrightarrow compound\ I + 2\ H_2O$$
$$compound\ I + AH_2 \longrightarrow AH° + compound\ II$$
$$compound\ II + AH_2 \longrightarrow AH° + peroxidase$$
$$AH° + AH° \longrightarrow AH_2 + A$$
$$or\ AH° + AH° \longrightarrow AH - AH$$
$$or\ (AH°)_n\ (AH-AH...)$$

In agreement with the mechanism indicated in eq. 4 to 9, the one-electron oxidation of 9-OH-E and 9-OH-NME$^+$ occurs in the presence of the horse radish peroxidase-hydrogen peroxide system (HRP H_2O_2). The free radical of the drugs primary generated can be detected at low temperature (110°K) (Fig. 15A). The radical of both 9-OH-E and 9-OH-NME$^+$, displayed a g factor value near 2.0042. The concentration of these radicals at the steady state was estimated to be lower than 10^{-7}M suggesting the presence of short-lived free radicals. Moreover, during the oxidation of 9-OH-NME$^+$ secondary free radical at g = 2.0050 can be detected at room temperature (Fig. 15B). The signal is related to the one provided by a steady state-radical occuring during the cationic polymerisation of the quinone 9-oxo-NME$^+$.

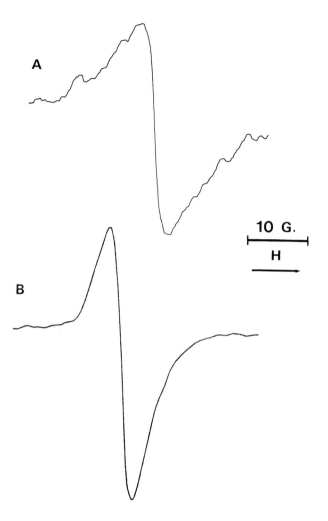

Fig. 15 :

EPR spectra 9-OH-E (A) and 9-OH-NME$^+$ (B) during their peroxidase catalyzed oxidation. Spectra were recorded at 110°K (spectrum A) or at room temperature (spectrum B), using a microwave frequency of 9.753 GH$_z$, 1 Gauss modulation and 250 mW microwave power. The mixtures were : 0.05 M phosphate buffer (pH 7.40) ; 10^{-4}M drugs 10^{-4}H$_2$O$_2$ and 2 x 10^{-9}M HRP. The mixture was frozen ten seconds after the addition of HRP in A or recorded two minutes after the addition of HRP at room temperature in B.

D I S C U S S I O N

9-hydroxylated ellipticine derivatives are oxidation prone compounds. This oxidation can be an one-electron process generating a neutral phenoxy radical, E-O˙ or an ellipticine radical cation, E-OH$^+$ depending on the pH. It occurs slowly and spontaneously in aqueous phase at neutral pH in presence of molecular oxygen. It generates superoxide anion, O_2^-, which dismutates into O_2 and H_2O_2, whereas the free radicals dismutate as well yielding the corresponding quinones, 9-oxo-ellipticines.

9-oxo ellipticine is a relatively stable compound which can be isolated ; 2-N-methyl 9-oxo ellipticinium is a very unstable one. The same quinones can be readily obtained by peroxydase action in a neutral pH range, the oxidizing agent being H_2O_2.

As shown on Fig. 16, the positive charge of the quinones derived from the 2-N alkylated elliptinium or from ellipticine derivatives at acidic pH can be delocalized after a reorganisation of the electron ring around these resonant heterocycles. This rearrangement induces the creation of an electrophilic center on the quinone imine ring : 8 and 10 carbon atom are equally possible candidates therefore. Adducts in position 10 have only been found when the electrophilic quinone imine reacts on different kinds of nucleophiles : pyridine, 2'-O of nucleosides, NH_2 of amino-acids or SH of cystine and glutathione. There is no available explanation for this C-10 regiospecificity of the nucleophilic attack. Even more puzzling is the regiospecificity of the nucleophilic attack of the adenine and guanine ribonucleoside which is restricted to the 2'-O, sparing other nitrogen nucelophilic centers of the purine ring. This reaction might be instructive for understanding some mechanism of enzymatic reactions, the specificity of which is also strictly restricted to the 2'-O-ribose (for general review see (31) : poly (ADP-ribose) polymerase (32) and oligoadenylate synthetase (33) carry out such reactions.

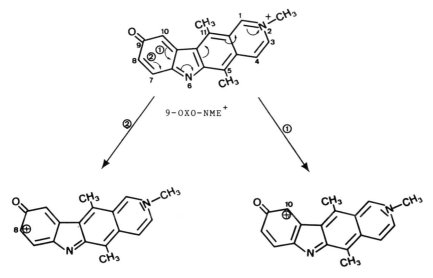

Fig. 16 :

The two possible sites of nucleophilic addition on
the 9-oxo-NME⁺

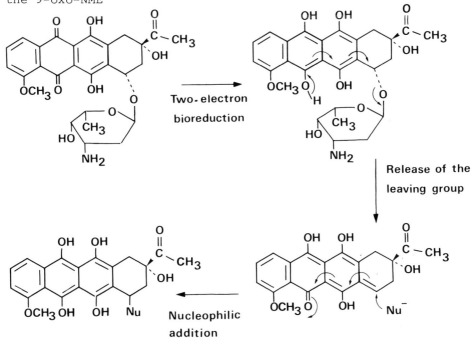

Fig. 17 :

Proposed mechanism of the cytotoxicity of antitumor
quinone anthracyclines according to Moore (16, 21).

The oxidative alkylation scheme described here is formally identical to the one which was proposed for other pharmacological quinones such as anthracyclines and mitomycine C (16, 21). After a first reductive step, these compounds generate quinone methides which make up electrophilic poles, analogues to the ones described here (Figure 17) (16, 21).

An essential question is the relevance of these in vitro observations for understanding the actual mechanisms of cytotoxicities due to the 9-hydroxy ellipticine derivatives. It should be reminded that no covalent adduct between anthracycline derivatives or mitomycine C and biomolecules has yet been isolated from cells exposed to these drugs. However, oxidative metabolism can lead to a secondary in vivo alkylation as shown for several drugs (see general review by S.D. NELSON (24)) and the antitumor agent, dacarbazine (25). Here, an important observation which presently lies only on preliminary data is the production of a glutathione adduct identical to the marker one obtained in vitro by an oxydation procedure. This adduct has been isolated from the bile of rats having received this drug. If confirmed, such a result would provide a compelling evidence that a bio-oxidative alkylation process capable of generating electrophilic intermediates in situ from 9-hydroxy ellipticine derivatives does exist. Whether such intermediates lead to detoxification and elimination of these derivatives or, on the contrary, are actual cytotoxic species inducing cell death, is an open question. However, it should be noted that ellipticine-amino acids which are not oxidation prone, at least in vitro and in usual conditions are yet highly cytotoxic compounds. One must therefore admit that biooxidation phenomenon described in this paper is not responsible for the pharmacologic action of 9-OH ellipticine derivatives or that the ellipticine-aminoacid adducts are endowed with peculiar properties which lead to a specific mechanism of cytotoxicity. Moreover, this picture can still be obscured by metabolic event which might very rapidly transform the ellipticine-aminoacid adducts into other species. A thiolytic process at the C-N bound level analogous to the one describes for some aminoacridines (34) is a likely hypothesis. The ellipticine-nucleoside adducts are good candidates for inhibiting enzymes which use ribose compounds as substrates : along this line, ribonucleoside reductase obviously deserves careful attention. Polynucleotide phosphorylase is partialy inhibited by such adducts (M. BLANDIN, unpublished results). Poly (ADP-ribose) polymerase and oligoadenylate synthetase have been above mentionned.

The production of an oxidation stress, i.e. the generation of O_2^- and derived toxic species is another possible mechanism of cytotoxicity of 9-hydroxy ellipticine derivatives suggested by our in vitro data ; this type of cytotoxic action has been proposed not only for anticancer anthracycline quinone agents, as before mentionned, but also for nitro-aromatics, such as misonidazole, a chemical radiosensitizer (35). However, a major difference between the mechanims of generation of O_2^- lies in the first step reduction of the anthraquinone or nitroaromatics as opposed to initial one electron oxidation step of the 9-hydroxy ellipticine compounds. Such an observation is in agrement with the published values for the respective electrochemical redox potentials at physiological pH of the quinone hydroquinone transition (36) (37) and the couples formed by 9-hydroxy ellipticine or 2-N methyl 9-hydroxy ellipticinium and their one electron polarographic oxidation products (semi quinone forms of the 9-oxo ellipticine and 9-oxo ellipticinium) (38) ; these values (versus normal hydrogen electrode) are respectively - 0,36 V to - 0,40 V for the anthracyclines and + 0,50 V and 0,60 V for the 9-OH ellipticine derivatives. However convincing biochemical cellular evidence has not been yet provided for supporting this oxidative stress mechanism of cytotoxicity of the 9-hydroxy-ellipticine drugs. This hypothesis is not supported by experiments on 9, 10 dioxo NME reported in this paper. This drug is unable to oxidatively generate electrophilic species whereas it is an active electron-carrier towards molecular oxygen. The last property does not produce neither any cytotoxic effect on L 1210 cells in vitro nor any antileukemic efficiency. Cardiotoxicity was not looked for in this case.

Finally, the production of organic free radical species as intermediate steps of oxidation of the 9-hydroxy ellipticine derivatives opens up a new way to comprehend the mode of expression of their toxicity. These very reactive oxidizing radicals might also covalently bind to molecular biostructures ; radicals have been detected in several series of drugs after an initial oxidation step (for instance, the hydrazine, Iproniazid (39), the amine methapyrilene (40) some alkenes and alkynes drugs (41).

ACKNOWLEDGMENTS

This work was supported by the Coordinating Council for Cancer Research, and by the Association pour le développement de la recherche sur le cancer (ADRC) and by INSERM grant PRC N° 119026.

B I B L I O G R A P H Y

1. DALTON L.K., DEMERAC S., ELMES B.C., LODER J.W., SWAN J.M., TEITEI T. (1967).
   Aust. J. Chem. 20, 2715.

2. LE PECQ J.B., DAT-XUONG N., GOSSE C., PAOLETTI C. (1974)
   Proc. Natl. Acad. Sci. USA 71, 5078.

3. PAOLETTI C., LE PECQ J.B., DAT-XUONG N., LESCA P., LECOINTE P. (1978).
   Curr. Chemother. 1195.

4. JURET P., TANGUY A., LE TALAER J.Y., ABBATUCCI J.S., DAT-XUONG N., LE PECQ J.B., PAOLETTI C. (1978).
   Eur. J. Cancer 14, 205.

5. PAOLETTI C., CROS S., DAT-XUONG N., LECOINTE P., MOISAND A. (1979).
   Chem. Biol. Interact. 25, 45.

6. FESTY B., POISSON J., PAOLETTI C. (1971).
   FEBS Lett. 17, 321.

7. KOHN K.W., WARING M.J., GLAUBIGER D., FRIEDMAN C.A. (1975).
    Canc. Res. 35, 71.

8. PAOLETTI C., LESCA C., CROS S., MALVY C., AUCLAIR C. (1978).
    Biochem. Pharmacol. 28, 345;

9. ZWELLING L.A., MICHAELS S., ERICKSON L.C., UNGERLEIDER R.S.,
    NICHOLS M., KOHN K.W. (1981).
    Biochemistry 20, 6553.

10. LECOINTE P., LESCA P., CROS S., PAOLETTI C. (1978).
    Chem. Biol. Interact. 20, 113.

11. PINTO M., GUERINEAU M., PAOLETTI C. (1982).
    Biochem. Pharmacol. 31, 2161.

12. MALVY C. (24 June 1982) Ph.D. Thesis - Paris VI University.

13. HODNETT E.M., PRAKASH G., AMIRMOAZZAMI J. (1978)
    J. Med. Chem. 21, 11.

14. DRISCOLL J.S., HAZARD G.F., WOOD H.B., GOLDIN A. (1974).
    Cancer Chemother. Rep. 4, 362.

15. LIN A.J., COSBY L.A., SARTORELLI A.C. (1974).
    Cancer Chemother. Rep. 4, 23.

16. MOORE H.W. (1977)
    Science 197, 527.

17. SINHA R.A.K. (1981)
    Chem. Biol. Interact. 36, 179.

18. SINHA B.K., GREGORY J.L. (1981).
    Biochem. Pharmacol. 30, 2626.

19. KELLER P.J., KOZLOWSKI J.F, HORNEMANN U. (1979)
    J. Am. Chem. Soc. 101, 7121.

20. TOMASZ M., LIPMAN R. (1981).
    Biochemistry 20, 5056.

21. MOORE H.W. (1981).
    Medicinal Res. Rev. 1, 249.

22. SATO S., IWAIZUMI M., HANDA K., TAMURA Y. (1977).
    Gann 68, 603.

23. BACHUR N.R., GORDON S.L., GEE M.V., KOHN H. (1979).
    Proc. Natl. Acad. Sci. USA 76, 954.

24. NELSON S.D. (1982).
    J. Med. Chem. 25, 753.

25. SKIBBA J.L., RAMIREZ G., BEAL D.D., BRYAN G.T. (1970).
    Biochem. Pharmacol. 19, 2043.

26. AUCLAIR C., PAOLETTI C. (1981).
    J. Med. Chem. 24, 289.

27. AUCLAIR C., HYLAND K., PAOLETTI C. (1982).
    J. Med. Chem. sous presse.

28. BACHUR L.R., GORDON S.L., GEE M.V. (1978).
    Cancer Res. 38, 1745.

29. PAN S.S., BACHUR N.R. (1980).
    Pharmacol. 17, 95.

30. MEUNIER G., MEUNIER B., AUCLAIR C., BERNADOU J., PAOLETTI C.
    Publication submitted to Tetrahedron Letter.

31. SMULSON M.E., SUGIMURA T. (1980).
    Developments in Cell Biol. 6.

32. KERR I.M., BROWN R. (1978).
    Proc. Natl. Ac. Sci. 75, 256.

33. JUSTESEN J., FERBUS D., THANG M.N. (1980).
    Proc. Natl. Ac. Sci. 77, 4618.

34. WILSON W.R., CAIN B., BAGULEY B.C. (1977).
    Chem. Biol. Interact 18, 163.

35. HODGSON E., BEND J.R., PHILPOT R.M. (1979).
    Reviews in Biochemical Toxicology 1, 151.

36. MOLINIER-JUMEL C., MALFOY B., REYNARD J.A., AUBEL-SADRON C.
    (1978).
    Biochem. Biophys. Res. Commun. 84, 441.

37. RAO G.M., LOWN J.W., PLAMBECK J.A. (1978).
    J. Electrochem. Soc. 125, 534.

38. MOIROUX J., ANNE A. (1981).
    J. Electroanal. Chem. 121, 261.

39. AUGUSTO O., ORTIZ DE MONTELLANO P.R., QUINTANILHA A. (1981).
    Biochem. Biophys. Res. Commun. 101, 1324.

40. HANZLIK R.P., KISHORE V., TULLMAN R. (1979).
    J. Med. Chem. 22, 759.

41. ORTIZ DE MONTELLANO P.R., KUNZE K.L. (1981).
    Biochemistry 20, 710.

42. BERNADOU J., MEUNIER G., PAOLETTI C., MEUNIER B. (1982).
    J. Med. Chem. in press.

DTIC: A SPRINGBOARD TO NEW ANTITUMOUR AGENTS

M.F.G. STEVENS

1. INTRODUCTION

Although the history of the development of 5-(3,3-dimethyl-triazen-1-yl)imidazole-4-carboxamide (DTIC; NSC 45388) has been fully documented (1-5) a definitive account of the mode of action of the drug has yet to appear. There are almost as many theories purporting to explain the mode of action of DTIC as there are chemists and biochemists who, ensnared by the apparent deceptive simplicity of the molecule, have responded to the challenge but abjectly failed in the task of unravelling its perverse secrets.

The reason for the prevailing confusion is very clear: with the possible exception of the nitrosoureas and procarbazine no antitumour agent of comparable modest molecular dimensions has such a devious chemistry. DTIC is capable of fragmenting by chemical or metabolic degradation into numerous cytotoxic moeities many of which have, at one time or another, been rated as strong contenders for the rôle of 'active' species. Even two decades of effort have shed little real light on the mode of action of the drug; accordingly, reviews on this aspect of DTIC (6-9) typically terminate in question marks rather than full stops. This present effort is no exception.

DTIC (I)   (II)

D.N. Reinhoudt, T.A. Connors, H.M. Pinedo & K.W. van de Poll (eds.), Structure-Activity Relationships of Anti-Tumour Agents.
© 1983, Martinus Nijhoff Publishers, The Hague/Boston/London. ISBN 90-247-2783-9.

In this Chapter recent studies on the chemistry and metabolism of DTIC (I) and its substituted 1-aryl-3,3-dialkyl-triazene counterparts (II) will be surveyed. In the final section attention will be focussed on some derivatives worthy of consideration as clinical candidates in the search for a second-generation triazene.

2. PHYSICAL AND CHEMICAL DEGRADATION OF DTIC AND 1-ARYL-3,3-DIMETHYLTRIAZENES

2.1. Photolytic degradation. Decomposition of DTIC under laboratory (non-metabolic) conditions has been shown to afford 5 different imidazoles (III-VII).

The most interesting — to a chemist — of these compounds is 5-diazoimidazole-4-carboxamide (Diazo-IC) (III) which is formed together with dimethylamine on photodecomposition of the drug (10): it is also the initial product formed when 5-aminoimidazole-4-carboxamide (AIC) is diazotised in the presence of excess nitrous acid (11). In contrast conventional diazotisation of AIC in the presence of excess of the amine leads to the imidazoazoimidazole (VI) (12) which is also formed in trace amounts when DTIC is stored at elevated temperatures.

Although liberation of Diazo-IC from DTIC may account for some of the effects of DTIC on bacteria (13) and tumour cells growing *in vitro* (14-16) reviewers of the biological properties of Diazo-IC are unanimous in the conclusion that it does not play a significant rôle in the *in vivo* antitumour action of the drug (2,4,6,8). Furthermore, although it has been claimed (17) that troublesome venous pain and other side effects elicited by DTIC in the clinic can be reduced by scrupulously shielding the drug from light at all times, it would be unjust to indict Diazo-IC as being culpable for these problems on such scant anecdotal evidence.

The early work on the photoconversion of DTIC to firstly Diazo-IC and thence 2-azahypoxanthine (IV) (10,18) has been extended recently (19) and the outcome shown to be crucially influenced by pH. Thus decomposition of the formulated drug (DTIC-Dome) at pH3 in diffuse light (Figure 1) yields a stable photoproduct ($\lambda_{max.}$ 236 and 275 nm) which is not 2-azahypoxanthine ($\lambda_{max.}$ 250 and 277 nm). This new photoproduct 4-carbamoylimidazolium-5-olate (V) is the stable imidazole derivative formed when DTIC is decomposed at spectroscopic concentration (0.01 mg ml^{-1}) in the pH range 2-5.2. At pH1 and pH 7.4 or above 2-azahypoxanthine is the product (Table 1). When the drug is photodecomposed at clinically-realistic concentrations (1 mg ml^{-1}) at pH 3-4 the solution goes pink and a dark maroon precipitate of the imidazoazoimidazolium olate (VII) rapidly forms (19): this coupling product arises by interaction between Diazo-IC (III) and the imidazolium olate (V).

186

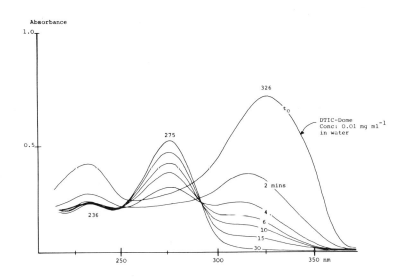

FIGURE 1.   Decomposition of DTIC-Dome at pH 3 in water in
diffuse light. (Adapted from reference 19).

The betaine (V) is the aglycone of the antitumour and
immunosupressant antibiotic bredinin (VIII) which is
elaborated by cultures of *Eupenicillium brefeldianum* M 2166
(20).   Although there is a salvage pathway in mammalian cells
whereby bredinin can be biosynthesised from its aglycone
precursor (21) it is unlikely that DTIC could ultimately give
rise to bredinin *in vivo* unless mammalian cells possess a
hitherto unrecognised capacity to effect the transformation
DTIC (I) ⟶ Diazo-IC (III) ⟶ imidazolium olate (V) which
cannot be mimicked in the laboratory except under photochemical
conditions.   Interestingly, 2-azahypoxanthine (IV) has been
identified as a transformation product of DTIC in Chinese
hamster ovary (CHO) cells even in the dark (16).

Because the formation of the imidazolium olate (V) from DTIC
via Diazo-IC is a purely photochemical event it has been suggested
that a reactive carbene species (IX) may be implicated as intermediate (12, 19);   when quenched with water this would yield
the imidazolium olate.   Independent evidence for this proposition
has been adduced from the U.V. photolysis of microcrystalline

Diazo-IC at 77K which affords a complex wide-field e.s.r. spectrum (22). A species of large D-value is generated which is probably the carbene in its triplet state (IXb). Diazo-IC also undergoes photoinduced C-H insertion reactions in alcohols (23) and the triplet carbene generated by photolytic degradation of 2-diazoimidazole (X) readily inserts into arenes to afford mixtures of o-, m- and p-substituted 2-phenylimidazoles (XI) (24).

Table 1. Stable imidazoles formed on decomposition of DTIC-Dome*, 5-(3,3-dimethyltriazen-1-yl)imidazole-4-carboxamide (Pure DTIC) and Diazo-IC at different pH values; conc. of substrate 0.01 mg ml^{-1}. (Adapted from references 12 and 19).

Substrate	Light conditions	pH 1	pH 2	pH 3	pH 5.2	pH 7.4	pH 8.5	pH 10.5	pH 12
DTIC-Dome	A	IV	V	V	V	IV	IV	IV	IV
DTIC-Dome	B	IV	V	V	V	IV	IV	IV	IV
DTIC-Dome	C	I	I	I	I	I	I	I	I
Pure-DTIC	A	IV	V	V	V	IV	IV	IV	IV
Pure-DTIC	B	IV	V	V	V	IV	IV	IV	IV
Pure DTIC	C	I	I	I	I	I	I	I	I
Diazo-IC	A	IV	V	V	V	IV	IV	IV	IV
Diazo-IC	B	IV	V	V	V	IV	IV	IV	IV
Diazo-IC	C	IV	IV	IV	IV	IV	IV	IV	IV

Light conditions. A: Direct sunlight
B: Natural light with no direct sunlight
C: In the dark

*DTIC-Dome is a freeze-dried preparation of DTIC containing mannitol and citric acid.

Diazo-IC could be an important synthon for the preparation of 5-(substituted)imidazole-4-carboxamides and examination of its photolytic and thermolytic degradation in a range of substrates would be a potentially rewarding study.

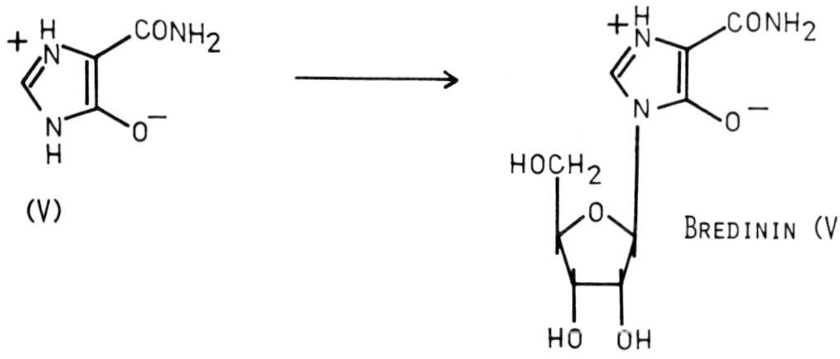

(V) → BREDININ (VIII)

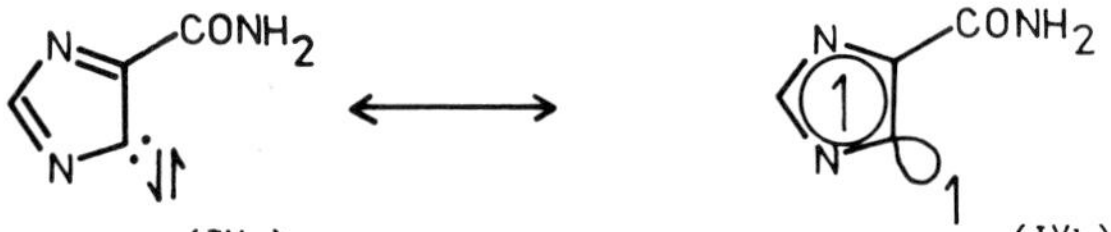

(IXa) ⟷ (IXb)

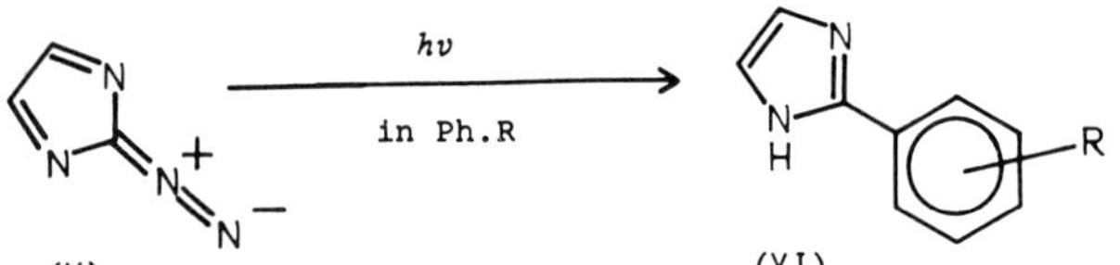

(X) → (XI)
$h\nu$ in Ph.R

2.2. Radiolytic and reductive degradation. Whereas photolysis of DTIC has been examined extensively, there is a dearth of information on the radiolysis of the drug. Radiolytic generation of reactive cytotoxic species within irradiated tumour masses is an attractive therapeutic prospect and presumably is the rationale behind recent efforts to demonstrate a radio-sensitising capability for DTIC. Rofstad *et al* (25) claim to have observed an increased effectiveness of DTIC combined with ^{60}Co γ-irradiation at delaying the onset of human malignant

melanoma regrowth in nude mice compared to the effects of
radiation alone.

Rauth and Mohindra (26) failed to demonstrate that DTIC has
radiosensitising activity against CHO and HeLa cells *in vitro*
and KHT mouse cells *in vivo*. However, high concentrations of
DTIC were approximately 5 times more effective at killing
hypoxic CHO cells (Figure 2) than killing aerobic cells over
drug exposure times of 0-12 hours; similar effects were
elicited against HeLa cells. Possibly the hypoxic cells can
effect a selective activation (reduction?) of the DTIC to a
hitherto undetected species distinct from those formed by
previously recognised chemical or metabolic processes.

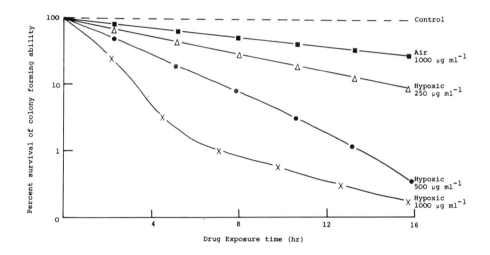

Figure 2. Effects of DTIC on aerobic and hypoxic Chinese
hamster ovary cells *in vitro*.(Adapted from reference 26).

Some measure of support for this hypothesis is provided by the
decomposition of the triazenyl-L-phenylalanine derivative (XII).
This triazene has pronounced activity against the TLX5 lymphoma
in vivo (27) and decomposes in aqueous solution at pH 1-7 in the
dark to afford *N*-acetyl-L-phenylalanine ethyl ester (XIII) in
high yield. It is difficult to envisage a mechanism for this
(formal) reduction process. The reaction conditions are
entirely wrong for a homolytic process (Gomberg reaction)

involving an intermediate aryl radical: on the other hand a
heterolytic process *via* an aryldiazonium ion and thence an aryl
cation, which is mechanistically more likely, would surely lead
to the production of the tyrosine analogue (XIV) rather than
the observed product. Moreover, no nitrogen is evolved at room
temperature and the fate of the dimethyltriazenyl fragment has
not yet been determined. It would be worthwhile to examine the
degradation of 3,3-dimethyl-1-*p*-tolyltriazene (XV) and other substituted tolyltriazenes for evidence of a comparable cleavage.
Interestingly, Pool (28) has claimed recently that phenylhydrazi?

(reduction product) is formed after incubating 1-phenyl-3,3-dimethyltriazene (II: X = H, R_1 = R_2 = H) with rat microsomes.

3. STRUCTURE-ACTIVITY RELATIONSHIPS IN ANTITUMOUR TRIAZENES

3.1. Lymphoid leukaemia L1210 and Sarcoma 180.

Because of the high efficiency of the coupling interaction between aromatic diazonium compounds and secondary amines many hundreds of variants of DTIC have been synthesised and screened for antitumour activity. It was inevitable that such bounty, particularly of 1-aryl-3,3-dialkyltriazenes (II), would attract the attentions of Hansch and his co-workers (29,30). In an analysis of QSAR in an extensive series of DTIC analogues evaluated for anti-tumour activity against L1210 in mice, Hansch (30) found that the imidazole carboxamide grouping conferred no special potency; it can be replaced by another π-excessive or π-deficient heterocyclic ring or by an aryl moeity. Optimum potency resides in derivatives with Log P ∿ 1.1. Aryldimethyltriazenes bearing an *ortho*-carboxamide function or other H-bonding group designed to mimic the intramolecularly bonded carboxamide revealed by a crystallographic analysis of DTIC (31) have no special merit.

Electron-releasing (+M) substituents in the aryl ring enhance activity of aryldimethyltriazenes against L1210 (30), but this is achieved at the price of increasing instability (32). Dunn and Greenberg (33) discerned a strong correlation between rate of hydrolysis of a series of aryldimethyltriazenes (XVI) to their diazonium cations (XVII) and inhibitory activity against Sarcoma 180 ascites tumour in mice. The rapid liberation of

(XVI)   (XVII)

diazonium cations from labile triazenes ($t_{\frac{1}{2}} < 2 \times 10^2$ min) also seems to be responsible for the induction of *local* tumours at the site of administration in rats (32).

3.2. <u>Antimetastatic activity of aryldimethyltriazenes.</u> A significant recent discovery has been the identification of specific *antimetastatic* activity in aryldimethyltriazenes. Giraldi and his colleagues studied the effects of three *para*-substituted phenyldimethyltriazenes and their monomethyl homologues on the primary tumour and lung metastasis formation in mice bearing the Lewis lung carcinoma (34). Against the primary tumour the stable derivatives bearing -M groups were the most active and the derivatives were ranked $NO_2 > CONH_2 > Me$. However the effects on lung metastasis formation were reversed (Table 2) and the unstable tolyltriazene had the greatest antimetastatic activity.

Because the corresponding monomethyltriazenes had, in general, less activity than dimethyltriazenes against the primary tumour and metastasis formation Giraldi concluded that metabolism does not play a major rôle in the action of the dimethyltriazenes against the Lewis lung tumour. Furthermore the triazene carboxylate salt (XVIII) which has potent anti-metastatic effects (35) apparently does not undergo microsomal demethylation (as adjudged by formaldehyde release).

$$K^+ \quad {}^-O_2C \diagdown \hspace{-0.3em} \bigcirc \hspace{-0.3em} \diagdown_{N \diagup\diagup N \diagdown_N \diagdown^{Me}_{Me}}$$

(XVIII)

It would be reasonable to interpret Giraldi's results as pointing to the involvement of two chemically distinct reactive intermediates, one active against the primary tumour and the other inhibiting spontaneous metastases.

Table 2. Effects of aryldimethyl- and arylmonomethyl-triazenes
on metastases of the Lewis lung tumour in mice.
(Adapted from reference 34).

X	R_1	R_2	Daily dose (mg kg^{-1})	Total number of metastases (mg)*	Total weight of metastases	$t\frac{1}{2}$ (min)[†]
NO_2	Me	Me	12.5	68.2 ± 11.6	75.6	2.32x10^5
$CONH_2$	Me	Me	15	56.5 ± 12.2	54.3	–
Me	Me	Me	12.5	42.9 ± 7.2	29.0	3.2 x10^1
NO_2	Me	H	12.5	105.9 ± 15.6	109.0	–
$CONH_2$	Me	H	12.5	73.1 ± 12.1	50.3	–
Me	Me	H	12.5	64.6 ± 10.0	49.1	–

* Values represent mean percent ratios (T/C) ± S.E. for groups
of 10 mice (treated) and 40 mice (controls) sacrificed on day
21 after tumour implantation.
[†] Determined by Kolar and Preussman (Ref. 32).

3.3. TLX5 lymphoma. The detailed study by Connors and his co-
workers (36) showed that the nature of the substituent in the
phenyl ring had absolutely no bearing on the activity of aryl-
triazenes against the TLX5 lymphoma in mice: the substituent can
by hydrophilic, hydrophobic, electron-withdrawing or -donating.
Crucially, however, at least one methyl group in aryldialkyl-
triazenes is required for *in vivo* activity against this tumour.
A similar conclusion was reached by Hansch (30) in his QSAR
analysis of L1210 results. Large alkyl groups depress activity
substantially and compounds with a *tert*-butyl group are inactive
even when the other alkyl substituent is methyl. These results
have been interpreted by Connors as follows: only those compounds
which can be metabolised to arylmonomethyltriazenes have anti-
tumour activity *in vivo* (at least against the TLX5). Thus
triazenes of general structure (XIX) are transformed by metabolic

activation to the corresponding monomethyl-triazenes (XX).

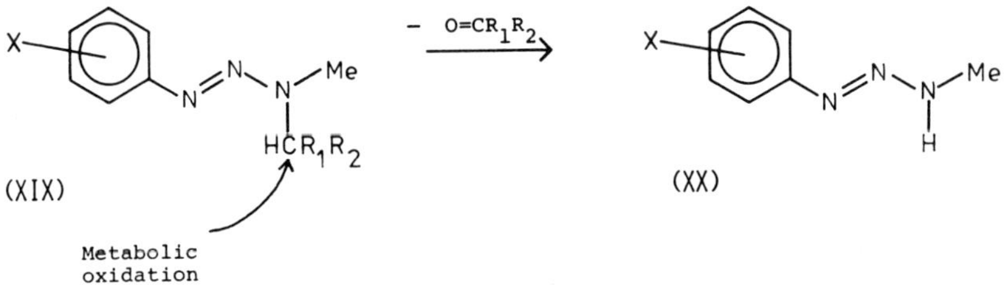

(XIX)

Metabolic
oxidation

(XX)

The inactivity of a methyl-*tert*-butyltriazene is explained by
the fact that the *tert*-butyl substituent has no α-CH group
amenable to metabolic oxidation and the derivative cannot be
metabolised to a monomethyltriazene (36).

3.4. Critical evaluation of test systems. QSAR conclusions
based on studies employing the L1210 and TLX5 lymphoma can be
criticised in that the results are unduly influenced by the
extreme responsiveness of these tumours to cytotoxic — as
distinct from antitumour — species. Thus the L1210 is
especially sensitive to electrophilic alkylating reactants
particularly of the β-chloroethyl type, and the TLX5 lymphoma
is exquisitely sensitive to those cytotoxic species generated
in vivo from dimethyltriazenes and nitrosoureas. [TLX5 cells
resistant to triazenes are, in fact, cross-resistant to
procarbazine and nitrosoureas (37)]. By their very nature
these tumours prejudicially respond *in vivo* to those triazenes
which undergo metabolic transformation to powerful electrophilic reactants — possibly monomethyltriazenes (but see

Section 4.2). It is premature to utterly dismiss the hypothesis that generation of weakly electrophilic diazonium ions may be crucial to antitumour activity, since it has been pointed out (33) that an externally administered diazonium compound (as opposed to one generated *in situ* within sensitive cells) would have only a remote prospect of entering target tumour cells.

Moreover, serious objections can be levelled at test systems like L1210 and TLX5 lymphoma since both tumour cells and drugs are introduced into the same body compartment. Perhaps a different story might have unfolded had metastasis inhibition in the Lewis lung tumour been employed for QSAR studies. Fundamentally different test systems — induction of long-term depression of immune responses (38) or inhibition of the low K_m form of cyclic AMP phosphodiesterase (39), properties which have been attributed to DTIC — would probably lead to fundamentally different conclusions.

4. METABOLIC GENERATION OF SELECTIVELY TOXIC SPECIES

4.1. <u>Activation of dimethyltriazenes.</u> Preussmann, von Hodenberg and Hengy (40) studied the *in vitro* metabolism of the carcinogen phenyldimethyltriazene (XXI) and proposed that a transient hydroxymethyl metabolite (XXII) was generated which eliminated formaldehyde to afford phenylmonomethyltriazene (XXIII): this potent alkylating agent would then methylate bionucleophiles; in the process aniline (XXIV) was formed. Methylation probably proceeds by an SN2 reaction and not *via* a 'free' methyl carbenium ion as so often reiterated.

This activation scheme has also been adopted to "explain" the antitumour properties of dimethyltriazenes. It has been claimed that many of the biological effects of DTIC, including methylation of DNA (41) can be accounted for by invoking a reactive monomethyl metabolite: the identification of 5-amino-imidazole-4-carboxamide (AIC) as the principle urinary metabolite of DTIC (42) lends further apparent support to the hypothesis.

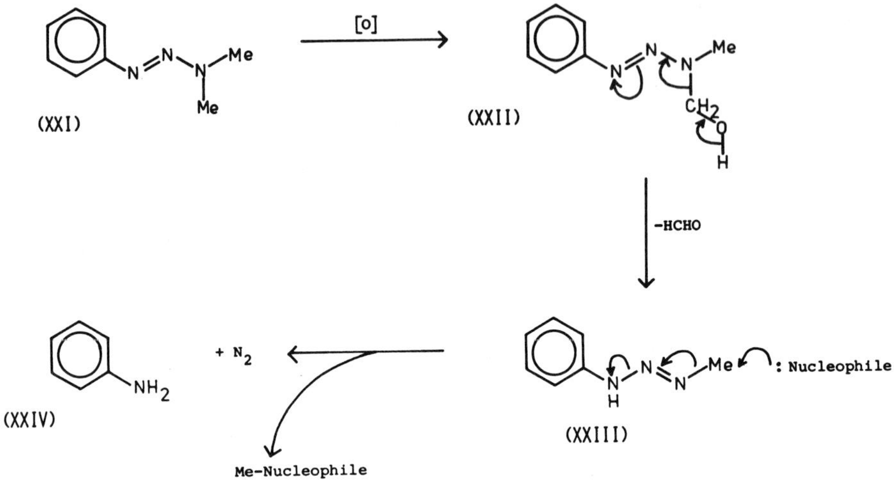

(XXI) (XXII)

−HCHO

(XXIV) + N₂

(XXIII) : Nucleophile

Me-Nucleophile

4.2. Methylation and selective antitumour effects. Hickman

(43) and Hansch, Hatheway, Quinn and Greenberg (44) have
summarised the evidence against the methylation hypothesis:

(i) The degree of de-methylation of dimethyltriazenes *in
vitro* (as measured by formaldehyde release) does not
correlate with cytotoxicity (45).

(ii) Diethyltriazenes are devoid of antitumour properties
in vivo (36) yet they are smoothly de-ethylated to
monoethyltriazenes. Monoethyltriazenes are potent
alkylating agents.

(iii) DTIC and aryldimethyltriazenes are active against a
tumour (TLX5 lymphoma) which is completely insensitive
to classical alkylating agents of the β-chloroethyl type
(e.g. cyclophosphamide) (37).

(iv) DTIC, which affects CHO cells principally in G_1 and early
S phases (15), differs from β-chloroethyl alkylating
agents in its marked effects on cycling as opposed to
resting cells (46).

(v)   Human melanoma cells are equivalently labelled with
^{14}C-methyl DTIC irrespective as to whether they are
sensitive or resistant to DTIC (14).

Hickman and his co-workers (47) have attempted to identify
the *selective* antitumour species generated from aryldimethyltriazenes *in vivo* by employing two mouse tumours — the TLX5(S)
lymphoma which is sensitive to dimethyltriazenes *in vivo* and the
TLX5(R) lymphoma which has been made resistant *in vivo*. As
expected two dimethyltriazenes were active *in vivo* against the
sensitive tumour but were inactive against the resistant variant
(Table 3). A monomethyltriazene also showed selectivity and
discriminated between the sensitive and resistant tumours.

Table 3.   Activity of triazenes against the mouse TLX5 lymphoma
           in vivo. (Adapted from reference 47).

| Compound | | | Tumour | Percent | Optimum dose |
X	R_1	R_2	[TLX5(S) or TLX5(R)]	ILS*	(mgkg^{-1} : 5 x daily)
Ac	Me	Me	(S)	56	40
Ac	Me	Me	(R)	6	40
CO_2Me	Me	Me	(S)	58	40
CO_2Me	Me	Me	(R)	0	40
CO_2Me	Me	H	(S)	87	5
CO_2Me	Me	H	(R)	4	20

Method: 2×10^5 TLX5 cells were injected s.c. into the inguinal
region on day 0. Animals were dosed daily from days 3 to 7.
*Percent ILS = percent increase in life span of test animals
compared with controls.

It was argued that if the selective species generated from
dimethyltriazenes *in vivo* are monomethyltriazenes then they
should show discriminating selectivity against the sensitive
tumour *in vitro*. This point was investigated in an *in vitro*

bioassay system in which TLX5(S) or (R) cells were incubated with drug for 2h at 37°. Cells were then reinjected into animals and the life span measured. The merit of this system resides in the possibility of incorporating a drug metabolic activation step which can be phased with the bioassay.

Table 4. Activity of dimethyl- and monomethyl triazenes against the mouse TLX5 lymphoma *in vitro*. (Adapted from references 47 and 48).

Compound X	R_1	R_2	Tumour [TLX5(S) or TLX5(R)]	With (+)* or without (-) metabolic activation	Concentration of drug (μg ml-1)	Percent ILS
Ac	Me	Me	(S)	(-)	500	0
Ac	Me	Me	(R)	(-)	500	0
Ac	Me	Me	(S)	(+)	500	38
Ac	Me	Me	(R)	(+)	500	23
CO_2Me	Me	Me	(S)	(-)	1000	0
CO_2Me	Me	Me	(R)	(-)	1000	0
CO_2Me	Me	Me	(S)	(+)	500	53
CO_2Me	Me	Me	(R)	(+)	500	17
Ac	Me	H	(S)	(-)	50	51
Ac	Me	H	(R)	(-)	100	47
CO_2Me	Me	H	(S)	(-)	250	52
CO_2Me	Me	H	(R)	(-)	250	Cures
CO_2Me	Et	Et	(S)	(-)	500	0
CO_2Me	Et	Et	(R)	(-)	500	0
CO_2Me	Et	Et	(S)	(+)	500	42
CO_2Me	Et	Et	(R)	(+)	500	60

Method: 2 x 10^6 TLX5 cells ml^{-1} were incubated with drugs for 2hr at 37°. 2 x 10^5 cells were injected into animals and the increase in life span compared with animals which received untreated cells.

* Mouse liver 9000g homogenate and cofactors.

The results (Table 4) show several points of interest. Firstly, the two dimethyltriazenes have no effect on TLX5 lymphoma *in vitro* in the absence of metabolic activation: when they are activated the cytotoxicity is more pronounced against the sensitive tumour line. This is entirely consistent with previous results (36). The monomethyltriazenes on the other hand do not require metabolic activation and are directly cytotoxic: moreover, they are non-selectively cytotoxic, being approximately equipotent towards sensitive and resistant cells. An unselective cytotoxic species can also be generated by metabolic activation of a diethyltriazene. This is surprising in view of the complete inactivity of diethyltriazenes *in vivo* (36). These results demonstrate that metabolism of dimethyl-triazenes generates a mixture of selective and non-selective metabolites and that the selective species are apparently *not* monomethyltriazenes. In arriving at this conclusion an important assumption must be made — that is, the addition of a monomethyl-triazene for 2 hours to cells *in vitro* is biologically equivalent to the cumulative production, by metabolism *in situ*, of the same agent over a 5 daily dose schedule. If this is not the case the foregoing conclusion is negated.

4.3. 1-Aryl-3-alkyl-3-hydroxymethyltriazenes.

So, if monomethyl-triazenes are not the selectively toxic species (against the TLX5 lymphoma),what are?

Attention has recently switched to hydroxymethyltriazenes as possible candidates. Compounds of this type, formerly considered only as metabolic transients (40), can be prepared simply by reacting aryldiazonium salts with methylamine-formal-dehyde mixtures (49, 50). Although hydroxymethyltriazenes with -M substituents are perfectly stable in non-polar solvents (49) they decompose in aqueous systems. Thus derivatives (XXV: X = p-Ac or p-CO$_2$Me) decompose in phosphate buffer (pH 7.4) at 37$^{\rm O}$ with $t_{\frac{1}{2}}$ ∿ 12±2 minutes as determined spectroscopically (51). The final products are the arylamines (XXVI) presumably arising by formaldehyde elimination and hydrolysis of intermediate monomethyltriazenes. Samples of hydroxymethyltriazenes also

decompose on silica gel or alumina adsorbents to yield diaryl-
triazenes (XXVII):   these latter products undoubtedly result
from 'diazo-migration' reactions (52).

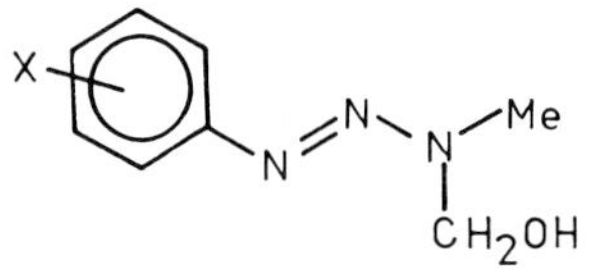

(XXV)

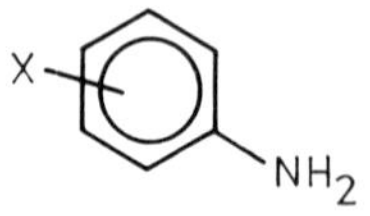

(XXVI)

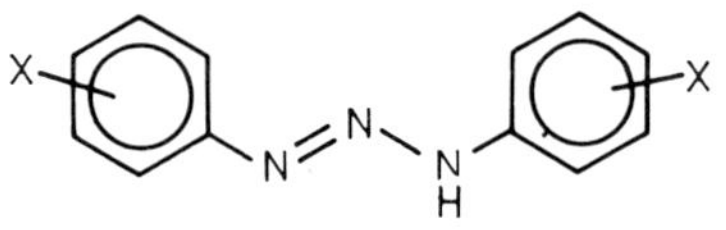

(XXVII)

X = p-Ac or p-CO$_2$Me

Hydroxymethyltriazenes have pronounced activity against
the TLX5(S) lymphoma *in vivo* (Table 5);   conjugation of the
hydroxy group with benzoic or glucuronic acids markedly reduces
their activity *in vivo* and *in vitro* (53).   Although the hydroxymethyltriazene (XXV: X = p-CO$_2$Me) shows selectivity *in vivo*,
closer examination of the biological properties of hydroxymethyltriazenes against TLX5 cells shows that they are simply acting
as prodrug modifications of monomethyltriazenes since they are
cytotoxic *in vitro*, but do not discriminate between the
sensitive and resistant tumours (54).   However, the persistence
of hydroxymethyltriazenes in biological fluids is undoubtedly
sufficient to allow them to diffuse from the liver, where they
are generated, to distant tumour sites.   There they could either
participate as the intact molecules in crucial molecular events
with unidentified target biomolecules, or decompose to reactive
electrophilic species with indiscriminate cytotoxicity.

Table 5. Antitumour activity of hydroxymethyltriazenes against
TLX5 lymphoma *in vivo*.

Compound		Tumour [TLX5(S) or TLX5(R)]	Percent ILS	Optimum dose (mg Kg^{-1}: 5 x daily)
X	R			
CO_2Me	Me	(S)	120	5
(benzoate ester)		(S)	31	20
CO_2Me	Me	(R)	0	5
Ac	Me	(S)	72	20
$CONH_2$	Me	(S)	62	20
CN	Me	(S)	54	160
CN	Et	(S)	0	160

For details of method see Table 3.

4.4. Stability of hydroxymethyltriazenes. Kolar has adduced
evidence which confirms that hydroxymethyltriazenes are long-
lived moeities *in vivo*. The *O*-glucuronide (XXIX) has been
identified as a urinary metabolite in rats treated with
1-(2,4,6-trichlorophenyl)-3,3-dimethyltriazene (XXVIII) (55) and
the unconjugated hydroxymethyl metabolite of DTIC (XXX) has
been tentatively identified in the urine of DTIC-treated rats
(56). The metabolite was chromatographically indistinguishable
from the product formed by reacting the monomethyltriazene (XXXI)
with formaldehyde in anhydrous methanol. An uncharacterised
polar metabolite excreted in the urine of dogs treated with
DTIC (57) might well also be the same hydroxymethyltriazene
(XXX) or a conjugate thereof.

Solution i.p. studies have confirmed that intramolecular
H-bonding stabilises the α-hydroxy derivative (XXXIII) formed
when the morpholinotriazene (XXXII) is oxidised by permanganate
or by a metabolic process (58): similar bonding in *N*-hydroxy-
methyltriazenes (XXXIV) could inhibit the facile elimination of

formaldehyde characteristic of other unstable carbinolamines.
Alternatively, one might argue that the lone pair of sp^2
electrons on the terminal azo nitrogen could initiate the
elimination by a neighbouring group effect (XXXV). The balance
between stabilisation and elimination should then be finely
tunable by modification of the aryl substituent X: electron-
donating substituents should encourage the elimination process,
whereas electron-withdrawing substituents should stabilise the
carbinolamine. Perhaps significantly, the most active aryldimethyltriazenes (against the TLX5 lymphoma) seem to be those
derivatives with -M substituents in the aryl group (36, 47) and
these are the very ones which form the most stable N-hydroxymethyl
derivatives (49).

(XXVIII)   (XXIX)

(I)   Rat metabolism   (XXX)   HCHO in MeOH   (XXXI)

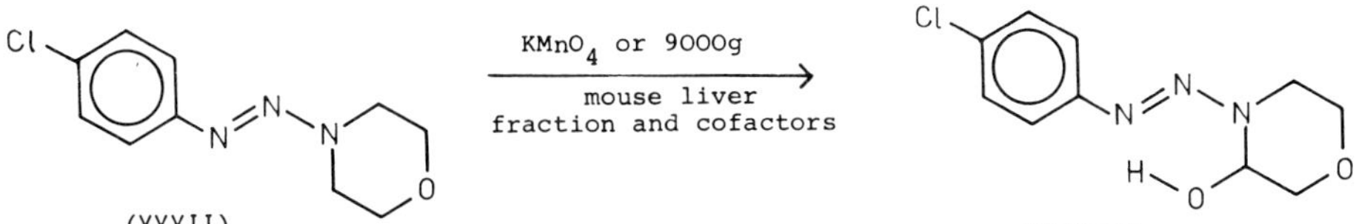

KMnO$_4$ or 9000g
mouse liver
fraction and cofactors

(XXXII)

(XXXIII)

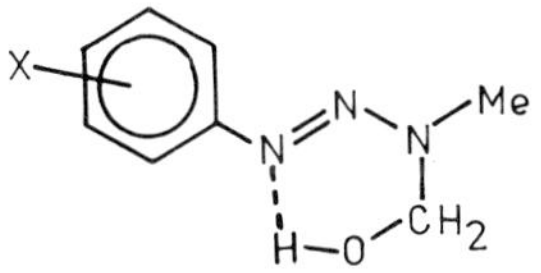

Me

(XXXIV)

Me

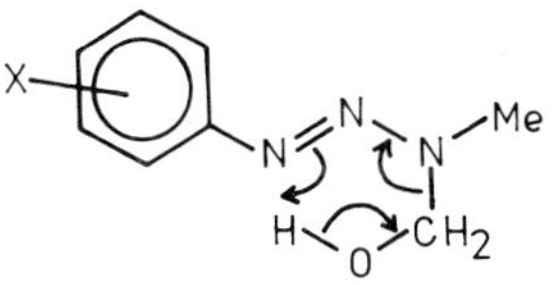

(XXXV)

4.4. Possible geometrical isomerism in 1-aryl-3-alkyl-3-hydroxymethyltriazenes.

No information is available on the solution conformations of *N*-hydroxymethyltriazenes but, surprisingly, a crystal structure determination of 1-(4-carbethoxyphenyl)-3-hydroxymethyl-3-methyltriazene shows that it exists as rotamer (XXXVI) (59) with the *N*-hydroxymethyl group in a *trans* arrangement with respect to the azo linkage (Figure 3). Within the unit cell the hydroxy group is intermolecularly H-bonded to the ester carbonyl group and there are strong stacking attractions between the benzene rings.

The temperature dependent n.m.r. spectra of a series of substituted 1-phenyl-3,3-dimethyltriazenes have been interpreted in terms of restricted rotation about the (formal) N_2-N_3 bond (XXXVII) (60). Free energies of activation for rotation in CDCl$_3$ range from 12.7 ± 0.4 (X = OMe) to 15.7 ± 0.2 k cal mol^{-1} when the negative charge can be delocalised by the aryl substituent (X = NO$_2$). Considerable double-bonded character of the comparable N-N bond of DTIC is evidenced by its short bond distance (1.305Å) and by the sp^2 character of the dimethylamino N atom (31). If the barrier to rotation about the N-N bond of *N*-hydroxymethyl-*N*-methyltriazenes in solution is sufficiently

enhanced by intramolecular bonding, there is a possibility
that discrete geometrical isomers of this type could exist.
The synthetic derivatives tested for antitumour properties
(Table 5) all presumably exist as intermolecularly bonded
rotamers (at least in the solid state): whether or not these
products are identical to the *N*-hydroxymethyltriazenes generated
from the metabolism of dimethyltriazenes *in vivo* is, at present,
unknown. A QSAR study based on molecular shape analysis (61)
predicts that the alternative rotamers (potentially intramolecularly bonded) would be the favoured metabolic products
[e.g. (XXV)].

(XXXVI)

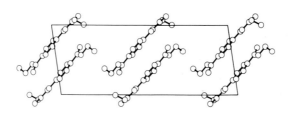

FIGURE 3. Crystal structure of 1-(4-carbethoxyphenyl)-3-
hydroxymethyl-3-methyltriazene (XXXVI). (Reproduced by
courtesy of Dr C H Schwalbe and Dr R J Simmonds).

(XXXVII)

4.5. Other possible activation processes.

Three further aspects of the metabolic activation of dimethyltriazenes deserve mention. The inactivity of an *N*-ethyl-*N*-hydroxymethyltriazene *in vivo* (Table 5) seems to indicate that hydroxymethyltriazenes *per se* are devoid of activity. Dimethyltriazenes are probably not acting as progenitors of cytotoxic formaldehyde and their mode of action is distinguishable from that of another *N*-methyl anti-tumour drug hexamethylmelamine which also produces a stable *N*-hydroxymethyl metabolite (62): in fact dimethyltriazenes have a different spectrum of antitumour activity to hexamethyl-melamine.

The possibility that *N*-hydroxymethyltriazenes might be substrates for further metabolic oxidation has been advanced (63). Chemical oxidation of 1-aryl-3,3-dimethyltriazenes with vanadium pentoxide and *tert*-butyl hydroperoxide in benzene affords a mixture of the *N*-formyltriazenes (XXXVIII) and the peroxides (XXXIX). Triazenes of the former type have never been detected as products of metabolic oxidation of dimethyltriazenes. Were they to be formed they might be expected to undergo heterolytic fission to the antitumour agent *N*-methylformamide (64). However, lack of cross-resistance of animal tumours to dimethyltriazenes and *N*-methylformamide does not support this hypothesis.

Recent studies on the metabolism of 1-(4-acetylphenyl)-3,3-dimethyltriazene (II: X = *p*-Ac, R_1 and R_2 = Me) *in vivo* in

mice have revealed the presence of the corresponding monomethyltriazene (II: X = p-Ac, R_1 = Me, R_2 = H) as a urinary metabolite
(48). HPLC analysis of the products of *in vitro* metabolism
confirmed the presence of the same monomethyltriazene metabolite
but in amounts insufficient to account for the observed cytotoxicity. The monomethyltriazene was itself rapidly bio-
transformed by a 9000g fraction of mouse liver homogenate
(Figure 4) and by isolated mouse hepatocytes (48); other monomethyltriazenes behaved similarly (65).

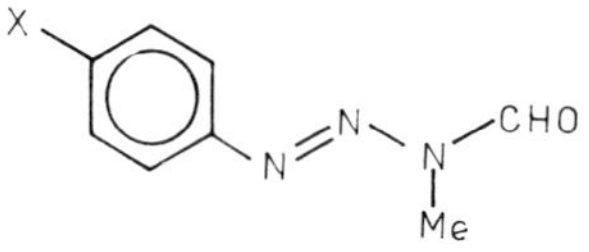

(XXXVIII) 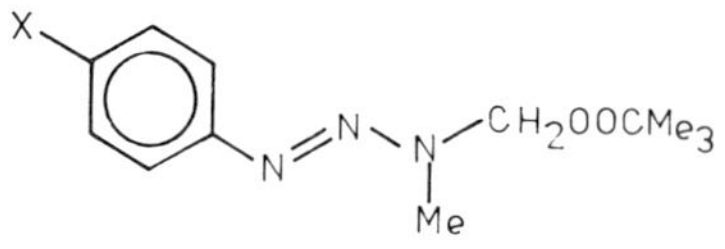   (XXXIX)

X = NO$_2$, Cl, Br or I

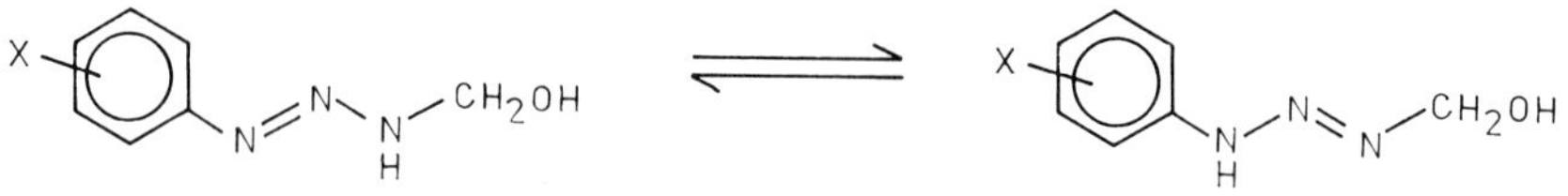

(XL)

Characterisation of these monomethyltriazene metabolites
has not yet been achieved. It is interesting to speculate that
these products could be hydroxymethylaminoazoarenes (XL). A
logical synthetic route to these novel triazenes would be by a
hydride ion or borane reduction of *N*-formyl- or *N*-alkoxycarbonyl-
triazenes and this is an important topic for synthetic effort.

Finally, it should be noted that the antitumour agent
procarbazine also affords hydroxymethyl-azo and -azoxy metabolites
(66). However, the cross-resistance observed in the actions of
procarbazine, DTIC and aryldimethyltriazenes against animal
tumours might also be attributable to the fact that these agents
all yield methylating species on metabolism.

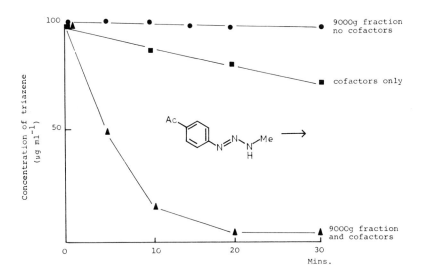

FIGURE 4.   Metabolism of 1-(4-acetylphenyl)-3-methyltriazene
by a 9000g fraction of mouse liver homogenate.

Only one tentative conclusion can be drawn at the present
time on the metabolic transformations of triazenes.   Oxidative
metabolism does appear to be a requirement for antitumour
activity against animal tumours, but it is unlikely that a
single reactive species can account for all the observed effects
against primary tumours and spontaneous metastases.   In the
specific case of DTIC it is possible that immunomodulatory
effects of the intact drug may enhance the cytotoxicity of the
reactive metabolites.   What is quite clear is that the clinical
use of DTIC as a "single agent" is nothing of the sort: DTIC,
like aryldimethyltriazenes, produces a cascade of reactive
moeities and patients treated with the drug are, in fact,
receiving combination chemotherapy.

5. NEW DTIC ANALOGUES AS CLINICAL CANDIDATES

In his extensive QSAR analysis of the triazene series of
drugs Hansch (30) was unable to identify an idiosyncratic result
which would act as a focus for imaginative drug design and recent
efforts which have concentrated on the synthesis of triazenes
bearing electron-withdrawing aryl substituents (67-71) have not
been rewarded by any biological breakthroughs. Moreover, the
prospect of minimising toxicity by molecular manipulation also
leads into a blind alley. The close correspondence of the QSAR
relating toxicity in mice (LD_{50}) and antitumour activity (L1210)
led Hansch and his colleagues (44) to conclude:

"Unless one had new biochemical or molecular biological
information suggesting that a new triazene might be more
effective in some specific way, we would not recommend
the synthesis and testing of new congeners".

Finding a reasonable excuse for rejecting this advice is
not difficult (see Section 3.4). QSAR studies based on the
highly proliferative mouse L1210 tumour certainly give an insight
into the biology of that popular tumour; however, they may
have only marginal relevance to an interpretation of the mode
of action of DTIC in the clinic against *human disease*. Supposing
that, for example, the clinical activity of the drug was
attributable to a specific ability to induce human interferon —
DTIC does product a flu-like syndrome recently recognised as a
characteristic side-effect of interferon (72) — this factor
would not have been revealed by animal screening results.

The imaginative chemist is not hard pressed to devise yet
more attractive molecules to extend the triazene lineage and a
second-generation drug would have to demonstrate only modest
clinical effects to supercede its calamitous parent.

5.1. Targeted triazenes. Interaction of aryldiazonium salts
with amino sugars (73,74) yields triazenes with novel physical
and chemical properties. Baki and Vaughan (75) have explored
the possibility of linking triazene moeities to dextran residues
(DEX) in the hope that the resultant conjugates would be (a)
water soluble; (b) photostable; and (c) more selective.
Conjugates (XLI - XLVII) were prepared and investigated for

activity against M21 tumour cells *in vitro* in comparison with
the monomethyltriazene (II: X = p-CO$_2$Me, R$_1$ = Me, R$_2$ = H). The
most active conjugate was the aryltriazenylalkyldextran (XLI).

(XLI)   DEX-O(CH$_2$)$_2$NH-N=NC$_6$H$_4$-CO$_2$Et(p)

(XLII)   DEX$\diagup^{O}_{O}\diagdown$C=N(CH$_2$)$_6$NH-N=NC$_6$H$_4$-CO$_2$Et(p)

(XLIII) DEX$\diagup^{O}_{O}\diagdown$C=NC$_6$H$_4$CH$_2$C$_6$H$_4$N=N-NMe$_2$

(XLIV)   DEX-NHC$_6$H$_4$CH$_2$C$_6$H$_4$N=N-NMe$_2$

(XLV)   DEX-NHC$_6$H$_4$CH$_2$C$_6$H$_4$N=N-NHMe

(XLVI)   DEX-NHC$_6$H$_4$CH$_2$C$_6$H$_4$N=N-N(Me)CH$_2$OH

(XLVII) DEX-NHC$_6$H$_4$CH$_2$C$_6$H$_4$N=N-N(CH$_2$CH$_2$Cl)$_2$

It is conceivable that the reactive monomethyl metabolite
of DTIC selectively inhibits an enzyme in *de novo* purine
biosynthetic pathways, although such a target enzyme has not yet
been identified. However, the incipient carbenium ion character
of monoalkyltriazenes has been exploited in the design of active-
site-directed irreversible enzyme inhibitors in the Baker mould
(76). The β-D-galactopyranosylmethyltriazene (XLVIII) inhibits
Na$^+$ and Mg^{2+} *E. coli* β-galactosidase (77), the inhibition being
quantitatively associated with attachment of the β-D-galacto-
pyranosylmethyl group to the protein. The monomethyltriazene
(II: X = p-CO$_2$Me, R$_1$ = Me, R$_2$ = H) similarly inhibits hog liver
esterase irreversibly (78).

The enzyme DHFR is an obvious target for drug design. The
dimethyltriazene derived from diethyl 4-aminobenzoyl-L-glutamate
(XLIX) is a very weak inhibitor of DHFR (I$_{50}$ > 10^{-4}M) and the
compound is only moderately effective against the Walker 256
carcinosarcoma (67). Potentially more interesting derivatives
can be prepared based on the 2,4-diaminopyrimidine moeity, which,
in its N-1 protonated form, binds effectively to the enzyme.
Thus, the dimethyltriazene (L) was conceived as a prodrug
designed to undergo metabolic demethylation *in vivo* to afford

a monomethyltriazene (LI) capable of locating and interacting
with the nucleophilic site adjacent to the diaminopyrimidine
binding locus (LII). The dimethyltriazene (L) shows weak
inhibitory activity against the TLX5 lymphoma and P388 tumours
in vivo (79) but the monomethyl analogue is inactive against
these tumours. Interestingly, the monomethyltriazene (LI)
displays untypical stability for a derivative of this class: it
can be recrystallised unchanged from boiling aqueous acetone.

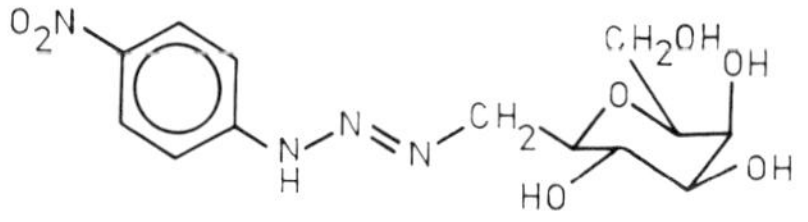

(XLVIII)

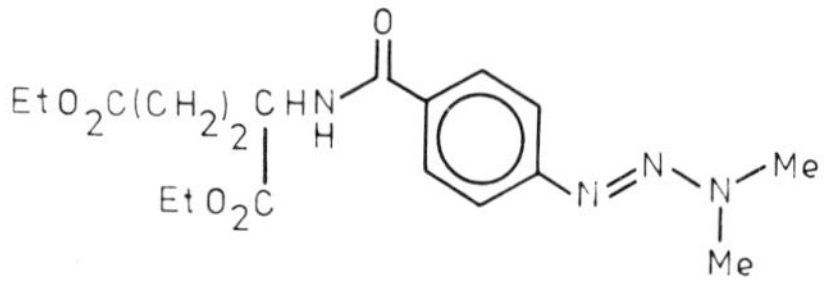

(XLIX)

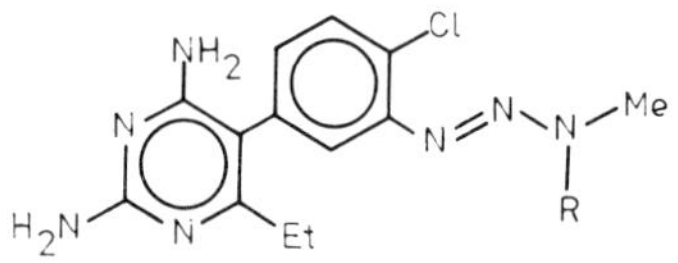

(L) R = Me
(LI) R = H

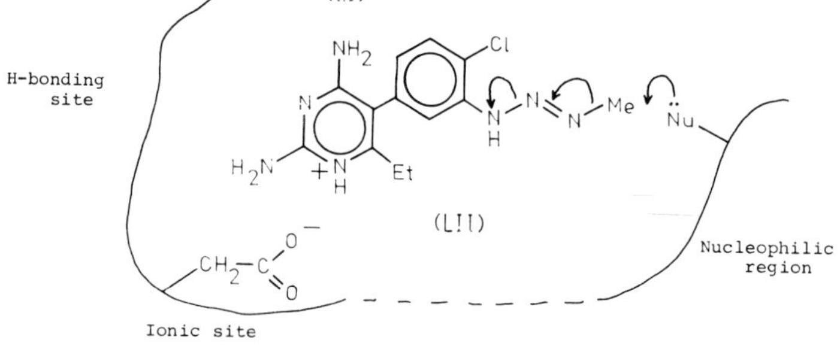

(LII)

H-bonding
site

Nucleophilic
region

Ionic site

DTIC finds its greatest application in the treatment of malignant melanoma (80). In an attempt to design drugs targeted to melanin Lin and Loo (81) prepared triazenes based on halogenated quinolines which exhibit marked affinity for pigmented tissues. With the exception of the derivative (LIII: X = 8-Cl) (% T/C 172) the triazenes were only marginally active,

(LIII)   X = 6-, 7-, or 8-Cl, -Br, or -I

or inactive, against P388, but most showed activity against L1210 comparable to that of DTIC. None of the compounds were active against the B16 melanoma although they exhibited a higher *in vitro* affinity for melanin than did DTIC.

Under normal physiological conditions phenylalanine is metabolised to tyrosine through the agency of the enzyme phenylalanine hydroxylase: tyrosine in turn is a precursor of melanin. Thus the triazenyl-L-phenylalanine derivative (XII) could afford reactive species which might concentrate in melanocytes. Because of its novel chemistry (see Section 2.2) and its pronounced activity against TLX5 lymphoma and L1210 *in vivo*, this triazene is an obvious candidate for further study.

5.2. Lipid-soluble triazenes. Efforts to improve penetration of triazenes into the CNS by incorporating lipophilic groups at various positions in the molecule have not been studied extensively. Although an optimum Log P of ∿ 1.1 is a requirement for activity against L1210 in mice attempts to improve lipid-solubility by incorporating +M methoxy substituents in the aryl moiety [e.g. aryldimethyltriazenes (LIV)] would probably lead to compounds so unstable (see Section 3.1) they would thwart the ingenuity of the most gifted pharmaceutical formulator. A more fruitful approach has been adopted by Wilman and Goddard (82) who prepared an homologous series of water-soluble triazenyl carboxylic acids and showed that activity against the TLX5 lymphoma reached a maximum in the pentyl derivative (LV: $X = CO_2H$). Significantly the corresponding carboxamide (LV: $X = CONH_2$) displays activity against intracerebrally-implanted human astracytoma xenografts (83) in mice and has the added advantage of being photostable.

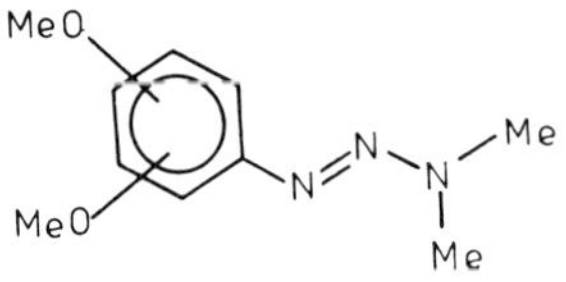

(LIV)

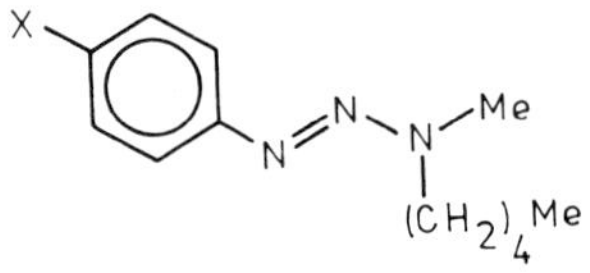

(LV)

$X = CO_2H, CONH_2$

5.3. Organometallic complexes of alkyltriazenes.

The nucleophilic character of alkyltriazenes readily lends itself to the formation of triazenido-metal bonds (7) particularly where the triazenido group acts as a bridging ligand between two metal atoms (LVI). Even the highly unstable 1,3-dimethyltriazene can be successfully complexed with copper (I) to form a novel arrange-ment of four dimethyltriazenido ligands bonded to four copper atoms in a sixteen-membered folded ring system (84). In the complex bis(triphenylphosphine)carbonylrhodiumcopperdimethyl-triazenidochloride (LVII) the three-co-ordinate Cu(I) is directly bonded to the five-co-ordinate Rh(I) with the Cu-Rh donor bond bridged by the triazenido link (85).

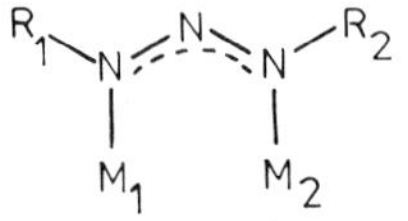

(LVI)

(LVII)

R_1, R_2 = Aryl, alkyl

M_1, M_2 = Metal atoms

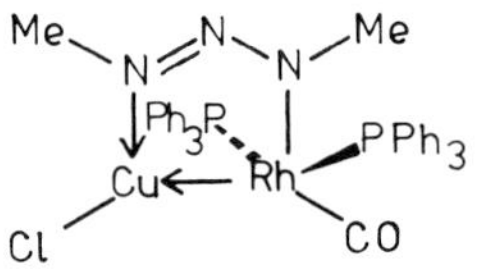

The stability of the molybdenum and tungsten complexes of 1-*p*-chlorophenyl-3-*iso*-propyltriazene in hydrochloric and acetic acids contrasts markedly with the reactivity of the uncomplexed triazene (86). Novel complexes such as these, and others (87, 88)

can be considered as potential drug combinations linking the cytotoxicities of methyltriazenes and transition metals within a stable drug-delivery entity. Although it is difficult to see how such complexes could achieve selectivity towards tumour cells they are structural novelties eminently worthy of biological evaluation.

5.4. DTIC analogues as radiosensitisers or hypoxic cell sensitisers.

The generation of reactive chemical intermediates from DTIC has been discussed in Sections 2.1 and 2.2. The triazene (LVIII) formed by coupling Diazo-IC (III) with 2,2,6,6-tetramethylpiperidine could potentially afford diazonium, diazo, carbene or radical species depending on its route of decomposition. If these species were generated selectively within the hypoxic areas of tumours a new therapeutic rôle for this type of triazene could be envisaged. The tetrasubstituted piperidino-triazene (LVIII) with α-carbon atoms blocked by methyl groups may be advantageous in that it could not be metabolically activated to a mutagenic or carcinogenic alkylating species (58). Similarly, azothioethers of type (LIX) formed by coupling Diazo-IC with thiols (89-91) cannot undergo the normal metabolic degradations of dialkyltriazenes but are potential precursors of a range of reactive chemical species.

(LVIII)

(LIX)

$$R = CH_2CH(NH_2)CO_2H$$
$$CH_2CH_2OH$$
$$CH_2CH_2NH_2$$

6. CONCLUSION

DTIC as a drug has proved to have only marginal efficacy in the clinic. DTIC as a molecule, however, exercises a powerfully addictive hold over many chemists and biochemists. The former will continue to be intrigued by the unique chemistry of the drug and it was the purpose of this chapter to focus their attention on interesting areas for further study. The biochemist determined to unravel the crucial molecular events responsible for antitumour action - if there are any - will be disappointed because the complexities have been detailed but not dispelled. Identification of the *active* chemical species responsible for selective antitumour effects in human disease, and dissection of these effects from the background competing cytotoxicity elicited by other metabolically-generated reactive moeities must be a priority in the future. Only then will enlightened design of a second-generation drug be possible, and only then will it be possible to answer the question: DTIC, a springboard to new antitumour drugs - or a flop?

The author would like to record his gratitude to his colleagues J A Hickman, A Gescher, K Vaughan, R J Simmonds, M D Threadgill and J K Horton whose work and ideas have been freely drawn upon in the production of this chapter.

REFERENCES

1. Schepartz SA. (1976) *Cancer Treatment Reports*, 60, 123-124.
2. Montgomery JA. (1976) *Cancer Treatment Reports*, 60, 125-134.
3. Venditti JM. (1976) *Cancer Treatment Reports*, 60, 135-140.
4. Bono VH. (1976) *Cancer Treatment Reports*, 60, 141-148.
5. Shealy YF. (1970) *J. Pharm. Sci.*, 59, 1533-1558.
6. Stevens MFG (1976) *Progr. Medicin. Chem.*, 13, 205-269.
7. Vaughan K, Stevens MFG. (1978) *Chem. Soc. Rev.*, 7, 377-397.
8. Kreis W. (1977) Cancer, a Comprehensive Treatise. Ed. Becker FF. Plenum Press, Vol. 5, pp. 489-519.
9. Julliard M, Vernin G. (1981) *Bull. Soc. chim. France II*, 150-159.
10. Shealy YF, Krauth CA, Montgomery JA. (1962) *J. Org. Chem.*, 27. 2150-2154.
11. Shealy YF, Struck RF, Holum LB, Montgomery JA. (1961) *J. Org. Chem.*, 26, 2396-2401.

12. Horton JK, Stevens MFG. (1981) *J.C.S. Perkin Trans.I,* 1433-1436.

13. Saunders PP, Schultz GA. (1970) *Biochem.Pharmacol.,* 19, 911-919.

14. Gerulath AH, Ti Li Loo, (1972) *Biochem. Pharmacol.,* 21, 2335-2343.

15. Gerulath AH, Barranco SC, Humphrey RM. (1974) *Cancer Res.,* 34, 1921-1925.

16. Saunders PP, Chao L-Y. (1974) *Cancer Res.,* 34, 2464-2469.

17. Baird GM, Willoughby MLN. (1978) *Lancet,* 681.

18. Shealy YF, Krauth CA, Clayton SJ, Shortnacy AT, Laster WR. (1968) *J. Pharm. Sci.,* 57, 1562-1568.

19. Horton JK, Stevens MFG. (1981) *J. Pharm. Pharmacol.,* 33, 808-811.

20. Mizuno K, Tsujino M, Takada M, Hayashi M, Atsumi K, Asano K, Matsuda T. (1974) *J. Antibiotics,* 27, 775-782.

21. Mizuno K, Yaginuma S, Hayashi M, Takada M, Muto N, (1975) *J. Ferment. Technol.,* 53, 609-619.

22. Ambroz HB, Golding BT, Kemp TJ. (1982) *J.C.S. Chem. Commun.,* 414.

23. Kang UG, Schecter H. (1978) *J. Amer. Chem. Soc.,* 100, 651-652.

24. Bru N, Vilarrasa J. (1980) *Chemistry Letters,* 1489-1492.

25. Rofstad EK, Brustad T, Johannessen JV, Mossige J. (1977) *Br. J. Radiol.,* 50, 314-320.

26. Rauth AM, Mohindra JK.(1981) *Cancer Res.,* 41, 4900-4905.

27. Stevens MFG, Simmonds RJ, Langdon SP. Unpublished results.

28. Pool BL. (1979) *J. Cancer Res. Clin. Oncol.,* 93, 221-231.

29. Hansch C, Smith N, Engle R, Wood H. (1972) *Cancer Chemother. Reports,* 56, 443-456.

30. Hatheway GJ, Hansch C, Kim KH, Milstein SR, Schmidt CL, Smith RN, Quinn FR. (1978) *J. Medicin. Chem.,* 21, 563-574.

31. Edwards SL, Sherfinski JS, Marsh RE. (1974) *J. Amer. Chem. Soc.,* 96, 2593-2597.

32. Kolar GF, Preussmann R. (1971) *Z. Naturforsch. B,* 26, 950-953.

33. Dunn WJ, Greenberg MJ, Callejas SS. (1976) *J. Medicin.Chem.* 19, 1299-1301.

34. Giraldi T, Guarino AM, Nisi C, Sava G. (1980) *Pharmacol. Res. Commun.*, <u>12</u>, 1-11.

35. Sava G, Giraldi T, Lassiani L, Nisi C. (1979) *Cancer Treatment Reports*, <u>63</u>, 93-98.

36. Connors TA, Goddard PM, Merai K, Ross WCJ, Wilman DEV. (1976) *Biochem. Pharmacol.*, <u>25</u>, 241-246.

37. Audette RCS, Connors TA, Mandel HG, Merai K, Ross WCJ. (1973) *Biochem. Pharmacol.*, <u>22</u>, 1855-1864.

38. Puccetti P, Giampietri A, Fioretti MC. (1978) *Experientia*, <u>15</u>, 799-800.

39. Haffner F, Christoffersen T. (1980) *Acta Pharmacol. et Toxicol.*, <u>47</u>, 93-97.

40. Preussmann R, von Hodenberg A, Hengy H. (1969) *Biochem. Pharmacol.*, <u>18</u>, 1-13.

41. Mizuno NS, Decker RW, Zakis B. (1975) *Biochem. Pharmacol.*, <u>24</u>, 615-619.

42. Skibba JL, Ramirez G, Beal DD, Bryan GT. (1970) *Biochem. Pharmacol.*, <u>19</u>, 2043-2051.

43. Hickman JA. (1978) *Biochimie*, <u>60</u>, 997-1002.

44. Hansch C, Hatheway CJ, Quinn FR, Greenberg N. (1978) *J. Medicin. Chem.*, <u>21</u>, 574-577.

45. Giraldi T, Nisi C, Sava G. (1975) *Biochem. Pharmacol.*, <u>24</u>, 1793-1797.

46. Pittillo RF, Schabel FM, Skipper HE. (1970) *Cancer Chemother. Reports*, <u>54</u>, 137-142.

47. Gescher A, Hickman JA, Simmonds RJ, Stevens MFG, Vaughan K. (1981) *Biochem. Pharmacol.*, <u>30</u>, 89-93.

48. Farina P, Gescher A, Hickman JA, Horton JK, D'Incalci M, Ross D, Stevens MFG, Torti L. *Biochem. Pharmacol.*, in press

49. Gescher A, Hickman JA, Simmonds RJ, Stevens MFG, Vaughan K. (1978) *Tetrahedron Letters*, 5041-5044.

50. Julliard M, Vernin G, Metzger J. (1980) *Synthesis*, 116-117.

51. Horton JK, Stevens MFG. Unpublished results.

52. H. Zollinger. (1961) Diazo and Azo Chemistry. Interscience New York, p.185.

53. Hickman JA, Simmonds RJ, Kolar GF, (1980) *Brit. J. Cancer*, <u>142</u>, 170.

54. Hickman JA. Unpublished results.

55. Kolar GF, Carubelli R. (1979) *Cancer Letters*, *7*, 209-214.

56. Kolar GF, Maurer M, Wildschütte. (1980) *Cancer Letters*, *10*, 235-241.

57. Ti Li Loo, Luce JK, Jardine JH, Frei E. (1968) *Cancer Res.*, *28*, 2448-2453.

58. Stevens MFG, Gescher A, Turnbull CP. (1979) *Biochem Pharmacol.*, *28*, 769-776.

59. Schwalbe CH, Simmonds RJ. Unpublished work.

60. Akhtar MH, McDaniel RS, Feser M, Oehlschlager AC. (1968) *Tetrahedron*, *24*, 3899-3906.

61. Hopfinger AJ, Potenzone R. (1982) *Mol. Pharmacol.*, *21*, 187-195.

62. Gescher A, Hickman JA, Stevens MFG. (1979) *Biochem. Pharmacol.*, *28*, 3235-3238.

63. Lassiani L, Nisi C, Sigon F, Sava G, Giraldi T. (1980) *J. Pharm. Sci.*, *69*, 1098-1099.

64. Clarke DA, Phillips FS, Sternberg SS, Barclay RK, Stock CC. (1953) *Proc. Soc. Exp. Biol. Med.*, *84*, 203-207.

65. Horton JK, Farina P, Gescher A, Hickman JA, Stevens MFG. *Br. J. Cancer*, in press.

66. Weinkam RJ, Shiba DA. (1978) *Life Sciences*, *22*, 937-946.

67. Ionescu D, Neagu V, Dobre V, Niculescu-Duvaz I. (1981) *Neoplasma*, *28*, 19-26.

68. Noyanalpan N, Özden S, Özden T. (1977) *Ankara Ecz. Fak. Mec.*, *7*, 104-110.

69. Giraldi T, Nisi C, Connors TA, Goddard PM. (1977) *J. Medicin. Chem.*, *20*, 850-853.

70. Dunn WJ, Greenberg MJ. (1977) *J. Pharm. Sci.*, *66*, 1416-1419.

71. Giraldi T, Goddard PM, Nisi C, Sigon F. (1980) *J. Pharm. Sci.*, *69*, 97-98.

72. Cowan DH, Bergsagel DE. (1971) *Cancer Chemother. Reports*, *55*, 175-181.

73. Tronchet JMJ, Rachidzadeh F. (1979) *Helv. Chim. Acta*, *62*, 971-977.

74. Larm O, Larsson K, Wannong M. (1977) *Acta Chem. Scand.*, *B31*, 475-478.

75. Baki Av, Vaughan K. *Carbohydrate Res.*, in press.

76. Baker BR. (1967) Design of Active-Site-Directed Irreversible Enzyme Inhibitors. John Wiley and Sons, Inc., New York.

77. Sinnott ML, Smith PJ. (1976) *J.C.S. Chem. Commun.*, 223-224.

78. Godin JRP, Llanos G, Vaughan K, Renton KW. (1981) *Can. J. Physiol. Pharmacol.*, 59, 1239-1244.

79. Stevens MFG. Unpublished results.

80. Comis RL. (1976) *Cancer Treatment Reports*. 60, 165-176.

81. Lin AJ, Ti Li Loo. (1978) *J. Medicin. Chem.*, 21, 268-272.

82. Wilman DEV, Goddard PM. (1980) *J. Medicin. Chem.*, 23, 1052-1054.

83. Wilman DEV. Personal communication.

84. O'Connor JE, Janusonis GA, Corey ER. (1968) *Chem. Commun.*, 445-446.

85. Kuyper J, Van Vliet PI, Vrieze K. (1975) *J. Organometallic Chem.*, 96, 289-299.

86. Pfeiffer E, Kuyper J, Vrieze K. (1976) *J. Organometallic Chem.*, 105, 371-378.

87. Kuyper J, Van Vliet PI, Vrieze K. (1976) *J. Organometallic Chem.*, 105, 379-387.

88. Van Vliet PI, Kuyper J, Vrieze K. (1976) *J. Organometallic Chem.*, 122, 99-111.

89. Iwata H, Yamamoto I, Muraki K. (1969) *Biochem. Pharmacol.*, 18, 955-956.

90. Iwata H, Yamamoto, Gohda E, Morita K, Nishino K. (1972) *Biochem. Pharmacol.*, 21, 2141-2144.

91. Iwata H, Yamamoto I, Gohda E. (1973) *Biochem. Pharmacol.*, 22, 1845-1854.

NITROSOUREAS

J.A. MONTGOMERY

INTRODUCTION

An understanding of the chemistry of the nitrosoureas is essential to an
understanding of their biologic activity, although their chemistry alone certainly does not explain their apparent specificity for neoplastic cells and the
resulting anticancer activity they display against both experimental animal neo-
plasms and human cancers. A variety of N-nitroso compounds with chemistry similar to that of the N-nitrosoureas show no anticancer activity (Table 1) even
though some of them are quite toxic, mutagenic, or carcinogenic and therefore
biologically active.[1] At the same time, none of the precursors of N-nitroso
compounds, including the ureas, are particularly active biologically, clearly
indicating the necessity for the N-nitroso group. Introduction of the N-nitroso
group labilizes the bond between the nitrosated nitrogen and the adjacent atom,
so that when the adjacent atom is a carbon double bonded to a heteroatom decomposition occurs spontaneously in aqueous media, the rate depending on the particular structure and the pH of the medium.[2,3] Breakage of this bond, regardless of the exact mechanism, gives rise to a diazotate (Fig. 1) capable of alkylating biologic molecules such as DNA under physiologic conditions of pH, ionic

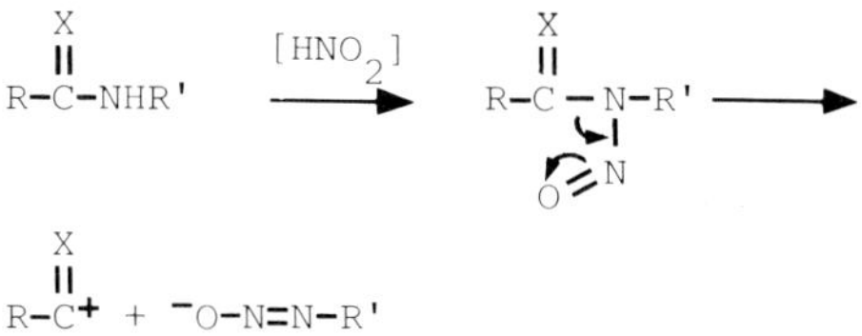

$$R-\overset{\overset{\displaystyle X}{\|}}{C}-NHR' \xrightarrow{[HNO_2]} R-\overset{\overset{\displaystyle X}{\|}}{C}-N-R' \longrightarrow$$

$$R-\overset{\overset{\displaystyle X}{\|}}{C}{}^{+} + {}^{-}O-N{\equiv}N-R'$$

Figure 1

strength, and temperature. In the case of the N-nitrosoureas the reaction may
be initiated by loss of a proton from the unnitrosated nitrogen (Fig. 2). In
support of this mechanism is the stability of the trisubstituted N-nitrosoureas,
which are not toxic to cells in culture and must be metabolized — dealkylating
in the liver — to show in vivo activity.[4] In the case of N-methyl-N-nitroso-

D.N. Reinhoudt, T.A. Connors, H.M. Pinedo & K.W. van de Poll (eds.), Structure-Activity Relationships of Anti-Tumour Agents.
© 1983, Martinus Nijhoff Publishers, The Hague/Boston/London. ISBN 90-247-2783-9.

Table I. Activity of Various N-Nitroso Compounds vs. Leukemia L1210 (10^5 cells, i.p.)

RN(NO)R'		Dose	Treatment	
R	R'	mg/kg/dose	Schedule	% ILS[a]
$H_2NC(=NH)-$	Me		Chronic	Inactiv
$O_2NHNC(=NH)-$	Me	16	Chronic	30
H_2NCO-	Me	12	Chronic	109
MeHNCS—	Me		Chronic	Inactiv
EtO_2C-	Me		Chronic	Inactiv
Me	Me		Chronic	Inactiv
$MeSO_2$	Me		Chronic	Inactiv
R''[f]	SO_2Me		Chronic	Inactiv
$O_2NHNC(=NH)-$	$(CH_2)_2Cl$	20	Chronic	189
R''HNCO—	$(CH_2)_2Cl$		Day 1	10/1
EtO_2C-	$(CH_2)_2Cl$		Chronic	Inactiv
R''CO—	$(CH_2)_2Cl$		Chronic	I to 65
$MeC_6H_4SO_2HNCO-$	$(CH_2)_2Cl$		Day 1	4/6
$MeC_6H_4SO_2-$	$(CH_2)_2Cl$		Chronic	I

[a] Increase in lifespan.
[b] Toxic.
[c] Carcinogenic.
[d] Cures/total number of animals.
[e] Highly toxic.
[f] R'' = alkyl

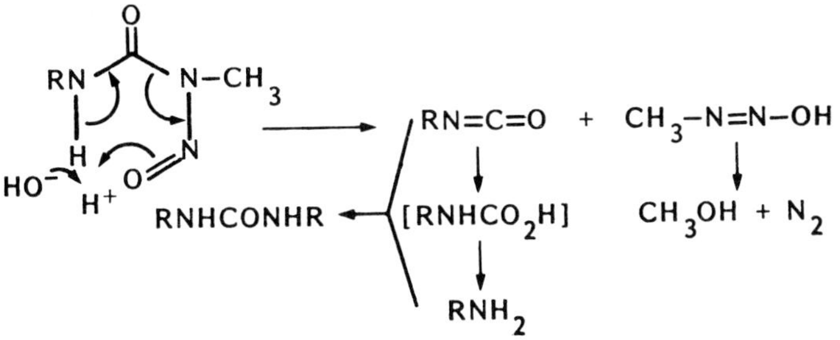

Figure 2. The Aqueous Decomposition of N-Methyl-N-Nitrosoureas

urea, the first nitrosourea found to have anticancer activity, this decomposition leads to methyldiazotate and isocyanic acid, compounds capable of methylating and carbamoylating biological macromolecules. Other N-nitroso compounds such as N-nitrosoamides and N-nitrosourethanes that produce alkylating moieties but not carbamoylating moieties have little or no anticancer activity (Table 1). At the same time, certain nitrosoureas that have little carbamoylating activity are quite active,[5] but nitrosoureas with no detectable alkylating activity are very weakly active or inactive (Table 2). Thus alkylating activity, but not carbamoylating activity, appears to be essential, although there is not a straight line correlation between alkylating and anticancer activity.[6,7] Carbamoylation has been associated with the inhibition by the nitrosoureas of the repair of DNA damaged by ionizing radiation or by alkylating agents[8,9] and thus may indirectly contribute to the cytotoxicity and anticancer activity of these compounds.

The data in Table 2 also show that the most active nitrosoureas in the L1210 system contain either the N-methyl-N-nitrosoureido or the N-(2-haloethyl)-N-nitrosoureido function. Table 3 compares these two structural types: the methyl vs. the 2-chloro- or 2-fluoroethyl. The 2-haloethyl compounds are two to twenty times as toxic as the methyl compounds, but are much more active against leukemia L1210, giving 50 to 100% cures with a single injection. The methyl compounds are two to nine times as stable and have only one-tenth to one-seventieth as much alkylating activity. The carbamoylating activity is more dependent on the nature of R than R'. The data also support the idea that alkylation is the most important factor to activity, with the 2-haloalkyl compounds being the best alkylating agents. The problem is more complicated than that, however, because the chemistry of the 2-haloalkyl compounds is more complex (Fig. 3), due to the lability of the carbon-halogen bond (Br > Cl > F). Kohn[10,11] has proposed that a two-step crosslinking of DNA (Fig. 4) is impor-

Table 2. The Relationship of Activity to Structure and Chemical Properties of Nitrosoureas

RNHCON(NO)R'		Leukemia L1210[a]		$T\frac{1}{2}$, min.	Alkylating Activity, A_{540}	Carbamoylating Activity dpm
R	R'	LD_{10} or OD (mg/kg) Single Dose	% ILS			
H	Me	12[b]	109	7.0	0.36	10,890
C_6H_{11}	Me	300	27	486	0.016	19,800
$(CH_2)_2Cl$	Me	150[b]	46	254	0.020	8,850
glucos-2-yl	Et	---	1[c]	46	ca. 0	low
Et	Et	400	44	202	0	13,730
$NC(CH_2)_2$	$(CH_2)_2CN$	150	55	32	0.04	7,000
C_6H_{11}	C_6H_{11}	---	1	5.6	0	36,540
$ClCH_2(Et)CH$	$CH(Et)CH_2Cl$	---	1	15	0.3	25,140
$ClCH(Me)CH_2$	$CH_2(Me)CHCl$	1000	140	41	0.04	10,290
C_6H_{11}	$CH_2(Me)CHCl$	750	87	53	0.013	26,270
R	$(CH_2)_2F$	6 – 89	Curative	9 – 68	0.6 to >3	0 – 49,000
R	$(CH_2)_2Cl$	4 – 600	Curative	1.3 – 61	0.3 to >3	800 – 42,000
R	$(CH_2)_2Br$	200 – 300	Curative	---	---	---
R	$(CH_2)_2I$	---	1	---	---	---

[a] 10^5 Cells, i.p.
[b] Chronic treatment.
[c] Inactive.

Table 3. Comparisons of N-Methyl- and N-(2-Haloethyl)-N-nitrosoureas

R	R'	Schedule	LD$_{10}$ or OD[a]	% ILS	Cures[b]	T$\frac{1}{2}$[c], min.	Alkylating Activity A$_{540}$[d]	Carbamoylating Activity dpm[e]
H	Me	Chronic	12	109	0	7.0	0.36	10,890
	⌒⌒Cl	Chronic	0.90	147	5–10[f]	1.3	3.0	8,560
⌒⌒X	Me	Chronic	150	46	0	250	0.02	8,850
	⌒⌒Cl	Chronic	8.0	187	5–10[f]	43	1.4	28,700
	⌒⌒F	Day 1	12	233	8	N.D.	1.3	19,800
	Me	Day 1	300	27	0	490	0.02	19,800
(cyclohexyl)	⌒⌒Cl	Day 1	48	---	10	53	0.52	42,000
	⌒⌒F	Day 1	34	---	5–10	68	0.64	49,100
(glucopyranosyl: HO, OH, OH, O ring)	Me	qd 1–9[g]	50	31		48	0.19	1,630
	⌒⌒Cl	Day 1	29	---	9	21	2.4	820
	⌒⌒F							

Leukemia L1210 (10^5 cells, i.p.)

[a] Optimal dose.

[b] Out of 10 treated animals.

[c] Half life.

[d] A$_{540}$ is a measure of concentration of alkylated 4-(p-nitrobenzyl)pyridine in an ethyl acetate extract of a mixture of the nitrosourea and the pyridine in acetate buffer (pH 6) incubated at 37° for 2 hours.

[e] The dpm is a measure of radioactivity present in unidentified reaction products obtained upon incubation of the nitrosourea with lysine-^{14}C in phosphate buffer (pH 7.4) at 37° for 6 hours.

[f] Cures from a single injection on day 1.

[g] Optimal schedule.

$$\log 1/C = -0.13\ (\pm0.07)\ \log P\ -0.014\ (\pm0.015)\ (\log P)_2\ -0.76\ (\pm0.15)\ I_1\ +0.33\ (\pm0.17)\ I_2\ -0.24\ (\pm0.11)\ I_3\ +1.78\ (\pm0.09)$$

$$n = 90;\ r = 0.868;\ s = 0.206;\ \log P_0 = -4.4\ (\pm8)$$

$$\log 1/LD_{10} = -0.041\ (\pm0.007)\ (\log P)^2\ -0.62\ (\pm0.15)\ I_1\ +1.01\ (\pm0.06)$$

$$n = 96;\ r = 0.829,\ s = 0.221,\ \log P_0 = 0\ (\pm8)$$

C = mol/kg of $RNHCON(NO)(CH_2)_2X$ required to kill 3 logs (99.9%) of L1210 leukemia cells (10^5 cells, i.p.; single dose drug, i.p.)

LD_{10} = dose that kills 10% of treated animals calculated from log-probit plots.

I_1 is assigned the value of 1 for nine cases of α-substitution on R

I_2 is given the value of 1 for thioethers

I_3 takes the value of 1 for X = F and O for Cl

Equations

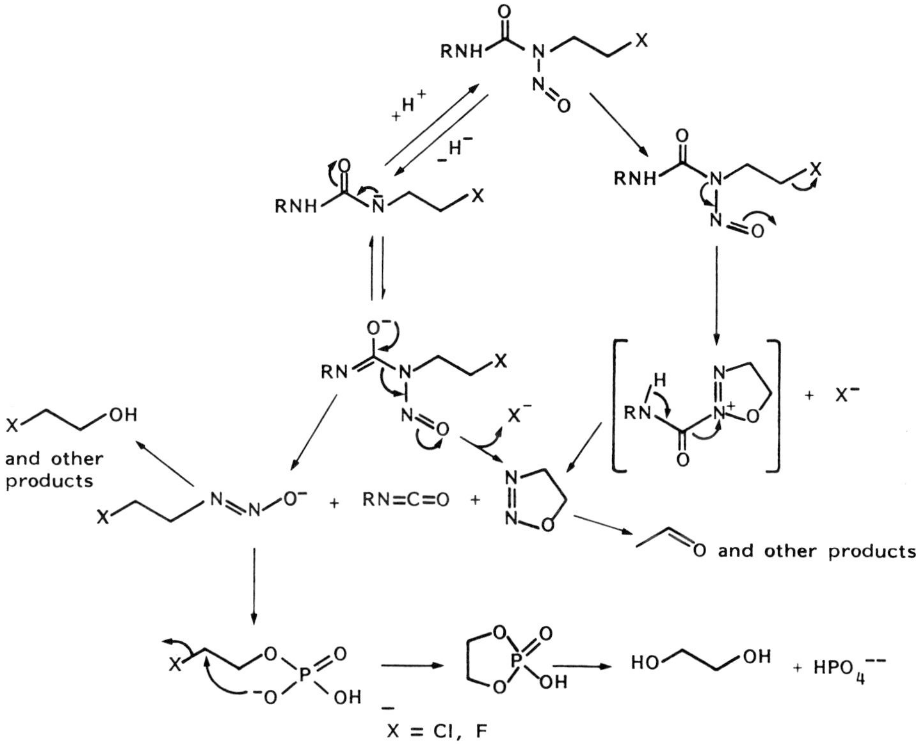

Figure 3.   The Aqueous Decomposition of the 2-Haloethylnitrosoureas

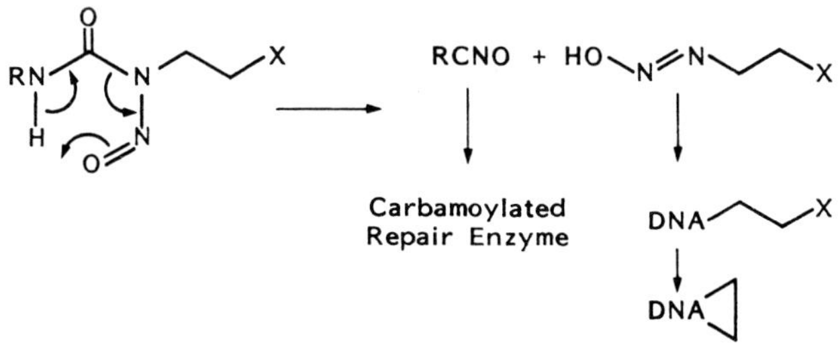

Figure 4.   The Important Reactions of the 2-Haloethylnitrosoureas

tant to the high level of anticancer activity of these compounds. This cross-
linking could occur by initial attack of the (2-haloethyl)diazotate on O^6 of a
guanine residue followed by displacement of the reactive halogen[12] by a nitrogen of a cytosine residue. Some evidence for the G-C crosslink has been
obtained.[13]

From a comprehensive study of 96 2-haloethyl nitrosoureas Hansch et al.[14]
derived equations relating activity, as judged by a 3-log kill of L1210 cells
in vivo, and toxicity, LD_{10}, to log P. Although the $\underline{r}$ and $\underline{s}$ values are reason
ably good for a study of this magnitude, no confidence limits could be placed
log P_0 for either activity or toxicity and, thus, there is no clear separation
of toxicity from activity as might be hoped. The most active compounds are al
the most toxic compounds, but at the same time they have the greatest therapeutic index. Furthermore, there is a log P_0 range for maximum activity even
though it is fairly broad.

SYNTHESIS

Most of the nitrosoureas that we have studied have been prepared by the
nitrosation of the corresponding ureas using anhydrous sodium nitrite, dinitro
gen trioxide, or dinitrogen tetraoxide; in most cases they were used in the
presence of an acid, hydrochloric, sulfuric, or undiluted formic (Fig. 5).

RNCO   + H_2NR' ⟶ RNHCONHR' ⟶ RN(NO)CONHR' + RNHCON(NO)R'
   or
RNHCON(NO)R''

Figure 5

These combinations generate the true nitrosating agents in situ: nitrous acid
nitrosyl chloride, and formyl nitrite.[1] The ureas to be nitrosated were prepared by the reaction of an isocyanate, usually methyl or 2-chloroethyl, with
amine. In some cases the isocyanate was generated in situ from the appropriat
nitrosourea. For example, N'-(2-chloroethyl)-N-methyl-N-nitrosourea is a good
source of 2-chloroethyl isocyanate. The method, however, has limitations: (a
sometimes mixtures of the undesired isomer is obtained, (b) functional groups
can interfere, and (c) some of the nitrosoureas formed are unstable in acid
media. To avoid these problems, and to make use of commercially available 2-
fluoroethylamine hydrochloride, we have applied the method of Kimura[15] to the
synthesis of the fluoro analogs of some highly active 2-chloroethylnitrosoure
such as chlorozotocin and PCNU (Fig. 6). Perhaps the most satisfactory

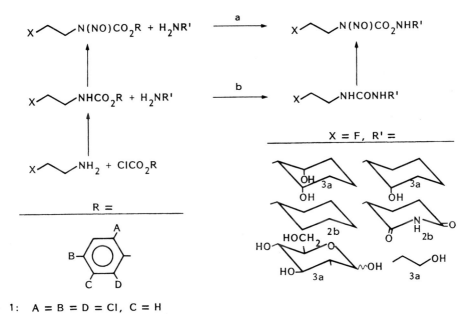

$$X \diagdown NHCO_2R + ClCO_2R$$

R =

1: A = B = D = Cl, C = H
2: A = B = C = Cl, D = H
3: A = NO_2, B = C = D = H
4: B = NO_2, A = C = D = H

Figure 6

activated urethane for this purpose is the 2,4,6-trichlorophenyl compound, which has also been used for the purpose by J. L. Imbach.[16]

RECENT BIOLOGICAL STUDIES

Interest in the 2-fluoroethylnitrosoureas was stimulated by the finding that, although the activity of these compounds is comparable to that of the 2-chloroethyl compounds (Table 4), the fluoroethyl compounds crosslink DNA poorly,[10,11] a result of the greater stability of the carbon-fluorine bond. I addition, the log P values are about 0.6 lower, meaning they are more hydrophilic. An examination of the chemical properties of fluoro and the chloro compounds shows little difference in half-life, alkylating activity, or carbamoylating activity, the alkylating activity being a measure of the reactivit of the (2-haloethyl)diazotates (Table 5).

There is, however, a significant difference in the toxicity of the fluoro and the chloro compounds, not in LD_{10} values, which are greater in some cases for the chloro compounds and in other cases for the fluoro compounds, but in median day of death, which varies from 6 to 27 days for the chloro compounds and from 2-5 days for the fluoro compounds (Table 6). This difference suggest fluoroacetate toxicity, since a significant amount of the fluoro compounds decomposes to 2-fluoroethanol,[2,3] which is readily oxidized via alcohol dehydr genase to fluoroacetate.[17] Sodium acetate in aqueous ethanol, which has been shown to reverse fluoroacetate toxicity in mice,[18] given 10 minutes after a single dose of N-cyclohexyl-N'-(2-fluoroethyl)-N'-nitrosourea (CFNU) raised it LD_{10} from 50 to 160 mg/kg (Table 7), but enhancement of its effectiveness against leukemia L1210 could not be demonstrated because the maximum tolerated dose of CFNU alone cured 10/10 animals (Table 8). Fluoroacetate toxicity reve sal and activity enhancement was observed in the treatment of SC B16 **melanoma** with the acetate of N-(2-fluoroethyl)-N'-[trans-4-(hydroxymethyl)cyclohexyl]-N nitrosourea and sodium acetate in aqueous ethanol (Table 9).

The kinetics of cell killing by the nitrosoureas, like that of other alkylating agents, is pseudo first order since the drug is always present in large excess (Fig. 7b). There is a small difference in the responsiveness of restir cells with dividing cells being two to three times as sensitive (Fig. 7A). Cells are essentially equisensitive in all phases of the cell cycle and cell killing is rapid. This behavior is in contrast to that of the antimetabolites such as 1-β-D-arabinofuranosylcytosine (ara-C), the cell killing by which is, above a certain minimum concentration, concentration dependent (Fig. 8).

Table 4. N-2-(Haloethyl)-N-nitrosoureas vs. Leukemia L1210
(i.p. 10⁵ cells, i.p. single dose)

RNHCON(NO)⁓X

R	LD₁₀, mmol/kg		ED₅₀, mmol/kg		LD₁₀/ED₅₀		Log 1/C		Log P	
X =	Cl	F	Cl	F	Cl	F	Cl	F	Cl	F
(structure)	0.19	0.043	0.093	0.036	2.0	1.2	1.0	1.5	1.5	0.33
Me (structure)	0.16	0.21	0.13	0.16	1.3	1.2	0.80	0.89	2.8	2.2
Et (structure)	0.17	0.19	0.073	0.11	2.3	1.7	1.1	0.97	3.3	2.7
(structure)	0.36	0.31	0.12	--	3.0	--	0.93	--	3.8	3.2
(structure)	0.26	0.28	0.11	0.14	2.4	2.0	0.96	0.87	3.0	2.4
(structure)	0.22	0.26	0.19	--	1.2	--	0.72	--	3.6	3.0
AcO (structure)	0.15	0.13	0.062	0.065	2.4	2.0	1.2	1.2	2.6	2.0
AcOH₂C (structure)	0.095	0.20	0.048	0.16	2.0	1.3	1.3	0.81	3.1	2.5
HO₂C (structure)	0.10	0.21	0.060	--	1.7	--	1.2	--	-1.1	-1.7
S (structure)	0.056	0.15	0.032	0.068	1.8	2.2	1.5	1.2	2.1	1.4
O₂S (structure)	0.060	0.12	0.029	0.037	2.1	3.2	1.5	1.4	0.19	-0.41
O₂S (structure)	0.14	0.24	0.026	0.088	5.4	2.7	1.6	1.1	-0.90	-1.5

Table 5. Some Properties of the N-(2-Haloethyl)-N-nitrosoureas[a]

RNHCON(NO)⌒X   X =

R	$T_{\frac{1}{2}}$		Alkylating Activity		Carbamoylating Activity	
	Cl	F	Cl	F	Cl	F
Me	100	128	100	123	100	117
Et	100	111	100	117	91	117
(S)	102	104	81	109	72	76
(O₂S)	62	64	350	403	33	32
(O₂S / SO₂)	42	36	456	> 577	27	26
(ring S)	15	17	> 577	> 577	0	0
(benzothiopyran)	116	113	256	354	37	41
X	81	---	266	242	68	47

[a]Expressed as % of the values for CCNU.

Table 6. Toxicity of Haloethylnitrosoureas

$RNHCON(NO)\sim X$

R	X =	Single Dose LD$_{10}$ (mg/kg)		Multiple of LD$_{10}$, Range		% Deaths		Median Day of Death	
		CI	F	CI	F	CI	F	CI	F
X~		41	8	1.1 – 2.4	1.3 – 3.2	30 – 100	40 – 100	6 – 10	2 – 4
Me		57	34	1.0 – 2.9	1.0 – 3.0	10 – 100	30 – 100	8 – 24	2 – 3
Et		44	42	1.3 – 3.3	1.4 – 3.1	30 – 100	30 – 100	7 – 27	2 – 3
HO_2C		94	75	1.6 – 4.0	1.2 – 5.0	40 – 100	10 – 100	6 – 7	2 – 5
HO_2C		27	56	1.1 – 3.4	1.2 – 1.8	60 – 100	30 – 80	7 – 22	4 – 4
AcO		26	29	1.2 – 2.4	1.6 – 3.4	30 – 100	40 – 50	7 – 20	4 – 4
S		45	36	1.7 – 5.6	1.0 – 3.4	60 – 100	10 – 100	6 – 16	2 – 2
S–S		14	35	1.1 – 3.3	1.0 – 2.3	0 – 100	10 – 100	7 – 8	3 – 4
O_2S		23	40	1.3 – 4.0	1.2 – 2.3	40 – 100	20 – 70	6 – 12	2 – 4
O_2S		17	32	1.2 – 2.7	1.2 – 1.8	70 – 100	35 – 100	7 – 12	5 – 2

Table 7. Reversal of Fluoroacetate Toxicity of
N-Cyclohexyl-N'-(2-fluoroethyl)-N'-nitrosourea (CFNU)

Single Dose (mg/kg)	Drug Alone		+NaAc (2 min. post)[a]		+NaAc (10 min. post)[a]	
	Deaths	Median Day of Death	Deaths	Median Day of Death	Deaths	Median Day of Death
500			10/10	2	10/10	2
400			10/10	2	10/10	2
300			10/10	2.5	10/10	5
200			10/10	2.5	10/10	6
112.5	10/10	2				
100		2	8/10	15	1/10	(29)
75	9/10	2				
50	9/10	2	5/10	16	0/10	––
33	0/10	–				
22	0/10	–				
	LD_{10} = ca. 50		LD_{10} = 120		LD_{10} = 160	

(Previously determined LD_{10}: 34)

[a] In ethanol-water. No toxicity reversal in water alone.

Table 8.   The Effect of Sodium Acetate Toxicity Reversal
on the Antileukemic Activity of CFNU[a]

Dose	Median Day of Death	% ILS	30-Day Survivors/ Total
0	7	--	0/10
50	2	Toxic	0/10
33	--	--	10/10
22	14	100	1/10
300[b]	2	Toxic	0/10
200[b]	6	-15	1/10
100[b]	16.5	135	8/10
50[b]	19.5	178	6/10
300[c]	2	Toxic	0/10
200[c]	7	0	0/10
100[c]	19	171	9/10
50[c]	15	114	9/10

[a] 10^5 L1210 Leukemia cell implanted IV with a single intraperitoneal injection of drug on day one.

[b] 65 mg Sodium acetate in 0.032 ml EtOH administered 2 min. post injection of drug.

[c] Administered 10 min. post injection.

Table 9. Treatment of SC B16 Melanoma with
the Acetate of Trans-N-(2-Fluoroethyl)-N'-
[4-(hydroxymethyl)cyclohexyl]-
N-nitrosourea[a]

Dose	Toxicity Control Survivors	% ILS	T-C (Days)
144	0/6	-79	--
+NaAc	2/6	89	22
108	1/6	-79	--
+NaAc	6/6	81	18
72	6/6	-63	--
+NaAc	6/6	116	16
48	4/6	83	19
+NaAc	6/6	62	7
32	6/6	56	6
+NaAc	6/6	13	3

[a]Treatment day 2 postimplant followed by
sodium acetate in ethanol 10 min. later;
calcd. LD_{10} = 42 mg/kg; with sodium
acetate 120 mg/kg.

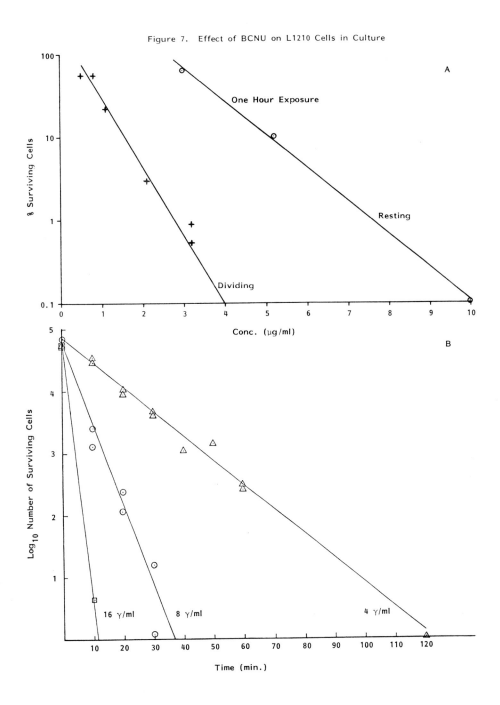

Figure 7.   Effect of BCNU on L1210 Cells in Culture

236

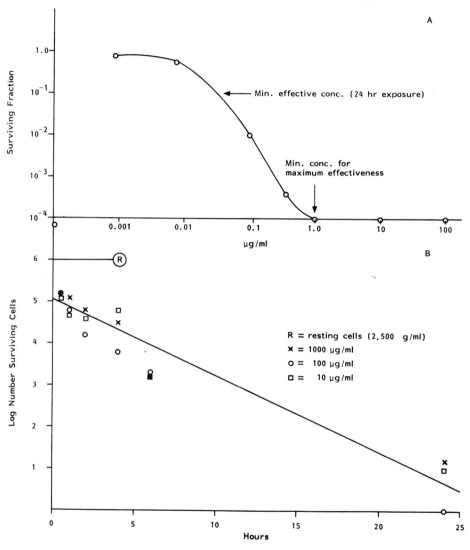

Figure 8. Effect of Ara-C on L1210 Cells in Culture

Table 10. Schedule Dependency in the L1210 Leukemia System

% ILS (Cures/Treated)[a]

	Single Dose, Day 2	q3h × 8, Days 2, 6, 10, and 14	qd 2-16	q2d, 2-16 Days	q4d, Days 2, 6, 10, and 14
BCNU	>100 (40/50)[b]	>100 (12/30)	50 (1/20)	>100 (5/10)	>100 (6/10)
CCNU	>100 (357/425)[b]	>100 (6/60)	33 (0/10)	>100 (5/10)	>100 (18/40)
Cyclophosphamide	>100 (44/79)[b]	20 (0/10)	38 (0/30)	60 (0/10)	>100 (0/10)
Daunomycin	33 (0/10)	25 (0/30)	27 (0/10)	16 (0/10)	33 (0/10)
Methotrexate	50 (0/30)	69 (0/30)	>100 (0/120)[b]	>100 (0/30)[b]	>100 (0/80)[b]
6-Mercaptopurine	39 (0/20)	46 (0/20)	60 (0/80)[b]	33 (0/10)	44 (0/10)
5-Fluorouracil	50 (0/20)	100 (0/30)	>100 (0/20)[b]	>100 (0/20)[b]	83 (0/10)
Ara-C	59 (0/20)	>100 (135/155)[b]	>100 (0/100)	>100 (0/20)	>100 (0/10)

[a]Median % increase in life span (excluding survivors) and cure rate for highest nontoxic dose for each schedule.

[b]Optimal schedule.

238

Ara-C is an S-phase specific agent requiring long exposure relative to BCNU for maximum cell kill. These differences are the basis for the schedule dependency of these agents in the treatment of mice inoculated with L1210 leukemia (Table 10). The nitrosoureas are most effective when given as a single dose, whereas ara-C must be given every three hours to realize its potential. Other antimetabolites, such as methotrexate, 6-mercaptopurine, and 5-fluorouracil, are maximally effective on a daily or every other day schedule.

REFERENCES

1. Montgomery JA. 1976. Cancer Treat. Rep. 60, 651-664.
2. Montgomery JA, James R, McCaleb GS, Johnston TP. 1967. J. Med. Chem. 10, 668-674.
3. Montgomery JA, James R, McCaleb GS, Kirk MC, Johnston TP. 1975. J. Med. Chem. 18, 568-571.
4. Cowens W, Brundrett R, Colvin M. 1975. Proc. Am. Assoc. Cancer Res. and ASCO 1975, 16, 100.
5. Johnston TP, McCaleb GS, Montgomery JA. 1975. J. Med. Chem. 18, 104-106.
6. Wheeler GP, Chumley S. 1967. J. Med. Chem. 10, 259-260.
7. Wheeler GP, Bowdon BJ, Grimsley JA, Lloyd HH. 1974. Cancer Res. 34, 194-200.
8. Kann Jr. HE, Schott MA, Petkas A. 1980. Cancer Res. 10, 50-55.
9. Kann Jr. HE, Blumenstein BA, Pethas A, Schott MA. 1980. Cancer Res. 40, 771-775.
10. Kohn KW. 1977. Cancer Res. 37, 1450-1454.
11. Ewig RAG, Kohn KW. 1977. Cancer Res. 37, 2114-2122.
12. Piper JR, Laseter AG, Johnston TP, Montgomery, JA. 1980. J. Med. Chem. 23, 1136-1139.
13. Ludlum D, personal communication.
14. Hansch C, Leo A. Schmidt C. Jow PYC, Montgomery JA. 1980. J. Med. Chem. 23, 1095-1101.
15. Kimura G. 1979. U.S. Patent 4,156,777.
16. Imbach JL, personal communication.
17. Williams RT. 1959. Detoxification Mechanisms, New York, John Wiley & Sons.
18. Tourllotte WW, Coon JM. 1949. Federation Proc. 8, 339.

OXAZAPHOSPHORINE CYTOSTATICS: STRUCTURE—ACTIVITY RELATIONSHIPS, SELECTIVITY AND METABOLISM, REGIONAL DETOXIFICATION*

N. BROCK

"Die idee ist nicnt so ohnmächtig,
es nur bis zur idee zu bringen"

G.W.F. Hegel

1. TRANSPORT FORM AND ACTIVE FORM AS A THERAPEUTIC PRINCIPLE IN THE CHEMOTHERAPY OF CANCER (1)

Progress in the field of chemotherapy of cancer depends decisively on whether we succeed in developing compounds with a higher selectivity of the antitumoral action and thus with a greater therapeutic range, i.e., less dangerous in clinical use. This has been the guiding principle in the work of the Asta research teams for over 30 years.

It all started with an idea. It was suggested by DRUCKREY (2) that a highly reactive drug should be administered not as an active compound but in a chemically masked, inactive "transport form". The compound should be so designed that it is transformed into the active form in the body and, if possible, preferentially in the tumour cells.

> We use the term "transport form" to designate compounds which are largely inactive pharmacologically and which are transformed by a metabolic process or at least by an enzymatically catalysed reaction before they develop a biological activity. We use the term "active form" (ultimate cytotoxic agent) to describe those compounds which react with the biological substrate spontaneously and directly. The biotransformation of the transport form into the active form may entail various intermediate products (metabolites), the properties of which are of decisive importance in shaping the profile of action of the drug. The structural identification and the pharmacological and pharmacokinetic characterisation of these metabolites are therefore of great importance for understanding the metabolism and the mechanism of action of the drug.

The first drug developed in the Asta Research Laboratories specifically

---

* Dedicated to Prof. Dr. Herbert Oelschläger for his 60th birthday. This work was supported by the Bundesministerium für Forschung und Technologie, Bonn.

D.N. Reinhoudt, T.A. Connors, H.M. Pinedo & K.W. van de Poll (eds.), Structure-Activity Relationships of Anti-Tumour Agents.
© 1983, Martinus Nijhoff Publishers, The Hague/Boston/London. ISBN 90-247-2783-9.

on the principle "transport form - active form" was fosfestrol (stilboestrol diphosphate) which was introduced in 1952 under the name of Honvan[R] for the therapy of metastasising prostatic carcinoma. Prostatic carcinoma and its metastases are characterised by high activity levels of acid phosphatase, an enzyme which cleaves phosphoric acid esters. Stilboestrol diphosphate is also split by acid prostatic phosphatase. The liberated stilboestrol, a diphenol, has a cytotoxic activity and accumulates transiently in the prostate and in the prostatic carcinoma tissue.

In the further course of development the Asta researchers investigated the question of whether perhaps the principle "transport form - active form" could be used to advantage in the chemotherapy of cancer in general. With most tumour types, however, the preconditions for a selective therapy are much more unfavourable than with prostatic carcinoma because we know of no fundamental biochemical differences between normal cells and tumour cells. We nevertheless tried to apply the principle of "transport form - active form", successfully proven in the case of fosfestrol, to the group of alkylating compounds, particularly of the nitrogen mustard type.

2. APPLICATION OF THE PRINCIPLE "TRANSPORT FORM - ACTIVE FORM" TO NITROGEN MUSTARD COMPOUNDS

Alkylating agents, with their high chemical reactivity, could not prima facie be expected to possess a selective action on tumour cells. Alkylating agents exert their oncocidal action by alkylation of nucleophilic centres of biomolecules which are responsible for cellular proliferation. It was thus found quite early that these compounds damage not only tumour cells but, at the same time, also normal host tissues, especially rapidly proliferating tissues. Great efforts were made in the ensuing decades to achieve a higher selectivity of the oncocidal action of these compounds, either by appropriate chemical modification ot the alkylating compounds themselves or, applying the carrier principle, by binding the functional groups to physiologically utilisable units such as amino acids or sugars. These efforts had a very modest success.

The starting compound in our own research was nitrogen mustard which has the drawback of a very narrow therapeutic range but presents the advantage of attacking and killing cancer cells of all types. The problem of applying the principle "transport form - active form" consisted of finding a way to inactivate the highly reactive nitrogen mustard compound by appropriate chemical binding and thus to convert it into a well-tolerated transport form. The solution was found with the help of the following considerations:

The biological efficacy of nitrogen mustard compounds is closely linked with the reactivity of the functional 2-chloroethylamino groups, and this in turn is linked to the basicity of the corresponding nitrogen atoms. The reactivity of the functional groups can thus be influenced by manipulating this basicity. It may be expected that an increase in the basicity of the nitrogen atom will be associated with an increase in reactivity and, conversely, a reduction in this basicity will be associated with a reduction in reactivity. The substitution of electrophilic groups at the amino nitrogen reduces the basicity and thus reduces the reactivity of the functional groups, whilst the introduction of nucleophilic groups has the opposite effects.

3. DEVELOPMENT OF NITROGEN MUSTARD OXAZAPHOSPHORINE CYTOSTATICS (3, 4)
Based on physiological considerations the phosphoryl group was chosen as the electrophilic group, and work was started on designing a molecule which would offer possibilities of attack for the body enzymes. The coupling of the mustard group to phosphoric acid was based on the assumption that the thus formed stable oxazaphosphorines would be inactive transport forms which would then be split in the organism to the active form with release of the active amine (3). The realisation of this idea made it possible in effect considerably to reduce the high reactivity and general toxicity of nitrogen mustard whilst retaining the chemotherapeutic efficacy, and thus to increase the antitumoral selectivity and the therapeutic range (4).

Amongst the over 1000 compounds which were synthetised, four compounds were found to possess particularly favourable properties. These compounds are cyclophosphamide, introduced in 1958 under the name of Endoxan[R], trofosfamide (1972, Ixoten[R]), ifosfamide (1977, Holoxan[R]) and sufosfamide which is a mixed-function oxazaphosphorine with interesting properties in the immunological field and which is still undergoing clinical trials.

3.1. <u>Chemotherapeutic characterisation of the nitrogen mustard</u>
<u>oxazaphosphorines</u> (5, 6)

The advances achieved with the introduction of oxazaphosphorines could
not have been achieved without the development of quantitative pharmacological test methods in appropriate animal models. These preconditions
have been considerably broadened in the last decades by the selection of
a suitable tumour spectrum, by the development of adequate model experiments for assessing both the chemotherapeutic and the toxic effects, by
extension of the range of more trenchant criteria of action, by the use
of quantitative test methods (especially of the dose-response analysis
method) and by the development of pharmacokinetic investigation methods.
The Asta researchers, jointly with H. DRUCKREY, Freiburg, and B. SCHNEIDER,
Hanover, have worked very intensively on these fundamental methodological
preconditions and have developed important parameters such as the Ehrlich
index (LD 5 : CD 95), the danger coefficient and the therapeutic unit
which make an exact and comprehensive evaluation of alkylating agents
both in screening tests and in specific pharmacotherapeutic characterisation
possible.

Cyclophosphamide is the prototype of oxazaphosphorines without a direct
alkylating action. It represents a new reaction type. Its chemical and
pharmacological behaviour differs markedly from that of the directly
alkylating nitrogen mustard compounds known formerly. The formerly known
nitrogen mustard compounds were either highly active chemically and
pharmacologically or largely inactive both chemically and pharmacologically,
like, e.g. the acyl derivatives of nitrogen-nor mustard. By contrast,
cyclophosphamide shows in vitro a low chemical reactivity and a correspon-
dingly low biological activity, whilst in vivo it shows a high oncocidal
efficacy. At the same time the organotoxic effects are attenuated, the
general toxicity is substantially reduced and the therapeutic range is
decisively increased.

To obtain accurate information on these various properties, the pharmacological test procedures had to be adapted to various reaction types and
appropriate tests had to be developed for determining the chemical and
the pharmacological activity in vitro and in vivo. In view of the importance
which attaches to pharmacological evaluation not only for the classification

of the individual compounds but also for the characterisation of various
metabolites, these tests are briefly discussed below.

3.1.1. Chemical reactivity

The chemical reactivity of a nitrogen mustard compound can be assessed
from its behaviour in aqueous solution. For this purpose the rate of
hydrolysis of alkylating nitrogen mustards is determined by means of the
4-(4'-nitrobenzyl)-pyridine (NBP) test by measuring the decrease in
alkylating activity in aqueous solution in the absence of other nucleophilic
partners. In contrast to the simple nitrogen mustard compounds, cyclophosphamide does not react with NBP directly but only after hydrolysis. For
a merely orienting determination of the chemical reactivity of alkylating
nitrogen mustards, it is also possible to measure the rate of chloride
ion release under physiological conditions of pH and temperature. The
ionisation rate of cyclophosphamide is much lower than that of simple
nitrogen mustard compounds (Fig. 1).

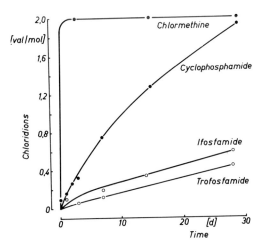

FIGURE 1. Chloride ion release of chlormethine, cyclophosphamide,
ifosfamide and trofosfamide (bicarbonate buffer solution pH 7.5;
0.026 M; 37° C)

3.1.2 Cytotoxic activity

The cytotoxic activity of a nitrogen mustard compound is assessed by
means of the combined incubation-transplantation test, in which cancer
cells with a known chemoresistance are incubated in vitro with an

244

increasing series of concentrations of the test compound. The test compound
is then washed out and the cells are tested for transplantability on untreated test animals. The mean effective concentration (EC 50) determined
in this manner provides a quantitative measure of the actual cytotoxic
activity of a compound, regardless of the possible concurrent presence of
potentially effective transport forms. This test is a good complement of
the chemical tests described above and has always been used by us in
parallel with the chemical tests in order to arrive at a more accurate
and more comprehensive characterisation of the individual compounds as
well as of their metabolites. In contrast to other nitrogen mustard compounds, cyclophosphamide shows no action in this test, even at very high
concentrations (Table 1).

Table 1. Cytotoxic concentration of ifosfamide, cyclophosphamide,
nor-nitrogen mustard, chlormethine-N-oxide and chlormethine in the
incubation test with Yoshida ascites cells in vitro

Compound	Yoshida ascites sarcoma in vitro (37°C, 1h) EC 50 [µg/ml]
Ifosfamide	> 1000
Cyclophosphamide	> 1000
Nor-nitrogen mustard	1,0
Chlormethine-N-oxide	0,5
Chlormethine	0,1

3.1.3 Therapeutic range

The therapeutic values of nitrogen mustard compounds are studied in
appropriate chemotherapeutic experiments on whole animals. These experiments are aimed at a quantitative assessment of the diverse chemotherapeutic and toxic components of action by determining the corresponding
dose-response relationships. The curative component of action is tested
on a range of various experimentally induced tumours, particularly of the
rat, the biological properties of which (including the particularly
important chemosensitivity) are well known and are checked at frequent

intervals. Analysis of the dose-response curves provides the decisive parameters for determining the therapeutic range. In the case of the so-called transport forms, demonstration of carcinotoxic (oncocidal) efficacy in vivo is considered proof of conversion into the active form in the organism and, in combination with the findings of the in-vitro experiments, as a kind of interim verdict regarding the underlying mechanism of action.

Table 2 presents, as an example, data on the high chemotherapeutic efficacy of cyclophosphamide against Yoshida's ascites sarcoma of the rat. It can be seen that the therapeutic index is up to 10-fold that of other alkylating agents.

Table 2. Indices of the curative and lethal effect of cyclophosphamide compared with chlormethine-N-oxide and nor-nitrogen mustard by i.v. administration to Yoshida's ascites sarcoma of the rat

Agent	LD50 [mg/kg]	Yoshida ascites sarcoma		
		CD 50		Therap. index $\frac{LD5}{CD95}$
		[mg/kg]	%LD50	
Cyclophosphamide	160	4,5	2,8	8,5
Chlormethine-N-oxide	50	5,4	10,9	2,2
Nor-nitrogen mustard	100	40	40	0,65

3.2 Relationships between the chemical constitution and the chemotherapeutic efficacy in the series of nitrogen mustard oxazaphosphorines (4, 8)

Most of the compounds synthetised in the Chemical Department of the Asta Werke are N-phosphorylation products of bis-(2-chloroethyl)-amine. Depending on the choice of the reaction components used in the synthesis, these products are triamides, diamido-mono-esters and mono-amido-diesters.

Applying the methods described here it proved possible to establish an unambiguous pharmacological characterisation of the various groups of nitrogen mustard phosphamides and thus to allocate the individual compounds to the reaction types described earlier. We shall now briefly consider certain structural peculiarities which were discussed in detail in a paper published in 1961 (4) and which are important for understanding the metabolism of cyclophosphamide.

Fig. 2 presents a plot of data points for various compounds, with the D 50 index (LD 50 : CD 50) plotted as ordinates against the release of chloride ions in 24 hours in a bicarbonate buffer solution (pH 7.5 at 37.5° C) plotted as abscissae. It can be seen that these data points cluster in three groups clearly corresponding to three reaction types. Two of the three groups lie near the axis of abscissae. These compounds have low index values and they exhibit different behaviours with respect to chemical reactivity. The group on the right, which includes the triamides, represents compounds with a high chemical reactivity whilst the compounds on the left, which include the mono-amido-diester compounds, have a low chemical reactivity. The third group of points represents the diamido-mono-ester compounds including cyclophosphamide, trofosfamide and ifosfamide. These compounds have index values of between 9 and 24, reflecting a greatly increased therapeutic range, and clearly occupy a special place amongst the some 1000 compounds studied.

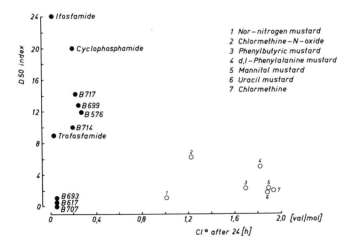

FIGURE 2. Relationship between chemotherapeutic effectiveness and chemical reactivity of some nitrogen mustard oxazaphosphorines compared with various highly reactive nitrogen mustard compounds.

The high tumour-selectivity of the diamido-mono-ester compounds is linked to a particular chemical structure (Fig. 3). A characteristic feature is the ring formed by the N-propylene group with an amide-like bond at one end and an ester bond at the other, closing the ring. This oxazaphosphorine ring is of decisive importance for the character of the action. Even minor deviations in the chemical structure abolish the characteristic selectivity of the antitumoral action.

Cyclophosphamide

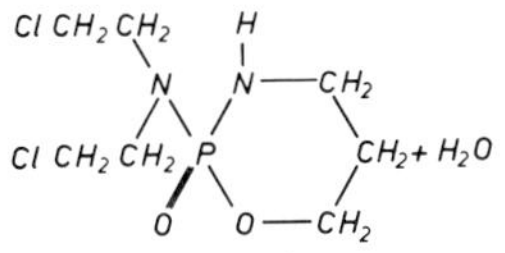

$$Cl\,CH_2\,CH_2 \quad H$$
$$Cl\,CH_2\,CH_2 \underset{N}{\diagdown} \quad N—CH_2$$
$$Cl\,CH_2\,CH_2 \underset{P}{} \quad CH_2 + H_2O$$
$$O \quad O—CH_2$$

Trofosfamide

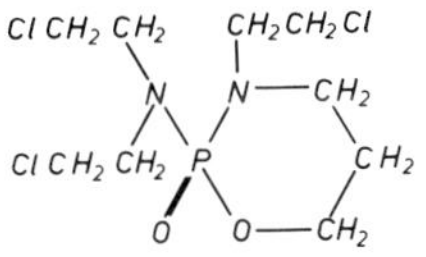

$$Cl\,CH_2\,CH_2 \quad CH_2\,CH_2\,Cl$$
$$N \quad N—CH_2$$
$$Cl\,CH_2\,CH_2 \underset{P}{} \quad CH_2$$
$$O \quad O—CH_2$$

Ifosfamide

$$Cl\,CH_2\,CH_2 \quad CH_2\,CH_2\,Cl$$
$$N \quad N—CH_2$$
$$H \underset{P}{} \quad CH_2$$
$$O \quad O—CH_2$$

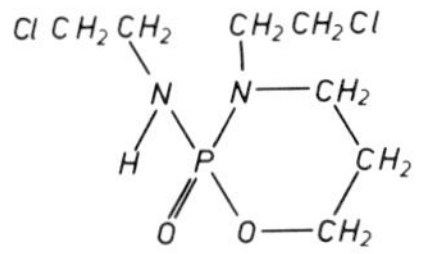

FIGURE 3. Structural formula of cyclophosphamide, trofosfamide and ifosfamide.

From the pharmacological viewpoint the development of cyclophosphamide appeared to signal the attainment of a certain optimum. It took extensive further work, entailing the synthesis of hundreds of new compounds, to develop the next generation compounds trofosfamide, ifosfamide and sufosfamide which, despite a certain overlap in the character of action, possess interesting peculiarities and more advanced therapeutic properties.

Trofosfamide differs chemically from cyclophosphamide by the introduction
of a third chloroethyl group. It is capable of curing therapy-resistant
tumours of the mouse which hardly react at all to cyclophosphamide.
Trofosfamide has relatively mild immunosuppressive side effects, which is
an advantage in so-called maintenance therapy.

Ifosfamide differs chemically from cyclophosphamide by the transfer of
one 2-chloroethyl group from the nitrogen mustard moiety of the molecule
to the cyclic phosphamide nitrogen atom of the oxazaphosphorine ring.
It differs pharmacologically from other comparable compounds mainly with
respect to the time constants of the curative versus the lethal components
of action (Fig. 4). Compared to cyclophosphamide, the cumulation of the
curative component of action is relatively strong whilst that of the
toxic component is reduced. Both these differences are desirable. By
virtue of these properties ifosfamide shows experimentally and clinically,
especially with fractionated administration, a greater therapeutic range
than most alkylating agents. This makes it possible to administer higher
total doses and to achieve beneficial effects in several types of tumour
formerly considered refractory to therapy.

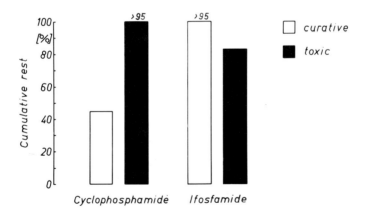

FIGURE 4. Cumulative rest of the curative and toxic effects of
cyclophosphamide and ifosfamide 24 hours after administration (cf. 6).

Sufosfamide is a mixed-function oxazaphosphorine differing from ifosfamide
in that the extracyclic 2-chloroethyl function has been replaced by a
mesyl-oxyethyl group. It is characterised by an extraordinary intensifi-
cation of the immunosuppressive component of action compared to the
carcinotoxic component. With this compound it has been possible to achieve
induction of a specific immune tolerance in models of humoral and cell-
bound antibodies (7).

In the discussion of relationships between the chemical constitution and
the biological efficacy of oxazaphosphorines, particular importance
attaches to methyl substitution in the hexacyclic ring. As evidenced by
the index values summarised in Table 3, the cyclophosphamide derivatives
monomethylated in position 4, 5 or 6 of the ring retain the specific
character of the parent compound. The D 50 index ranges between 12 and
14.4.

Table 3. Monomethylation at the carbon atoms of the oxazaphosphorine
ring of cyclophosphamide (comparison of the D 50 indices).

Agent	$CI-CH_2CH_2$ $\diagdown N$ H $N-$ $CI-CH_2CH_2$ $\diagup P \diagup$ O $O-$	$\dfrac{LD\ 50(1)}{CD\ 50(4)}$
Cyclophosphamide	$-CH_2$ $_4\ _5CH_2$ $-CH_2$ ^{6}	20,0
B 717	$-CH_2$ $\diagup CHCH_3$ $-CH_2$	14,4
B 699	$-CHCH_3$ $\diagup CH_2$ $-CH_2$	12,5
B 576	$-CH_2$ $\diagup CH_2$ $-CHCH_3$	12,0

More interesting is the behaviour of disubstituted homologues, particularly the double methyl substitution at the carbon atom 4, 5 or 6 of
the ring. Double methyl substitution at the carbon atom 4 or 5 results
in the total loss of biological efficacy, especially of the curative
efficacy. By contrast, double methyl substitution at the carbon atom 6
does not alter the special character of the parent compound (Table 4).

Table 4. Dimethylation at the carbon atoms of the oxazaphosphorine ring of cyclophosphamide (comparison of the D 50 indices)

Agent	$Cl\text{-}CH_2CH_2$ ... N — ... $Cl\text{-}CH_2CH_2$ ... P ... O ... O—	$\dfrac{LD\ 50\,(1)}{CD\ 50\,(4)}$
B 707	$-CH_2$ CH_3 / C / $-CH_2$ CH_3	<0,1
B 617	$-C\text{-}CH_3$ / CH_3 / CH_2 / $-CHCH_3$	0,5
B 693	$-CH_2$ CH_3 / C / $-CHCH_3$ CH_3	1,0
B 714	$-CHCH_3$ / CH_2 / $-C\text{-}CH_3$ / CH_3	10,0

This peculiar pharmacological behaviour of the monomethyl compounds and the consequences of dimethylation at a carbon atom of the oxazaphosphorine ring are largely understandable in the light of our current understanding of the metabolism of cyclophosphamide. The disubstitution at carbon atom 4 prevents hydroxylation in this position, and the introduction of 2 methyl groups at the carbon atom 5 inhibits the splitting off of an unsaturated aldehyde (similar to the liberation of acrolein in the case of cyclophosphamide) and thus prevents toxification to the alkylating nitrogen mustard phosphoric acid diamide.

4. ON THE QUESTION OF THE SELECTIVITY OF NITROGEN MUSTARD OXAZAPHOSPHORINES
   (literature see 9)

We had initially tried to explain the high selectivity of the nitrogen mustard oxazaphosphorines by the "transport form - active form" mechanism. In the last 15 years, however, we have found that the actual conditions are more complex than could be expected on the basis of our working hypothesis. Despite its undoubted heuristic value in the development of the aforementioned oxazaphosphorine compounds, the "transport form - active form" principle can in the last analysis shed no light on the actual basis of the relatively high carcinotoxic selectivity of these compounds.

4.1. Relationship between selectivity and metabolism

Cyclophosphamide and other nitrogen mustard oxazaphosphorines differ from directly acting alkylating agents in that they require biotransformation before they can exert their alkylating and carcinotoxic (oncocidal) properties. The key to the understanding of the relative selectivity of these compounds may lie in these metabolic changes. With this in mind together with HOHORST we started studies on the metabolism of cyclophosphamide very early, a task which also attracted many research teams throughout the world. We found in 1962 that, in warm-blooded animals, the biotransformation of cyclophosphamide to cytotoxically active metabolites takes place mainly in the liver and not in the tumour cells, as had originally been expected on the basis of our working hypothesis.

The metabolism of cyclophosphamide can be divided into three major steps, namely, activation, toxification and deactivation (detoxification).

4.1.1. The activation

The initial step in the biotransformation of cyclophosphamide is a "mixed-function" hydroxylation, by means of which the inactive transport form is activated to yield metabolites which exert their alkylating and cytotoxic action without further enzymatic conversion (Fig. 5). This hydroxylation occurs at carbon atom 4 of the oxazaphosphorine ring which thus attains the oxidation level of an aldehyde.

The activation products, namely, 4-hydroxy-cyclophosphamide and its tautomeric open-ring product aldophosphamide, are the carriers of the special alkylating and cytotoxic properties of cyclophosphamide in vivo. They can be detected in the serum and in the urine. Other N-2-chloro-ethylamido-oxazaphosphorines, such as ifosfamide and trofosfamide, probably follow the same pattern of enzymatic activation in vivo.

4.1.2. The toxification

The increased reactivity caused by enzymatic hydroxylation at carbon atom 4 of the oxazaphosphorine ring leads to spontaneous release of a 3-carbon compound (acrolein) with formation of the directly alkylating nitrogen

252

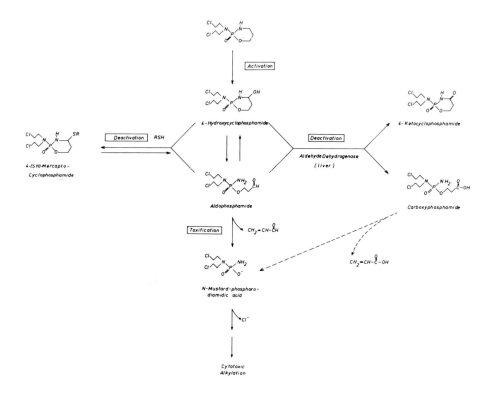

FIGURE 5. Metabolism of cyclophosphamide: routes of deactivation and toxification of 4-hydroxy-cyclophosphamide.

mustard phosphoric acid diamide. This reaction is a ß-elimination which we have called "toxification" and which determines the spontaneous breakdown rate of 4-hydroxy-cyclophosphamide.

Toxification results from resonance stabilisation of the reaction product acrolein. Whenever the possibility of resonance stabilisation of the breakdown product is reduced, as for instance after dehydrogenation of the oxo function of aldophosphamide yielding a carboxyl group (carboxyphosphamide), the toxification reaction is markedly slowed down. Thus, the deactivated cyclophosphamide derivatives such as carboxyphosphamide or 4-keto-cyclophosphamide have little or no alkylating activity under physiological conditions of pH and temperature.

4.1.3 The deactivation (detoxification)

The sequence of enzymatic activation followed by spontaneous rate-determining toxification of N-2-chloroethylamido-oxazaphosphorines allows possibilities of interactions at the oxazaphosphorine ring in vivo, which may partly or completely deactivate the activated metabolites and thus delay or even abolish the toxification process. In contrast to other alkylating cytostatics, this detoxification resulting from deactivation is due not to reactions of the alkylating moiety, i.e., of the nitrogen mustard group in the case of cyclophosphamide, but to reactions at the oxazaphosphorine ring. Consequently, the resulting deactivation products (detoxification products) retain their alkylating potency, as evidenced by the fact that after acid hydrolysis they are able to alkylate 4-(4'-nitrobenzyl)-pyridine in the NBP test. By contrast, in the case of nitrogen mustard derivatives not possessing an oxazaphosphorine ring detoxification, e.g., by sulfhydryl compounds, is invariably followed by a complete loss of alkylating capacity.

Enzymatic deactivation by dehydrogenation of activated cyclophosphamide to 4-keto-cyclophosphamide or to carboxyphosphamide is known to take place in the organism, particularly in the liver and the kidneys. It is catalysed by aldehyde dehydrogenases and/or by aldehyde oxidases. This enzymatic dehydrogenation is irreversible under in-vivo conditions and represents the main route by which activated N-2-chloroethylamido-oxazaphosphorines are eliminated from the body.

Another deactivation reaction which may, under physiological conditions of pH and temperature, delay or even prevent the toxification of activated N-2-chloroethylamido-oxazaphosphorines is the substitution of the crypto-aldehyde group at carbon atom 4 of the oxazaphosphorine ring by sulfhydryl compounds. In the case of 4-hydroxy-cyclophosphamide this substitution yields thioglycoside-like 4-(S-R)-mercapto-cyclophosphamide derivatives according to the following scheme:

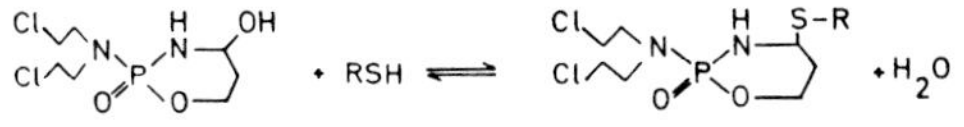

Some compounds of this type have been synthetised (10). In contrast to the
unstable and therefore less manageable 4-hydroxy-cyclophosphamide, the
4-(S-R)-mercapto-cyclophosphamides in crystalline form are relatively
stable at room temperature and only decompose in aqueous solution by
rapid equilibration to form 4-hydroxy-cyclophosphamide and breakdown
compounds.

The reaction of activated cyclophosphamide with sulfhydryl compounds is
of great interest for the elucidation of the cytotoxic specificity of
N-2-chloroethylamido-oxazaphosphorines. Owing to its higher reaction rate
compared to that of the toxification reaction, sulfhydryl-deactivation
offers the possibility of controlling the alkylating and cytotoxic activities of N-2-chloroethylamido-oxazaphosphorines at the level of their
activated metabolites, i.e., before the toxification step.

In a similar way to low molecular weight thiols, free sulfhydryl groups
of proteins also react by substitution at the oxazaphosphorine ring. In
addition, the reaction with sulfhydryl groups of proteins leads to fixa-
tion of the cyclophosphamide metabolite to the biomolecule, so that the
toxification of 4-hydroxy-cyclophosphamide to the ultimate alkylating
phosphamide mustard cannot take place. By this mechanism a large proportion
of the activated cyclophosphamide which has permeated into cells is
initially bound in the form of 4-(S-protein)-sulfido-cyclophosphamide
and thus temporarily deactivated. It will be shown that this binding and
temporary deactivation is an important precondition for the understanding
and elucidation of the cytotoxic specificity in vitro and of the carcinotoxic selectivity in vivo.

4.2. Specificity and selectivity of cyclophosphamide metabolites

Having largely clarified the individual biotransformation steps to which
cyclophosphamide is subjected in the organism of warm-blooded animals,
and having identified the structure of the metabolites, the next task
was to identify the metabolites which retain the high specificity and
high selectivity of the parent compound and those which have lost these
chemotherapeutically decisive properties. Before we approach this
question, however, we should define the concepts of specificity and
selectivity more precisely than they have been defined so far in pharmacology and particularly in chemotherapy.

We use the term <u>selectivity</u> to designate that property of a drug which enables it, in the organism, to act on cells of one particular type without affecting any other cells. We determine selectivity in experiments on whole animals by establishing the dose ratio between the carcinotoxic (oncocidal) efficacy on the one hand versus the organotoxic or lethal potency on the other. Important parameters in this field are the therapeutic index and the danger coefficient.

We define cytotoxic <u>specificity</u> as the biological potency of the alkylating reaction which is decisive for the cytotoxic effect. It is characterised by the cytotoxic activity in vitro referred to the chemical reactivity (the solvolysis rate) of the compound concerned. Specificity is thus independent of the special in-vivo conditions and it is only one amongst various factors which may influence the selectivity of a cytostatic agent in vivo. High specificity of a cytotoxic nitrogen mustard compound may, but need not necessarily, entail high selectivity in vivo.

4.3. Cytotoxic activity and specificity

We are now in a position to determine the cytotoxic activity and the cytotoxic specificity and to compare these two parameters to each other. Table 5 shows that a comparison of the cytotoxic <u>activity</u> of various nitrogen mustard and oxazaphosphorine compounds reveals differences of over 2 orders of magnitude. As far as the cytotoxic <u>specificity</u> is concerned, the data ratios are shifted. The simple nitrogen mustard compounds show cytotoxic specificity indices ranging between 2 and 40, with only relatively minor deviations. It is particularly striking that the very high cytotoxic activity of the N-methyl mustard is accompanied by a relatively low cytotoxic specificity. By contrast, the group of activated nitrogen mustard oxazaphosphorines, hydroxylated or peroxidised at carbon atom 4 of the oxazaphosphorine ring, shows a cytotoxic specificity higher by a factor of about 10 to 100. It may also be noted that 4-keto-cyclophospha-mide and carboxyphosphamide are almost totally inactive under in-vitro conditions.

4.4. Therapeutic range and selectivity

Table 6 summarises the therapeutic indices of various metabolites and nitrogen mustard compounds calculated from their curative and lethal doses.

Table 5. Cytotoxic activity and specificity of nitrogen mustards and N-2-chloroethylamido-oxazaphosphorines. Cytotoxic activity as determined in the incubation/transplantation test on Yoshida ascites sarcoma cells in rats (strain Sprague-Dawley). For definition see (9).

$$\text{Cytotoxic specificity} = \frac{\text{Cytotoxic activity}}{\text{Alkylating activity}}$$

The alkylating activity is measured by determining the hydrolytic rate of the various nitrogen mustards.

Compound	Cytotoxic Activity CU/µmol	Cytotoxic Specificity $[(CU/\mu mol) \cdot min] \cdot 10^{-2}$
N-methyl-mustard	138	40
Chlorambucil	14	10
Nor-N-mustard	1.4	10
N-oxide-mustard	1.5	2
N-mustard phosphoro-diamidic acid	7.5	8
4-Hydroxy-cyclophosphamide	63	225
4-Hydroperoxy-cyclophos-phamide	63	315
4-Hydroxy-ifosfamide	63	700

Table 6. Carcinotoxic selectivity (margin of safety) of various nitrogen mustards and N-2-chloroethylamido-oxazaphosphorines (Sprague-Dawley rats Asta; tumour: Yoshida ascites sarcoma AH 13)

Compound	LD 50 (mg/kg)	CD 50 (mg/kg)	D 50-Index (LD 50/CD 50)
Cyclophosphamide	220	1.25	175
Ifosfamide	305	1.5	204
Trofosfamide	124	1.25	99
4-Hydroxy-cyclophosphamide	150	1.25	120
4-Hydroperoxy-cyclophosphamide	97.5	1.25	78
Nor-N-mustard	100	40	2.5
N-methyl-mustard	1.1	0.25	4.4
N-oxide-mustard	60	5	12
N-mustard phosphoro-diamidic acid	61	20	3.1
Carboxyphosphamide	~ 800	~ 200	~ 4
4-Keto-cyclophosphamide	>800	>800	-

The first group comprises oxazaphosphorine compounds as transport forms. The second group comprises the oxazaphosphorine compounds arising from these transport forms in vivo by hydroxylation at carbon atom 4 of the oxazaphosphorine ring and some perhydroxylated oxazaphosphorine compounds (taking cyclophosphamide as an example) obtained by chemical synthesis. The third group comprises nitrogen mustard compounds not bound to an oxazaphosphorine ring. The fourth group comprises deactivated or toxified metabolites of cyclophosphamide.

The compounds of the first two groups differ from those of the last two groups by their comparatively high selectivity in vivo. They have D 50 indices ranging between 78 and 204 thus exceeding the corresponding indices of the simple nitrogen mustards and those of the toxified or deactivated cyclophosphamide metabolites by up to two orders of magnitude.

The data presented in this table illustrate two important findings: Firstly, taking cyclophosphamide as an example, the selectivity of the so-called transport forms of oxazaphosphorine compounds matches almost exactly that of their primary activation products, i.e., of the metabolites hydroxylated at carbon atom 4 of the oxazaphosphorine ring. Secondly, further metabolic dehydrogenation of the primary activation products to 4-keto-cyclophosphamide or to carboxyphosphamide, as well as spontaneous decomposition to the directly alkylating nitrogen mustard phosphoric acid diamide, results in loss of selectivity.

The primary activation products thus appear to be the sole carriers of the selectivity of the oxazaphosphorine cytostatic drugs.

4.5 Carcinotoxic selectivity (therapeutic range) in vivo and cytotoxic specificity in vitro

According to the findings presented in Tables 5 and 6 is should be possible to describe in greater detail the relationships between the cytotoxic specificity in vitro and the carcinotoxic selectivity in vivo both for the activated N-2-chloroethylamido-oxazaphosphorines and for the simple nitrogen mustard compounds. With this in mind we have brought these two parameters for the biological reactivity, which are in principle quite independent of each other, together in the same diagram (Fig. 6). It can be seen that these two parameters vary essentially parallel to one another.

258

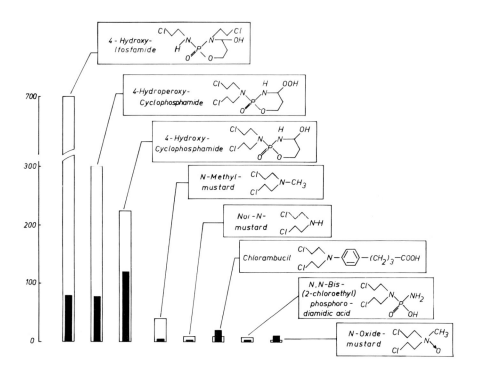

FIGURE 6. Selectivity in vivo and specificity in vitro of N-mustards and of activated N-2-chloroethylamido-oxazaphosphorines. Carcinotoxic selectivity (LD 50 : CD 50). Cytotoxic specificity (CU/µmol·min)·10^{-2}

The high therapeutic indices of the nitrogen mustard oxazaphosphorines are matched by high levels of cytotoxic specificity of their active metabolites in vitro. Simple nitrogen mustard derivatives on the other hand, including those with a high chemical reactivity such as N-methyl-mustard, show not only a low selectivity in vivo but also a low cytotoxic specificity.

This striking parallelism, which can be explained neither by peculiarities of the pharmacokinetics nor by the "transport form - active form" principle or the carrier principle, clearly points to a causal link. According to this causal link hypothesis the selectivity of the afore-mentioned oxaza-phosphorines in vivo is based mainly, and possibly even exclusively on the high cytotoxic specificity of the primary metabolites as well as on the particular reactivity of the oxazaphosphorine ring hydroxylated at carbon atom 4, and not on the alkylating activity of the nitrogen mustard moiety of the molecule. In other words, the oxazaphosphorine ring should be considered as the carrier of the carcinotoxic selectivity and of the cytotoxic specificity of the compounds of this group.

We were for a long time unable to identify the ultimate mechanism responsible for the high cytotoxic specificity and high carcinotoxic selectivity of these compounds. In particular, we did not know how the alkylating agent responsible for the cytotoxic activity is released from the deactivated protein-fixed 4-(S-protein)-sulfido-oxazaphosphorines. An important advance in this area was recently achieved by HOHORST et al. (11). They have demonstrated the existence of an enzyme which cleaves not only 4-hydroxy-cyclophosphamide and 4-hydroperoxy-cyclophosphamide but also 4-(S-protein)-sulfido-cyclophosphamide and in this process releases nitrogen mustard phosphoric acid diamide as the alkylating agent. This enzyme is a 3'-5'-exonuclease closely related to DNA-polymerase. This enzyme can cleave the phosphordiester bond of 4-(S-protein)-sulfido-cyclophosphamide and thus release the ultimate alkylating and cytotoxic agent. Although several points of detail still require clarification, this important research finding of the HOHORST team represents a major step in support of the thiol hypothesis for explaining the phenomenon of carcinotoxic specificity of the oxazaphosphorine cytostatics.

4.6. Stabilised primary metabolites of cyclophosphamide with high cytotoxic specificity and carcinotoxic selectivity requiring no enzymatic activation (12)

Amongst the metabolites of oxazaphosphorine cytostatics, the activated 4-hydroxy-compounds play a key rôle with reference to antitumour properties. 4-Hydroxy-cyclophosphamide has in common with the parent compound a high cytotoxic specificity in vitro and a high carcinotoxic selectivity in vivo. Unlike cyclophosphamide, it requires no enzymatic activation in the liver because toxification takes place owing to the inherent chemical reactivity of the compound depending on the milieu conditions. With these different properties it became of interest to develop 4-hydroxy-cyclophosphamide as a cancer chemotherapeutic, but this proved impossible because this compound has a low chemical stability and is therefore not amenable to galenic processing. Even experimental investigations of 4-hydroxy-cyclophos-

phamide can only be conducted under the most stringent safety precautions.
The 4-hydroperoxy-cyclophosphamide first synthetised by TAKAMIZAWA (lit.
see 9), which releases 4-hydroxy-cyclophosphamide in aqueous solution, is
also not sufficiently stable even though it has been used occasionally
in experiments and even clinically.

We therefore set ourselves the task to stabilise 4-hydroxy-cyclophosphamide
by chemical means. We were looking for a compond which would be stable in
crystalline form at room temperature but would, in aqueous solution, release
4-hydroxy-cyclophosphamide spontaneously and at a sufficiently high rate.
We approached this problem by chemical substitution of various thio-alkane
sulfonates at the crypto-aldehyde function of the oxazaphosphorine ring.
A prototype of this class of compounds is ASTA Z 7557 (Fig. 7). This
compound readily forms crystallising salts which are chemically stable and
which allow galenic processing. ASTA Z 7557 is readily soluble in water
and hydrolyses in aqueous solution, depending on the pH and the temperature,
with release of 4-hydroxy-cyclophosphamide.

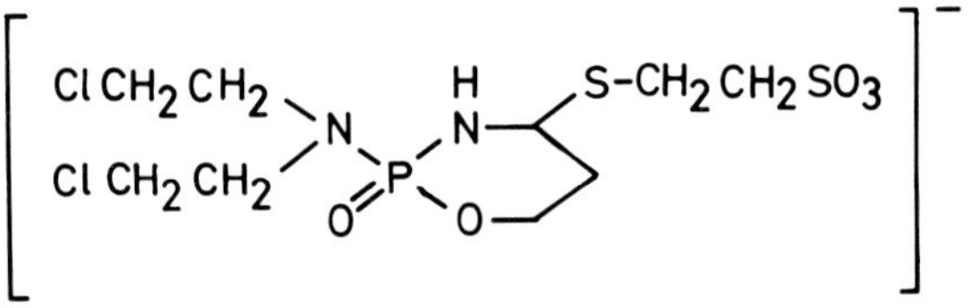

FIGURE 7.   Structural formula of ASTA Z 7557

In the incubation test against Yoshida 's ascites sarcoma cells, the
efficacy of ASTA Z 7557 is about the same as that of 4-hydroxy-cyclophos-
phamide itself. The two compounds also match with respect to cytotoxic
activity and specificity. ASTA Z 7557 is also highly active chemotherapeutically against several experimental tumours such as leukaemia L5222
of the rat, Yoshida's ascites sarcoma AH 13, Walker's carcinosarcoma 256,
DS-carcinosarcoma of the rat and the leukaemias L1210 and P388 of the
mouse.

The acute toxicity of ASTA Z 7557 in the mouse is relatively low, with
an LD 50 of about 300 mg/kg i.p. as against 100 mg/kg for 4-hydroxy-
cyclophosphamide.

On the strength of its spectrum of action described above, ASTA Z 7557
seems to offer considerable promise in local and regional as well as in
systemic chemotherapy. In the field of pre-clinical oncology ASTA Z 7557
has been found effective in human tumour stem cell assays, in bone marrow
cleaning in autologous transplantation for the treatment of leukaemia,
and in regional perfusion of malignant tumours. By virtue of its pharmacokinetic properties we may hope that the range of tumours responding to
oxazaphosphorine cytostatics may possibly be extended by ASTA Z 7557 in
systemic clinical use.

5. REGIONAL DETOXIFICATION OF UROTOXIC OXAZAPHOSPHORINE CYTOSTATICS BY SULFHYDRYL COMPOUNDS (13, 14, 15)

5.1 Introduction and methods

Despite all the advances achieved with the development of oxazaphospnorine
cytostatics, the selectivity and consequently the therapeutic range of
these drugs are still unsatisfactory. As with other important cytostatics,
the therapeutic use of these drugs is burdened with side effects some
of which are quite specifically limited to certain organs. In the case of
cyclophosphamide and ifosfamide the most important therapy-limiting factor
is their urotoxicity which manifests itself mainly as haemorrhagic cystitis.

We therefore set ourselves the task of solving the problem of organ-
specific detoxification of the oxazaphosphorine cytostatics in order to
obviate the urotoxic side effects and thus achieve a further increase in
selectivity and, consequently, also in the therapeutic range.

The urotoxicity of cyclophosphamide and ifosfamide is due to the renal
elimination of aggressive metabolites, and its severity depends on the
concentration of these metabolites in the urine. The problem was to find
a systemically administrable antidote which would not impair the chemotherapeutic efficacy of the oxazaphosphorines against the tumour, but
would reliably prevent damage to the kidneys and the urinary bladder
(regional detoxification).

The development of this uroprotector took place in three phases. In the
first phase we studied the mechanisms of urotoxicity of alkylating compounds,
particularly the relationships between the chemical constitution and the
urotoxic potency. In the second phase we studied experimentally the

the uroprotective efficacy of compounds of various structural classes,
with particular emphasis on mercapto compounds. In the third phase we
studied the pharmacotherapeutic properties of the only compound which
had shown itself as a suitable uroprotector, namely, sodium 2-mercapto-
ethane sulfonate (Uromitexan[R], INN: mesna, Fig. 8).

We first developed an experimental model for urotoxicity which makes a
rapid and reliable quantitative assessment of the bladder inflammation
phenomena following systemic administration as well as following local
instillation of the test compounds into the bladder possible. We found the
rat to be a suitable test animal for this purpose. In the rat, the inflammation symptoms in the bladder and the kidneys are fully developed within
24 hours after intravenous administration of cyclophosphamide. The criteria
of a urotoxic action are the macroscopically demonstrable inflammation
signs swelling and bleeding, as well as increased capillary permeability
which manifests itself as a blue coloration of the bladder after intravenous injection of trypan blue (extravasation of trypan blue). The
increase in the moist weight of the bladder as a measure of the swelling,
and the intensity of the blue coloration of the bladder as a measure of
the capillary permeability, are quantifiable on appropriate scoring scales
and thus provide the basis for a scaled macroscopic evaluation.

In the systemic testing of urotoxicity the test compounds were administered
in increasing doses by i.v. or i.p. injection or, with intravesical
application, by direct instillation into the bladder of female rats. The
methodological data have been described in detail elsewhere.

5.2 Urotoxicity of oxazaphosphorines

With systemic administration only a few of the alkylating agents tested
were found to possess urotoxic potency. This includes above all the
oxazaphosphorine cytostatics themselves as well as their primary metabolites
(the 4-hydroxy-compounds). Systemically administered, the direct alkylating
nitrogen mustard phosphoric acid diamide has only a low urotoxic potency,
and the simultaneously formed acrolein has none. The metabolic end products
4-keto-cyclophosphamide and carboxyphosphamide are also not urotoxic.
With intravesical instillation the transport form cyclophosphamide, as
expected, causes no inflammation, whilst the 4-hydroxy metabolites do cause

inflammation of the bladder, the severity of which depends on their concentration. By far the most potent urotoxic agent with intravesical instillation is acrolein. The urotoxic potency of acrolein is higher than that of 4-hydroxy-cyclophosphamide by a factor of between 5 and 10. All the other metabolites have hardly any urotoxic potency.

The only carriers of the specific urotoxicity of the oxazaphosphorine cytostatics are thus their primary 4-hydroxy metabolites and especially the acrolein which they release.

5.3 Uroprotective efficacy of mercapto compounds

An effective uroprotective antidote should be capable of intercepting the metabolites responsible for the urotoxicity regionally, i.e., in the kidneys and the efferent urinary tract. This means that such an antidote should either stabilise the 4-hydroxy metabolites, thus preventing the release of acrolein or should detoxify the acrolein directly, as soon as it is released. The investigations were centred mainly on mercapto compounds of which it was expected that they might fulfil this double requirements.

To summarise the extensive investigations very briefly, most of the test compounds studied were incapable of ensuring a regional detoxification of the urotoxic oxazaphosphorine cytostatics. Protection of the kidneys and of the bladder could be achieved with a few of the thio compounds tested, but only with doses in the toxic or even in the sub-lethal range. This also applies to N-acetyl-cysteine which has occasionally been recommended for regional uroprophylaxis.

A special position is occupied by the group of mercaptoethane sulfonic acids. The archetypal compound of this group, sodium 2-mercaptoethane sulfonate (INN: mesna) fulfils the requirements defined above well-nigh ideally.

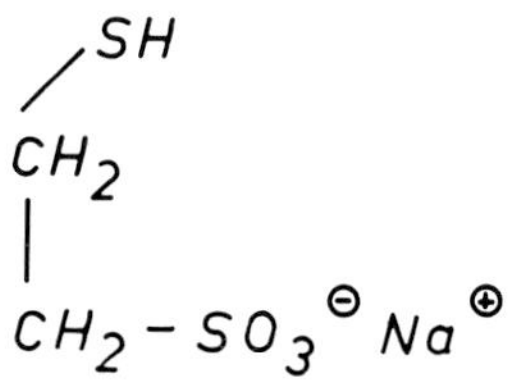

$$\begin{array}{l} \diagup SH \\ CH_2 \\ | \\ CH_2 - SO_3^{\ominus} \; Na^{\oplus} \end{array}$$

FIGURE 8.   Structural formula of mesna

It can be seen from Table 7, that the urotoxic potency of 68.1 mg/kg cyclophosphamide is totally abolished by simultaneous intravenous administration of 31.6 mg/kg mesna. In these experiments the protective effect of mesna could not only be demonstrated mascroscopically but could also be impressively confirmed histologically.

Table 7. Protective action of mesna against urotoxic side-effects of cyclophosphamide (i.v. injection)

Cyclophosphamide mg/kg	Mesna mg/kg	No. of rats	Assessment of Urinary Bladder	
			Inflammation Score	Bleeding %
68.1	—	40	2.6	45
68.1	10.0	10	2.3	20
68.1	14.7	10	2.6	0
68.1	21.5	10	1.1	0
68.1	31.6	10	0	0
68.1	68.1	5	0	0

5.4. On the pharmacology and pharmacokinetics of sodium 2-mercaptoethane sulfonate (mesna)

The intrinsic pharmacological and toxicological activities of mesna are quite weak. An important observation is that the curative efficacy of oxazaphosphorines is not impaired by mesna even in high doses.

The pharmacological action profile of mesna, particularly its uroprotective properties, are determined by its pharmacokinetic behaviour. In the organism mesna is rapidly oxidised to the biologically inactive mesna disulfide. The disulfide remains in the intravasal space and is rapidly eliminated through the kidneys. After glomerular filtration mesna disulfide is picked up by the renal epithelia and is partly reduced again to the free thiol compound. This free mesna reacts chemically in the urine with the urotoxic oxazaphosphorine metabolites and detoxifies them. An important rôle in the reduction of mesna disulfide to mesna in the renal epithelia is played by the reaction of the disulfide with glutathione. We have worked on this problem jointly with the team of ORRENIUS, Stockholm (16). ORRENIUS suggests the following three-step reaction sequence:

$$MSSM + GSH \longrightarrow MSSG + MSH$$

$$MSSG + GSH \longrightarrow GSSG + MSH$$

$$GSSG + NADPH + H^+ \longrightarrow 2\,GSH + NADP^+$$

where MSH = mesna, GSH = glutathione.

In this sequence the first two reactions are catalysed by thiol-transferase, the third is catalysed by glutathione-reductase.

In the detoxification process the first and most important chemical step is the addition of mesna to the double bond of acrolein. The addition compound formed in this reaction is a stable thio-ether which has been detected in the urine chromatographically and has been confirmed by synthesis. In a second mode of action mesna reduces the breakdown rate of the 4-hydroxy-metabolites, e.g., of 4-hydroxy-cyclophosphamide, in the urine. The product of this reaction is a relatively stable and non-urotoxic condensation product of 4-hydroxy-cyclophosphamide and mesna. By this stabilisation reaction mesna prevents the breakdown of 4-hydroxy-cyclophosphamide and thus formation of acrolein. This temporary deactivation product has also been detected in the urine by chromatography (17).

5.4 Clinical prospects

The experimental findings of reliable protection against the urotoxic side effects of oxazaphosphorine cytostatics have been fully confirmed in extensive studies. The elimination of vesical and renal damage has made it possible to administer these cytostatics in higher doses and thus markedly to increase their therapeutic efficacy (18). It has also been shown in an animal experimental study together with SCHMÄHL and HABS (19) that, besides preventing cystitis as an acute side effect of treatment with cyclophosphamide, the use of mesna can apparently also obviate the occurrence of bladder cancer in old age as a late sequel of an otherwise successful chemotherapeutic treatment with cyclophosphamide (20).

In the introduction to his book "A Review of Cyclophosphamide" (1975) Donald L. HILL writes: "The study of cyclophosphamide has contributed very much to cancer research" (21). The validity of this statement is confirmed by over 13'000 scientific publications. The development of stabilised primary metabolites of the oxazaphosphorine cytostatics and the solution of the problem of organ-specific detoxification with mesna have contributed important new advances of considerable promise for the therapeutic treatment of cancer patients.

REFERENCES

1. Brock, N. Chem.Exp.Technol. 3, 441 - 448 (1977)

2. Druckrey, H, Raabe, S. Klin.Wschr. 30, 882 - 884 (1952)

3. Arnold, H, Bourseaux, F, Brock, N. Nature 181, 931 (1958)

4. Arnold, H, Bourseaux, F, Brock, N. Arzneim.-Forsch. (Drug Res.) 11, 143 (1961)

5. Brock, N. Experimental Basis of Cancer Chemotherapy. In: K. Hellmann and T.A. Connors (Eds), Chemotherapy Vol. 7, 1976, Plenung Publishing Corp., New York, p.19

6. Brock, N. Pharmakologische Grundlagen der Krebs-Chemotherapie. In: A. Georgii, Verhandlungen der Deutschen Krebsgesellschaft,Band 1, 1978, Gustav Fischer Verlag, Stuttgart - New York, p. 15

7. Brock, N, Potel, J. Arzneim.-Forsch. (Drug Res.) 24, 1149 (1974)

8. Brock, N. Cancer Treat.Rep. 60, 301 - 307 (1976)

9. Brock, N, Hohorst, HJ. Z. Krebsforsch. 88, 185 - 215 (1977)

10. Peter, G, Wagner, T, Hohorst, HJ. Cancer Treat.Reports 60, 429 - 435 (1976)

11. Hohorst, HJ, Bielicki, L, Voelcker, G.The Mode of Action of Cyclo-phosphamide. 9th Int. Symposium on the Biological Characterization of Human Tumours, 1981, Bologna.

12. Brock, N, Niemeyer, U, Pohl, J, Scheffler, G. Stabilised primary metabolites of oxazaphosphorine cytostatics with high cytotoxic specificity and cancerotoxic selectivity needing no enzymatic activation. Third NCI-EORTC Symposium on New Drugs in Cancer Therapy, 1981, Brussels

13. Brock, N, Pohl, J, Stekar, J. Europ.J.Cancer 17, 595 - 607 (1981)

14. Brock, N, Pohl, J, Stekar, J. Europ.J.Cancer Clin. Oncol.17, 1155 - 1168 (1981)

15. Brock, N, Pohl, J, Stekar, J, Scheef, W. Europ.J.Cancer Clin.Oncol. 1982 in print

16. Ormstad, K, Orrenius, S, Lastbom, T, Uehara, N, Pohl, J, Brock, N. 1982 in print

17. Brock, N, Stekar, J, Pohl, J, Niemeyer, U, Scheffler, G. Arzneim.-
    Forsch. (Drug Res.) 29, 659 - 661 (1979)

18. Pohl, J, Brock, N, Stekar, J. Toxicology, Pharmacology and Interactions
    of Sodium 2-mercaptoethane sulfonate (Mesna). 12th int. Chemotherapy
    Congress, 1981, Florence

19. Habs, M, Schmähl, D, Brock, N. Prevention of urinary bladder tumors
    in cyclophosphamide-treated rats by additional medication with the
    uroprotectors sodium 2-mercaptoethane sulfonate (mesna) and disodium
    2,2'-dithio-bis-ethane sulfonate (dimesna). 13th Int. Cancer Congress,
    1982, Seattle

20. Kaufmann, B, Wegmann, W. Schweiz.med.Wschr. 111, 540 - 545 (1981)

21. Hill, D.L. A review of cyclophosphamide. 1975. Charles C. Thomas
    Publ., Springfield, Ill.

Address for reprints: Prof. Dr.Dr. Norbert Brock, Asta-Werke AG
Degussa Pharma Gruppe, Abt. Tumorforschung, D-4800 Bielefeld 14

STUDIES ON ANTITUMOUR ANTIBIOTICS, LOW MOLECULAR WEIGHT IMMUNO—MODIFIERS AND THEIR ANALOGS AND DERIVATIVES

H. UMEZAWA

1. INTRODUCTION

Antibiotic research has been expanded to low molecular weight inhibitors of enzymes and immuno-modifiers, and continuous progress is being made in the screening, biosynthesis, and understandings of the mechanism of action of antibiotics, and the development of their useful derivatives.

In order to cure cancer, tumors may be macroscopically eliminated by surgery, radiation or chemotherapy, and minimal residual tumors after these treatments should be completely eliminated by the action of the host defense system or additional chemotherapy. Moreover, the immunity reduced in cancer patients should be restored. In addition, the treatment of patients with a compound which inhibits the action or generation of suppressor cells should enhance the effects of radiation, chemotherapy, and immunity-enhancing agents, because suppressor cells have a strong action to suppress host defenses. For example, IMC carcinoma grows slightly in CDF_1 mice immunized against this tumor, but the resistance to this tumor is eliminated by transfer of 10^7 spleen cells from mice bearing this tumor. It is possible that some cytotoxic compounds may inhibit the action or generation of suppressor cells more strongly than that of effector cells. Such effects against suppressor cells in mice have been observed with cyclophosphamide, aclacinomycin (1), adriamycin, etc. Thus, research in the field of antitumor antibiotics is also being extended to those compounds inhibiting the action or generation of the suppressor cell system.

In this paper, I will review our studies with my colleagues on new antitumor antibiotics with potential usefulness, bleomycin, new anthracyclines, low molecular weight immuno-modifiers

D.N. Reinhoudt, T.A. Connors, H.M. Pinedo & K.W. van de Poll (eds.), Structure-Activity Relationships of Anti-Tumour Agents.
© 1983, Martinus Nijhoff Publishers, The Hague/Boston/London. ISBN 90-247-2783-9.

and their derivatives.

2. NEW ANTITUMOR ANTIBIOTICS —— BACTOBOLIN, SPERGUALIN, NEOTHRAMYCIN

The screening of microbial culture filtrates is still leading to the finding of new types of antitumor antibiotics.

2.1. Bactobolin

In 1979, we found a new antitumor antibiotic and elucidated its structure (Fig. 1) (2). We named this antibiotic bactobolin because it is produced by Pseudomonas sp. and is structurally related to actinobolin produced by actinomycetes. Bactobolin was also discovered independently by two other Japanese research groups. Bactobolin has a strong activity in inhibiting L-1210 leukemia, affecting the B lymphocytes more strongly than T cells. Its intraperitoneal injection at the time of immunization of mice to sheep red blood cells did not affect either the number of antibody-forming cells in the spleen or delayed-type hypersensitivity. However, its injection 1, 2, or 3 days after immunization markedly decreased the number of antibody-forming cells without affecting the hypersensitivity response. Its activity of inhibiting mouse T cell type leukemia (EL4 leukemia) was significantly weaker than that against L-1210 leukemia. Therefore, we imagined that bactobolin might be worth testing on human leukemia. The N.C.I. (U.S.A.) subjected this antibiotic to a human stem cell assay and observed a wide spectrum of effects against various human tumor cells.

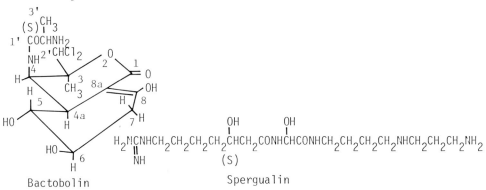

Bactobolin   Spergualin

FIGURE 1. Bactobolin and spergualin.

2.2. Spergualin

We were interested in screening microbial culture filtrates for the activity which inhibited focus formation in chicken fibroblasts exposed to Rous sarcoma virus. The products from streptomyces strains selected by this screening were identified as daunomycin. The other strain selected by this screening was classified as Bacillus laterosporus. Intraperitoneal injection of its culture filtrate had a strong toxicity and caused death of mice; and it did not show any antitumor effect against L-1210 leukemia. But the culture filtrate did inhibit the growth of B. subtilis. Therefore, this antibacterial antibiotic was extracted and purified. To our surprise, this antibacterial antibiotic had a strong activity in inhibiting L-1210 leukemia. We determined the structure of this antibiotic as shown in Fig. 1 (3). This structure was confirmed by total synthesis of this antibiotic (4). As shown by the structure, this antibiotic has a spermidine moiety and guanidine group; thus, we named this antibiotic "spergualin".

Spergualin inhibits the growth of cultured L-1210 cells (5×10^4 cells/ml), with a 50% inhibition at 2 μg/ml. As shown in Table 1, daily intraperitoneal injection of spergualin showed a strong inhibition against L-1210 leukemia which had been kept in the

Table 1. Antitumor effect of spergualin against 2 lines of L-1210.[*]

Dose (mg/kg/day)	Against L-1210 in IMC		Against L-1210 from NCI	
	T/C (%)	Survivor (60 days)	T/C (%)	Survivor (30 days)
50	295	0/8	250	0/6
25	334	0/8	—	—
12.5	586	4/8	233	0/6
6.25	732	8/8	—	—
3.13	441	3/8	214	0/6
1.56	301	1/8	—	—
0.78	107	0/4	160	0/6

[*]Indicated dose of spergualin was intraperitoneally injected daily for 9 days starting from day 1 after the intraperitoneal inoculation of 10^5 L-1210 cells to CDF_1 mice.

Institute of Microbial Chemistry. About one half of the mice treated with 3.13 or 12.5 mg/kg daily survived 60 days after the inoculation of 10^5 tumor cells, and in case of 6.25 mg/kg daily all mice survived. The surviving mice rejected a second inoculation of L-1210 cells. However, another line of L-1210 cells supplied by the N.C.I. (U.S.A.) to the Cancer Institute (Tokyo) was more resistant to spergualin as shown in Table 1. In this case, the survival period was markedly prolonged by 0.78, 3.13, 13.50 or 50 mg/kg daily, but none of mice survived more than 30 days after the tumor cell inoculation.

The LD_{50} by intraperitoneal injection was about 150 mg/kg and by subcutaneous injection it was a little higher than 150 mg/kg. It is characteristic of spergualin to have a very low cumulative toxicity. All mice survived after 25 mg/kg daily for 20 days.

As shown in Table 1, in the experiment testing the effect against L-1210 kept in the Institute of Microbial Chemistry, none of the mice treated with 50 or 25 mg/kg of spergualin daily survived 60 days after inoculation. The death of these mice was due to the delayed growth of the ascites tumor. In the other experiment, 5 out of 6 mice treated with 25 mg/kg daily and 3 out of 6 treated with 50 mg/kg daily died. The recurrent cells were collected from the ascites of one of mice treated with 50 mg/kg and inoculated intraperitoneally into 6 new mice. The resulting tumors were much more resistant to spergualin treatment than the tumor in the original L-1210.

Spergualin does not inhibit synthesis of DNA, RNA, or protein. The mechanism of action of this antibiotic, the resistance induced by high doses in vivo, and derivatives and analogs with improved antitumor activity are being studied.

2.3. Neothramycin

Neothramycin shown in Fig. 2 is one of antitumor antibiotics which we found (5) and is being studied clinically. Before our finding of neothramycin, as shown in Hurley's review in 1977 (6), anthramycin, tomaymycin and sibilomycin (Fig. 2) had already been reported; and Korman et al. (1964) (7) had reported on their clinical study of anthramycin. After neothramycin, we found another one and named it "mazethramycin" (Fig. 2) (8).

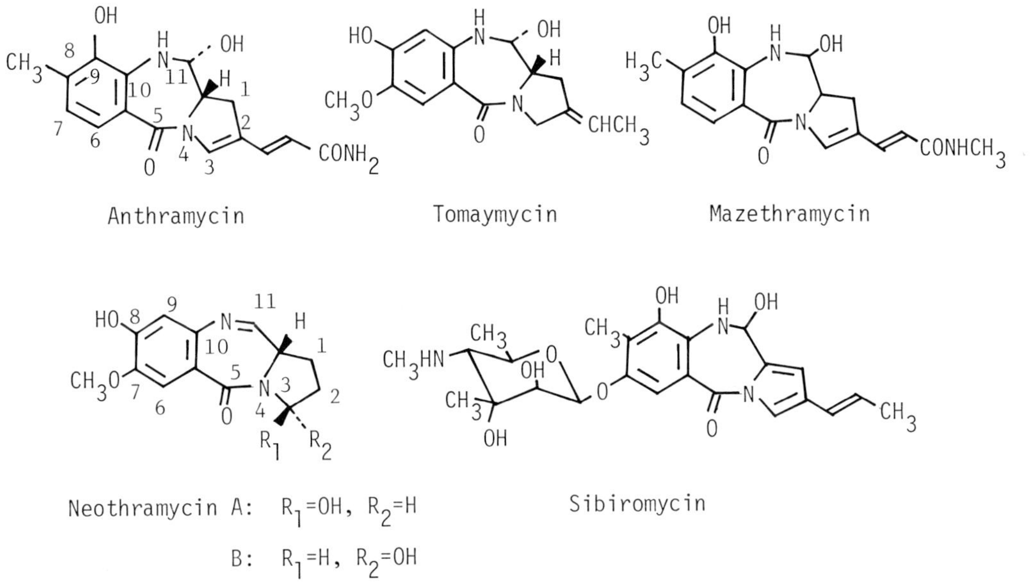

Anthramycin   Tomaymycin   Mazethramycin

Neothramycin A: R_1=OH, R_2=H   Sibiromycin

B: R_1=H, R_2=OH

FIGURE 2. Pyrrolo(1,4)benzodiazepine antitumor antibiotics.

The discovery of a new antitumor antibiotic is always followed
by the difficult problem of deciding whether or not this antibiotic is worthy of preclinical study. First we were interested
in the low toxicity of neothramycin compared with other pyrrolo-
(1,4)benzodiazepine antibiotics and next in its antitumor spectrum
against mouse and rat tumors.

The LD_{50} of neothramycin by intravenous injection was 17.5
mg/kg in male mice, 22.0 mg/kg in female mice, 10.2 mg/kg in male
rats and 11.9 mg/kg in female rats. These LD_{50} values indicate
that neothramycin has 10 to 1,000 times lower toxicity than
other pyrrolo(1,4)benzodiazepine antibiotics; for example, the
LD_{50} of anthramycin in mice was reported to be 0.2 mg/kg; of
tomaymycin, 3 mg/kg; of sibiromycin, 0.058 mg/kg; of mazethramycin, 0.8 mg/kg.

Neothramycin has a unique antitumor spectrum (5,9). It shows
only slight inhibition against Ehrlich carcinoma which are susceptible to most antitumor antibiotics produced by streptomyces.

It exhibits a strong inhibition against sarcoma 180, mouse L-1210 leukemia, and Yoshida rat sarcoma. Some mice were alive even 60 days after the inoculation of Yoshida rat sarcoma cells. Having the lowest toxicity among pyrrolo(1,4)benzodiazepine antibiotics, its unusual antitumor spectrum suggested that neothramycin was worthy of further study. In a test done by the N.C.I. (U.S.A.), it showed a strong inhibition against Novikoff hepatoma (see Table 2).

Table 2. Antitumor effect of neothramycin against Novikoff hepatoma (N.C.I. data).

Dose (mg/kg/day)	Median survival days	T/C (%)	Survivor (60 days)
2	60.0	674	6/6
1	60.0	674	5/6
0.25	60.0	674	4/6
0.12	60.0	674	3/6
0.06	10.0	11.2	1/6
Control	8.9	—	—

Animal: Random bred albino rat (female); Tumor inoculation: ip; Drug administration: ip; Administration schedule: Day 1-9; Parameter: Median survival time.

Neothramycin has a low cumulative toxicity. Electrocardiograms were normal in dogs and hamsters after intravenous injection of 50 mg/kg and 10 mg/kg, respectively. In 1978, a clinical study was started in Japan. Phase I study has indicated that 40 mg/m^2 or more could be administered intravenously. Moreover, intravenous injections of 30 mg/m^2 (daily or twice weekly) did not cause any serious side effects except for nausea and vomiting. Neothramycin does not have any cardiac toxicity and has no bone marrow toxicity in either animals or cancer patients. Daily injection in mice of a quarter of an LD_{50} dose 4 days decreased neither delayed-type hypersensitivity nor the number of antibody-forming cells. Its intraperitoneal injection (0.3, 1.2, 5.0, or 20 mg/kg) at the time of immunization increased the number of antibody-forming cells in mouse spleen. Its addition

(1.5 ng/ml) to mouse spleen cells at the start of the culture increased the number of antibody-forming cells. The addition at not less than 0.062 µg/ml inhibited lectin-induced blastogenesis, suggesting the inhibition of the induction of suppressor cells. It also enhanced macrophage phagocytosis at doses of 1.25 or 5 mg/kg.

Neothramycin inhibits the growth of L-1210 cells and Yoshida rat sarcoma cells, with 50% inhibition at 0.28 and 0.065 µg/ml, respectively. It inhibits RNA synthesis more strongly than DNA synthesis (10).

If neothramycin solution is irradiated at 316 nm, fluorescence at 420 nm is produced. This fluorescence is enhanced by double-stranded DNA. The interaction of neothramycin with DNA has been studied by fluorospectrometry (11). The results indicate that its interaction with poly[dG-dC] is stronger than that with poly[dI-dC] and poly[dA-dT]. The interaction with poly[dG] is much weaker than with poly d[dG-dC]. The fluorescence increase is caused neither by heat-denatured calf thymus DNA nor by tRNA. The enhancement of the fluorescence by double-stranded DNA indicates the intercalation of the 8-hydroxy-7-methoxybenzene moiety of neothramycin between bases of DNA. 3-O-methyl and 3-O-butylneothramycin A (Fig. 2, R_1=O-alkyl, R_2=H) are more stable than 3-O-methyl and 3-O-butylneothramycin B (Fig. 2, R_1=H, R_2=O-alkyl) in aqueous solution; that is, the 3-O-alkyl groups of B are easily replaced by the hydroxyl group of water. Probably for this reason, the 3-O-alkylneothramycin B fluorescence is enhanced by DNA, whereas 3-O-alkylneothramycin A is not (11). These results suggest the involvement of the 3-carbon in the binding to double-stranded DNA.

In 20% aqueous dimethylsulfoxide, neothramycin reacts with 2'-deoxyguanosine and produces two reaction products. The major product was isolated and determined to be the aminal linkage compound in which the amino group of 2'-deoxyguanosine is bound to the 3-carbon of neothramycin (12). This also suggests the possible involvement of the 3-carbon in the interaction with DNA. However, the fluorescence of 10,11-dihydroneothramycins A and B was not enhanced by DNA. This may be due to a conformational

276

change in the neothramycin molecule or the involvement of the 11-carbon in the interaction with DNA. Hurley (6) has proposed the aminal linkage at the 11-carbon of anthramycin.

The blood level in cancer patients after the intravenous infusion of 40 mg/m^2 of neothramycin at a constant rate for 60 minutes has been measured by high pressure liquid chromatography. The results indicate that the maximum blood level at the end of the infusion goes down rapidly for 30 minutes and thereafter more slowly.

3. DERIVATIVES AND ANALOGS OF ANTITUMOR ANTIBIOTICS WHICH HAVE BEEN USED IN CANCER TREATMENT —— BLEOMYCIN, ANTHRACYCLINE

In addition to the new types of antitumor antibiotics found by screening, anticancer agents with potential usefulness have been found by study of derivatives and analogs of antitumor antibiotics which have been used in cancer treatment.

3.1. Bleomycin and its derivatives and analogs

With colleagues in my institute and in the laboratories of Nippon Kayaku Co., I am still continuing the study of bleomycin, its derivatives, and analogs.

We determined the structure of bleomycin in 1978 as shown in Fig. 3 (13). In 1981, we were successful in total synthesis of the peptide part (14). Finally, we were also successful in the total synthesis of bleomycin A2 (15).

Cleomycin, phleomycin, tallysomycin, YA-56X (zorbamycin), YA-56Y, zorbonomycin, platomycin, and victomycin are members of the bleomycin group of antibiotics. We determined the structure of cleomycin (16) and phleomycin (13,17). Cleomycin contains the amino acids, cleonine, shown in Fig. 4 instead of the threonine found in bleomycin. Phleomycin does not contain the bithiazole group, but has the dihydrobithiazole group shown in Fig. 4. Phleomycin D1, E, and G have the same terminal amines as bleomycin B2, B4, and B6, respectively. D1 and E were oxidized to B2 and B4, respectively. The strong renal toxicity of phleomycin is due to E and G which contain two or more guanidine groups (18). From a consideration of the structures of bleomycin and phleomycir

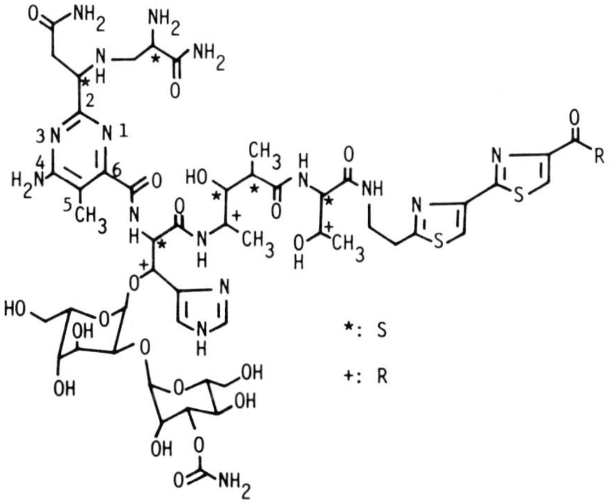

Various bleomycins: A1 (R=NH-(CH$_2$)$_3$-SO-CH$_3$),

Demethyl-A2 (R=NH-(CH$_2$)$_3$-S-CH$_3$), A2 (R=NH-(CH$_2$)$_3$-S$^+$$\overset{CH_3}{\underset{CH_3}{}}$),

A2'-a (R=NH-(CH$_2$)$_4$-NH$_2$), A2'-b (R=NH-(CH$_2$)$_3$-NH$_2$),

A2'-c (R=NH-(CH$_2$)$_2$-⟨N...N⟩), A5 (R=NH-(CH$_2$)$_3$-NH-(CH$_2$)$_4$-NH$_2$),

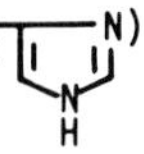

A6 (R=NH-(CH$_2$)$_3$-NH-(CH$_2$)$_4$-NH-(CH$_2$)$_3$-NH$_2$), B1' (R=NH$_2$),

B2 (R=NH-(CH$_2$)$_4$-NH-$\overset{NH}{\overset{\|}{C}}$-NH$_2$), B4 (R=NH-(CH$_2$)$_4$-NH-$\overset{NH}{\overset{\|}{C}}$-NH-(CH$_2$)$_4$-NH-$\overset{NH}{\overset{\|}{C}}$-NH$_2$)

and Bleomycinic acid (R=OH)

Peplomycin: R=NH-(CH$_2$)$_3$-NH-$\overset{CH_3}{\underset{H}{C}}$-⟨phenyl⟩

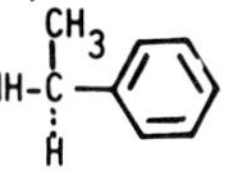

BAPP: NH-(CH$_2$)$_3$-NH-(CH$_2$)$_3$-NH-(CH$_2$)$_3$-CH$_3$

A5033: NH-(CH$_2$)$_3$-NH-(CH$_2$)$_4$-NH-CO-(CH$_2$)$_2$-COOH

FIGURE 3. Natural bleomycins, bleomycinic acid, peplomycin, BAPP, and A5033.

the structures of tallysomycin and YA-56X have been proposed (19).

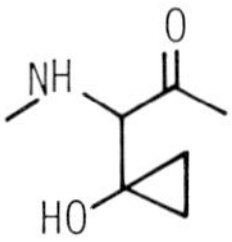

Cleonine moiety
in cleomycin

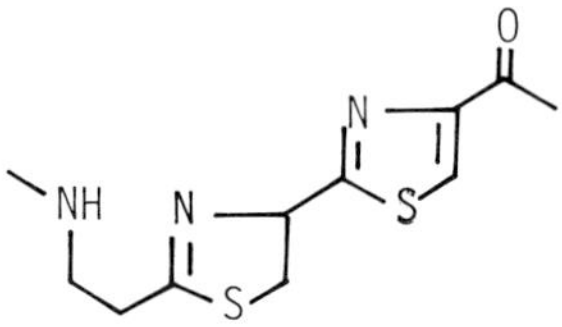

Dihydrobithiazole moiety
in phleomycin

FIGURE 1. The structural parts of cleomycin and phleomycin
which differ from bleomycin.

One of the amino acid moieties of bleomycin has a pyrimidine
ring; consequently, we named this amino acid "pyrimidoblamic
acid" and have chemically synthesized it (20). A bleomycin
analog which lacks the methyl group in the pyrimidoblamic acid
moiety has also been found in culture filtrates of actinomycetes.

As we report for the first time in this paper, incorporation
studies of labeled amino acids into the pyrimidoblamic acid
moiety of bleomycin suggest that this amino acid moiety is biosynthesized from serine and asparagine and that the methyl group
is derived from methionine. It appears that the α-aminopropionyl
group in the side chain of pyrimidoblamic acid is derived from
serine, and the other part of the pyrimidoblamic acid moiety
except for the methyl and amino groups is biosynthesized from
2 molecules of asparagine. The 2'-(2-aminoethyl)-2,4'-bithiazole-
4-carboxylic acid moiety was shown to be biosynthesized from 3-
aminopropionic acid and 2 molecules of cysteine. The methyl
group of methionine is introduced into the 2-methyl group of the
4-amino-3-hydroxy-2-methylpentanoic acid moiety.

The following peptides were isolated from culture filtrates
of bleomycin (19), suggesting the following biosynthetic pathway
for the biosynthesis of the peptide part of bleomycin:

Demethylpyrimidoblamylhistidine ⟶ demethylpyrimidoblamyl-
histidylalanine ⟶ demethylpyrimidoblamylhistidyl-(4-amino-3-
hydroxy-2-methyl)-pentanoic acid [4-amino-3-hydroxy-2-methyl-
pentanoic acid is abbreviated as AHP] ⟶ demethylpyrimidoblamyl-
histidyl-AHP-threonine ⟶ pyrimidoblamylhistidyl-AHP-threonyl-
[2'-(2-aminoethyl)-2,4'-bithiazole-4-carboxylic acid] (this

bithiazole carboxylic acid is abbreviated as BTC) $\longrightarrow$ pyrimido-blamyl-β-hydroxyhistidyl-AHP-Thr-BTC (β-hydroxyhistidine is abbre-viated as β-OH-His) $\longrightarrow$ pyrimidoblamyl-β-OH-His-AHP-Thr-BTC-(3-aminopropyl)dimethylsulfonium (deglycobleomycin A2).

Bleomycin binds with Cu(II) and an equimolar bleomycin-Cu(II) complex is formed. X-ray crystallographic analysis of demethyl-pyrimidoblamylhistidylalanine and the chemical study of the bleomycin-Cu(II) complex indicate the structure of the complex as shown in Fig. 5 (21). Although the structure of bleomycin-Fe(II) complex which we proposed (21) has not yet been completely proved, there are no experimental data which conflict with this structure (22). Generation of active oxygen species from the oxygen adduct of bleomycin-Fe(II) has been observed by ESR using a spin trap reagent (23). Moreover, the active form of the

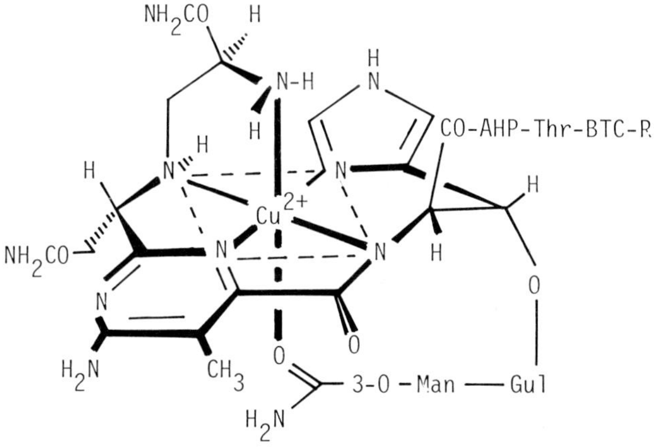

AHP=4-amino-3-hydroxy-2-methylpentanoyl; Thr=threonyl; BTC=2'-(2-aminoethyl)-2,4'-bithiazole-4-carboxyl; R=terminal amine; Man-Gul=2-0-(α-D-mannopyranosyl)-α-L-gulopyranosyl

FIGURE 5. Bleomycin-copper complex.

bleomycin-iron-O_2 complex which embodies its DNA cleaving activi-ty has been suggested to be bleomycin-Fe(III)-^-O_2H (24). The mode of oxygen activation by the bleomycin-iron complex has also been studied by Peisach (25).

The products of DNA fragmentation caused by bleomycin-iron-O_2

complex were isolated by Grollman and Takeshita (26). On the basis of these reaction products, the DNA fragmentation reaction caused by bleomycin can be described as shown in Fig. 6.

Reaction of Bleomycin (BLM) with DNA, Resulting in DNA Strand Scission

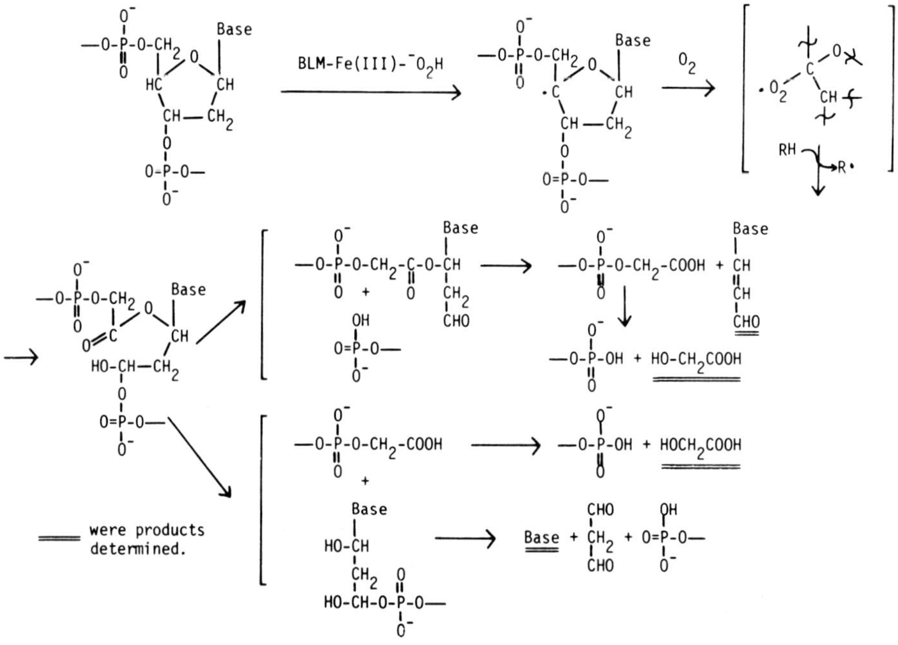

FIGURE 6. Reaction of bleomycin (BLM) with DNA, resulting in DNA strand scission.

The extinction of fluorescence indicates the binding of bleomycin to the guanine moiety of DNA (27). The terminal amine of bleomycin is also involved in the binding to DNA. Bleomycin intercalates between bases of double-stranded DNA (28). The bleomycin-Fe(III)-^-O_2H complex binding to DNA abstracts the hydrogen radical from the 4-carbon of the 2-deoxyribose moiety, leaving a 4-carbon radical. This radical then reacts with molecular oxygen. As a result of this reaction, the 4-carbon is oxygenated, and the furanose ring is opened between the 4- and 3-carbons. This ring cleavage is followed by cleavages of phosphate and ester bonds in various ways as shown in Fig. 6. The cleavage which yields thymine and other bases also occurs. Although more studies are necessary to know the complete reaction, we wrote the most plausible reaction sequence as seen in Fig. 6.

Bleomycin causes double-strand scission, but its mechanism still remains to be solved. In this connection, it is interesting that phleomycin which has the dihydrobithiazole moiety neither intercalate with DNA (29), nor causes double-strand scission. It causes single strand scission (30).

After penetrating into cells, the Cu(II) of bleomycin-Cu(II) complex is reduced to Cu(I) by reducing agents such as cysteine, etc. in the cells, and the Cu(I) is transferred to a cellular protein which can bind selectively to it (31). Cu(II)-free bleomycin thus formed undergoes reaction with bleomycin hydrolase which hydrolyzes the α-aminocarboxamide bond of the pyrimidoblamyl moiety of bleomycin (32). This enzyme is widely distributed in human and animal cells. Cu(II)-free bleomycin which escapes this enzymic action reaches nuclei, binds, and reacts with DNA as described above. Knowledge of the mechanism of action thus elucidated is very useful for designing studies of derivatives or analogs with improved therapeutic activities. One of the reasons why bleomycin exhibits a therapeutic effect against squamous cell carcinoma is due to the low content of bleomycin hydrolase in this type of tumor (33).

A side effect caused by bleomycin occurs in the lungs. Therefore, bleomycin derivatives which have lower pulmonary toxicity than bleomycin can exhibit stronger therapeutic action than the latter against tumors susceptible to bleomycin treatment. Various bleomycins are different from one another in the terminal amine moiety (Fig. 3). The degree of pulmonary or renal toxicity is different among these bleomycins (18).

We have established fermentation and chemical processes for the preparation of various bleomycins (18). By the addition of many kinds of amines to the fermentation medium, various bleomycins containing the added amines are produced. We found acyl agmatine hydrolase in Fusarium sp., and this enzyme hydrolyzes

the terminal peptide bond of bleomycin B2, yielding bleomycinic
acid (34). Bleomycinic acid was also obtained by reaction of
cyanogen bromide with bleomycin demethyl A2 (35). Various bleomycins were synthesized from bleomycinic acid.

A method of testing the pulmonary toxicity of bleomycins in
mice was developed by Matsuda et al. (37) and bleomycin 5033
(Fig. 3) was first selected for testing. The pulmonary toxicity
index in mice of this bleomycin shown by Matsuda's method was
0.22, taking the index of bleomycin clinically used as 1.0. In
about 1974, bleomycin 5033 was clinically studied and its pulmonary toxicity was shown by a pulmonary function test to be
lower than that of bleomycin clinically used. Thus, it was shown
that Matsuda's method for testing pulmonary toxicity was useful
in selecting bleomycin derivatives and analogs worthy of the
clinical test. Bleomycin PEP (peplomycin) and bleomycin BAPP
(Fig. 3) were selected as those which have lower pulmonary toxicity and a strong antitumor activity. The pulmonary toxicity
index of PEP was 0.25 and that of BAPP was 0.22 (36). They were
as effective in inhibiting Ehrlich carcinoma and squamous cell
carcinoma induced by methylcholanthrene in mouse skin as bleomycin clinically used. In high doses they showed therapeutic
effects against adenocarcinoma induced by N-methyl-N'-nitro-N-
nitrosoguanidine in rat stomach (37). Bleomycin clinically
used did not inhibit this adenocarcinoma.

We named bleomycin PEP "pepleomycin"; however, this name was
changed by instruction of the Japanese Welfare Ministry to
"peplomycin". Peplomycin has been studied clinically since 1975
and marketed since 1981. The clinical study suggested that
peplomycin was more effective against carcinomas in the head,
neck, and skin and had lower pulmonary toxicity than bleomycin.
Peplomycin was also confirmed to be effective against prostatic
carcinoma.

Radioactive metal complexes of bleomycin are taken up by
tumors, especially in lung cancer and are useful for diagnosis
(38). Therefore, the bleomycin analogs and derivatives which
are resistant to bleomycin hydrolase can be assumed to have a
wider anticancer spectrum than bleomycin. Modification of the

α-aminocarboxamide part of the bleomycin molecule gives such derivatives.

As already described, bleomycin hydrolase hydrolyzes the carboxamide of the α-aminocarboxamide moiety, and the product of this hydrolysis can be used as the starting material for the modification of the α-aminocarboxamide moiety. In this paper, I will report two examples of such derivatives, PEP-PEP and DBP-PEP, shown in Fig. 7. Both were resistant to bleomycin

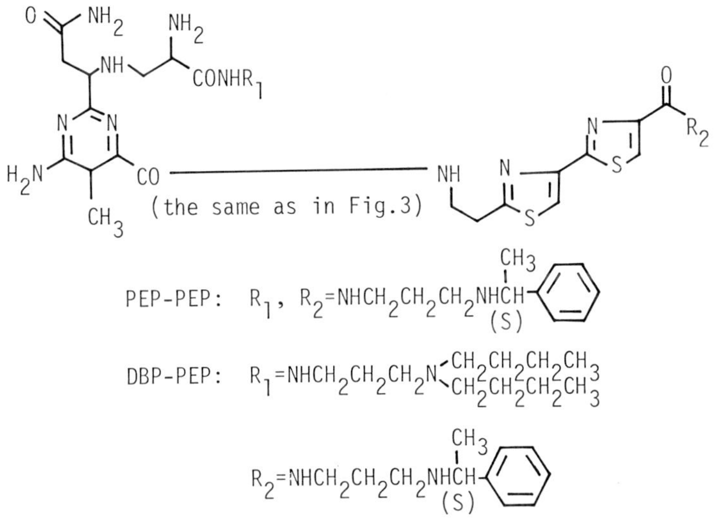

FIGURE 7. New bleomycin analogs resistant to bleomycin hydrolase.

hydrolase, and their 50% inhibition concentration against HeLa cells was around 0.9 µg/ml. The index of pulmonary toxicity was 0.05 for PEP-PEP and 0 for DBP-PEP. The interesting thing is that their therapeutic index against Ehrlich carcinoma is as high as that of bleomycin. We are selecting such derivatives which have a wide spectrum against mouse tumors, low pulmonary toxicity, and low renal toxicity. It is certain that bleomycin analogs and derivatives which are more useful in cancer treatment than the present bleomycins will be developed.

3.2. Anthracyclines

As written in this book, a great many studies have been done by Arcamone and his associates for development of anthracyclines which have improved activities. In the last 10 years, with colleagues in my institute and in the Institute of Sanraku-Ocean Co., I have also continued the study of anthracyclines.

Aclacinomycin A (Fig. 8) which we found has been clinically studied (39). Aclacinomycin was found by Dantchev et al. to have significantly lower cardiac toxicity than adriamycin in hamster (40), and this low cardiac toxicity has been confirmed by clinical study. It showed therapeutic effect against leukemia, lymphoma, stomach carcinoma, and some other solid tumors.

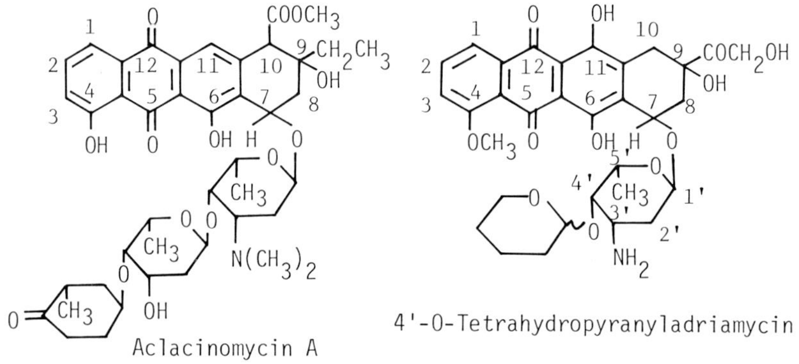

Aclacinomycin A

4'-O-Tetrahydropyranyladriamycin

FIGURE 8. Structures of anthracyclines clinically used or under clinical test.

We studied the biosynthesis of anthracyclines and obtained various mutants which produce neither red nor yellow pigments and convert aglycones to anthracyclines. In addition, we found a mutant which produces 2-hydroxyaklavinone (aklavinone is the aglycone of aclacinomycin). Adding 2-hydroxyaklavinone to the culture medium and culturing a pigmentless mutant of an aclacino-mycin-producing strain, we isolated 2-hydroxyaclacinomycin (41). It is the first finding of 2-hydroxyanthracycline. 2-Hydroxy-aclacinomycins A and B showed higher therapeutic indices against L-1210 leukemia than aclacinomycins A and B.

We have also found baumycins (42). Baumycin A1 showed a strong action against L-1210 in my laboratories. Therefore, we started the synthesis of 4'-O-glycosidic derivatives of adriamycin

and daunomycin. Among about 50 4'-O-glycoside derivatives synthesized, one of two stereoisomers of 4'-O-tetrahydropyranyl-
adriamycin (Fig. 8) showed a stronger effect against L-1210 than
adriamycin and daunomycin (43). This derivative was confirmed
to have a lower cardiac and skin toxicity than adriamycin in
hamsters (40). The degree of cardiac toxicity in hamsters was
the same as, or lower than, aclacinomycin. This derivative,
abbreviated as THP-ADM, was recognized to be worth studying clinically. In phase I study, 60 mg/patient every 3 weeks has shown
therapeutic effects in the treatment of Hodgkin's lymphoma,
reticulosarcoma, ovarial carcinoma, etc. Its side effects of
causing hair loss and stomach irritation are very weak. It is
certain that the study of anthracyclines will lead to the development of very effective cancer chemotherapeutic agents.

4. SMALL MOLECULAR WEIGHT IMMUNO-MODIFIERS —— BESTATIN, ETC.

As discussed already, in order to destroy minimal residual
tumors and to obtain a complete cure, it would be advantageous
to have immunity-enhancing agents to restore the immune resistance which is reduced in cancer patients. With my colleagues,
I initiated the screening of low molecular weight enzyme inhibitors, reporting the first work in 1969; at present, I have discovered about 45 enzyme inhibitors and elucidated their structures
(44,45,46). Furthermore, I extended the study of enzyme inhibitors to include immunity-enhancing agents with potential usefulness in cancer treatment (47).

In 1972, we found that the administration of coriolins, antitumor antibiotics produced by Coriolus consor and their derivative, diketocoriolin B, (Fig. 9), increased the number of mouse
spleen cells producing antibody to sheep red blood cells (48).
On the other hand, we found that diketocoriolin B inhibits Na^+-
K^+-ATPase (49). Therefore, I thought that the binding of diketocoriolin B or coriolin to ATPase in cell membranes caused the
blastogenesis of lymphocytes producing antibody. Later, we
confirmed that the increase in the number of antibody-forming
cells by diketocoriolin B was due to its interaction with B
lymphocytes (50).

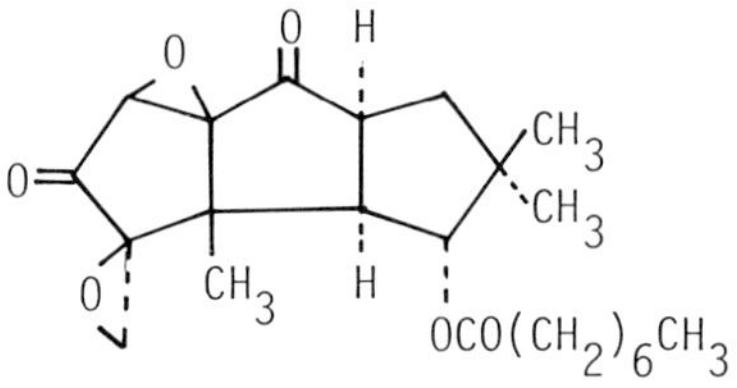

FIGURE 9. Structure of diketocoriolin B.

I assumed that the screening of compounds which bind to cell membranes or surfaces would result in the finding of immuno-modifiers: so, with my colleagues, I began a search for inhibitors of enzymes on cell surfaces or membranes. We first found that all aminopeptidases are not only in cells but also located on their surfaces (51). These enzymes are not released extra-cellularly. Alkaline phosphatase and esterase were also found to be located on cell surfaces. Searching for inhibitors of these enzymes, we found bestatin (47,52), inhibiting aminopepti-dase B and leucine aminopeptidase; amastatin (47,53), inhibiting aminopeptidase A and leucine aminopeptidase; forphenicine (47,54), inhibiting chicken intestine alkaline phosphatase; and esterastin (47,55) and ebelactone (47,56), inhibiting esterase. Their structures are shown in Fig. 10. All these inhibitors except for esterastin enhanced immune responses.

A low dose (1-100 µg/mouse) of bestatin enhanced delayed-type hypersensitivity (DTH) to sheep red blood cells and, at higher doses (1 mg/mouse), it increased the number of antibody-forming cells in spleen. Amastatin increased the number of antibody-forming cells. Forphenicine (1-100 µg/mouse) enhanced DTH and also increased the number of antibody-forming cells (10-1,000 µg/mouse). Ebelactone enhanced DTH. But esterastin suppressed DTH and reduced the number of antibody-forming cells. The Ki value for esterastin was about 10^{-10}M, whereas those of the others ranged from about 10^{-6} to 10^{-8}M.

We have synthesized all stereoisomers of bestatin (47). Those isomers which have the same configuration (S) as bestatin at the carbon adjacent to the carbonyl group of the 3-amino-2-hydroxy-4-

phenylbutyryl moiety showed similar activity as bestatin in
inhibiting aminopeptidase B and enhancing DTH, but the other
isomers having the R configuration at this carbon atom had
neither activity.

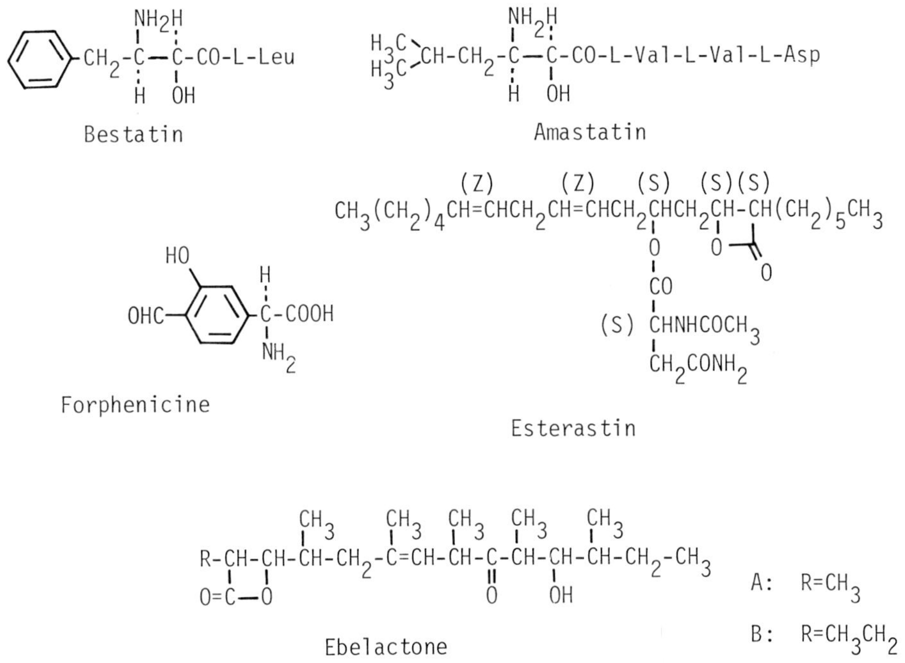

$$\text{C}_6\text{H}_5\text{-CH}_2\text{-}\overset{\overset{\displaystyle NH_2}{|}}{\underset{\underset{\displaystyle H}{|}}{C}}\text{-}\overset{\overset{\displaystyle H}{}}{\underset{\underset{\displaystyle OH}{|}}{C}}\text{-CO-L-Leu}$$

Bestatin

$$\overset{\displaystyle H_3C}{\underset{\displaystyle H_3C}{>}}\text{CH-CH}_2\text{-}\overset{\overset{\displaystyle NH_2}{|}}{\underset{\underset{\displaystyle H}{|}}{C}}\text{-}\overset{\overset{\displaystyle H}{}}{\underset{\underset{\displaystyle OH}{|}}{C}}\text{-CO-L-Val-L-Val-L-Asp}$$

Amastatin

Forphenicine

$$\text{OHC-C}_6\text{H}_3(\text{HO})\text{-}\overset{\overset{\displaystyle H}{}}{\underset{\underset{\displaystyle NH_2}{|}}{C}}\text{-COOH}$$

$$CH_3(CH_2)_4\overset{(Z)}{CH}=CHCH_2\overset{(Z)}{CH}=CHCH_2\overset{(S)}{CHCH_2}\overset{(S)}{CH}-\overset{(S)}{CH}(CH_2)_5CH_3$$

Esterastin

(S) CHNHCOCH$_3$
CH$_2$CONH$_2$

$$R-\overset{}{\underset{\underset{\displaystyle O=C-O}{|}}{CH}}-CH-\overset{\overset{\displaystyle CH_3}{|}}{CH}-CH_2-\overset{\overset{\displaystyle CH_3}{|}}{C}=\overset{\overset{\displaystyle CH_3}{|}}{CH}-\overset{\overset{\displaystyle CH_3}{|}}{CH}-\overset{}{\underset{\underset{\displaystyle O}{||}}{C}}-\overset{\overset{\displaystyle CH_3}{|}}{CH}-\overset{}{\underset{\underset{\displaystyle OH}{|}}{CH}}-CH_2-CH_3$$

A: R=CH$_3$

B: R=CH$_3$CH$_2$

Ebelactone

FIGURE 10. Low molecular weight immuno-modifiers.

Forphenicine inhibits chicken intestine alkaline phosphatase,
but its action against other alkaline phosphatases is very weak.
The type of inhibition of chicken intestine alkaline phosphatase
by forphenicine is very interesting; that is, it is uncompetitive
with the substrate. Its derivative, forphenicinol, in which
the aldehyde group of forphenicine is reduced to alcohol, does
not inhibit alkaline phosphatase, but it does bind to animal
cells including lymphocytes. As I will report for the first time
in this paper, forphenicinol has been found to enhance DTH when
given at 0.1-100 µg/mouse by intraperitoneal injection or 0.1-
1,000 µg/mouse by oral administration.

The effects of bestatin on immune responses in mice can be

summarized as follows (47):   (1) bestatin (1-100 µg/mouse given
orally) enhanced delayed-type hypersensitivity (DTH) to sheep red
blood cells in aged (older than 8 weeks) CDF_1 mice; bestatin
(1,000 µg/mouse) increased the number of antibody-forming cells
in CDF_1 mouse spleen; (2) bestatin (10 µg or 1,000 µg/mouse given
orally) restored DTH to oxazolone in mice whose cellular immunity
had been reduced by cyclophosphamide treatment, or bestatin (0.1,
10 or 1,000 µg/mouse given orally) restored DTH which had been
depressed by inoculation of Ehrlich carcinoma cells; (3) 5, 10 or
50 mg/kg of bestatin given intraperitoneally increased markedly
(about 3 times compared with the control) ^{3}H-thymidine incorporation into DNA of T cells but not of B cells; it enhanced the
activity of DNA polymerase α in T cells but not polymerase β;
it activated terminal deoxyribonucleotidyl transferase in bone
marrow cells; the exposure of L-5178Y cells (T-cell lymphoma line)
to bestatin (1-50 µg/ml) increased the amount of polysomes (47,57)
(4) bestatin in vitro (0.001-0.1 µg/ml) or in vivo (10 µg/mouse)
increased the number of colony-forming units in bone marrow
cultures; (5) daily bestatin treatment (0.05, 0.5 or 5.0 mg/kg)
given orally for 5 days to mice which had received subcutaneous
inoculations of 10^6 tumor cells 8 or 14 days earlier showed a
marked suppression of the growth of IMC-carcinoma or Gardner
lymphosarcoma; (6) bestatin (1, 10 or 100 µg/mouse) enhanced
the antitumor effect of bleomycin or adriamycin; (7) bestatin
(10 or 100 µg/mouse given daily) retarded the induction of skin
cancer by 20-methylcholanthrene; and (8) 100 µg/mouse of bestatin
given intraperitoneally every week showed a significant reduction
in spontaneous tumors. As first described in this paper,
bestatin has been found to increase the production of both inter-
leukin 1 and 2.

   Bestatin given orally is well-absorbed. In human, when given
30 mg daily by oral administration, more than 80% is excreted in
urine and 5-15% is metabolized to p-hydroxybestatin. This metabolite is more than 5 times more active than bestatin in inhibiting aminopeptidase B and has the ability to enhance DTH as well
as bestatin. It has a stronger activity than bestatin in increasing the number of antibody-forming cells.

Daily oral administration of bestatin produces no toxicity.
In the last 3 years of the clinical study, the effect on T cell
percentage and NK cell activity in cancer patients and the effect
of daily various doses on T cell percentage were studied in Japan,
Sweden, and France. The results of the clinical study can be
summarized as follows (47): (1) bestatin, when given at 30, 60,
or 100 mg daily, restored the reduced T cell percentage and absolute number of T cell in cancer patients; (2) 30 or 60 mg daily
enhanced NK cell activity; bestatin increased NK cell activity
also in vitro; (3) IgG production by healthy human lymphocytes
is inhibited by sera of cancer patients, and this inhibition is
eliminated by bestatin in vitro or by its administration to
cancer patients; (4) 30 mg daily enhanced the activity of helper
T cells for IgG production; 30 mg daily normalized mitomycin C-
sensitive suppressor cells which were increased in cancer patients; antigen-dependent killer T cell activity was increased by
30 mg daily (58); (5) bone marrow cell populations in cancer
patients were improved by 30 mg daily; (6) skin reactions in
anergy patients turned to positive after daily oral administration of 30 mg.

Oral administration of forphenicinol, as first described in
this paper, also restored the reduced T cell percentage in cancer
patients and enhanced NK cell activity. Forphenicinol enhances
macrophage phagocytic activity toward yeast.

The effects of bestatin in eliminating minimal residual tumors
are being studied under a randomized schedule. This study is
being conducted in various kinds of tumors such as melanoma,
head and neck carcinomas, bladder carcinoma, stomach cancer, etc.

5. CONCLUSION

The screening of microbial culture filtrates is still leading
to the discovery of new antitumor antibiotics with potential usefulness in cancer treatment. Bactobolin and spergualin may be
worth a clinical study. Neothramycin may contribute to cancer
treatment. It is also certain that the studies of derivatives
and analogs of bleomycin, adriamycin, etc. are leading to compounds more effective than their parent compounds.

It is possible that compounds which inhibit the action or generation of suppressor cells will be found among cytotoxic antibiotics.

Moreover, low molecular weight immuno-modifiers have been discovered and their usefulness in cancer treatment has been suggested by the clinical study of bestatin.

The study of antitumor antibiotics and low molecular weight immuno-modifiers will contribute to its progress in cancer treatment and an increase in the rate of its cure.

REFERENCES

1. Ishizuka M, Takeuchi T, Masuda T, Fukasawa S, Umezawa H. 1981. Enhancement of immune responses and possible inhibition of suppressor cells by aclacinomycin A. J. Antibiotics 34, 331-340.
2. Kondo S, Horiuchi Y, Hamada M, Takeuchi T, Umezawa H. 1979. A new antitumor antibiotic, bactobolin produced by Pseudo-monas. J. Antibiotics 32, 1069-1071.
3. Umezawa H, Kondo S, Iinuma H, Kunimoto S, Ikeda Y, Iwasawa H, Ikeda D, Takeuchi T. 1981. Structure of an antitumor antibiotic, spergualin. J. Antibiotics 34, 1622-1624.
4. Kondo S, Iwasawa H, Ikeda D, Umeda Y, Ikeda Y, Iinuma H, Umezawa H. 1981. The total synthesis of spergualin, an antitumor antibiotic. J. Antibiotics 34, 1625-1627.
5. Takeuchi T, Miyamoto M, Ishizuka M, Naganawa H, Kondo S, Hamada M, Umezawa H. 1976. Neothramycins A and B, new antitumor antibiotics. J. Antibiotics 29, 93-96.
6. Hurley LH. 1977. Pyrrolo(1,4)benzodiazepine antitumor antibiotic. Compared aspects of anthramycin, tomaymycin and sibilo-mycin. J. Antibiotics 30, 349-370.
7. Korman S, Tendler MP. 1965. Clinical investigation of cancer chemotherapeutic agents for neoplastic diseases. J. New Drugs 5, 275-285.
8. Kunimoto S, Masuda T, Kanbayashi N, Hamada M, Naganawa H, Miyamoto M, Takeuchi T, Umezawa H. 1980. Mazethramycin, a new member of anthramycin group antibiotics. J. Antibiotics 33, 665-667.
9. Hisamatsu T, Uchida S, Takeuchi T, Ishizuka M, Umezawa H. 1980. Antitumor effect of a new antibiotic, neothramycin. Gann 71, 308-312.
10. Maruyama IN, Suzuki H, Tanaka N. 1978. Mechanism of action of neothramycin. I. The effect on macromolecular syntheses. J. Antibiotics 31, 761-768.
11. Maruyama IN, Tanaka N, Kondo S, Umezawa H. 1979. Mechanism of action of neothramycin. II. Interaction with DNA. J. Antibiotics 32, 928-934.
12. Maruyama IN, Tanaka N, Kondo S, Umezawa H. 1981. Structure of neothramycin-2'-deoxyguanosine adduct. Biochem. Biophys. Res. Commun. 98, 970-976.

13. Takita T, Muraoka Y, Nakatani T, Fujii A, Umezawa Y, Naganawa H, Umezawa H. 1978. Chemistry of bleomycin. XIX. Revised structures of bleomycin and phleomycin. J. Antibiotics 31, 801-804.
14. Takita T, Umezawa Y, Saito S, Morishima H, Umezawa H, Muraoka Y, Suzuki M, Otsuka M, Kobayashi S, Ohno M. 1981. Total synthesis of deglyco-bleomycin A2. Tetrahedron Letters 22, 671-674.
15. Takita T, Umezawa Y, Saito S, Morishima H, Tsuchiya T, Miyake T, Umezawa H, Muraoka Y, Suzuki M, Otsuka M, Ohno M. 1982. Total synthesis of bleomycin A2. Tetrahedron Letters 23, 521-524.
16. Umezawa H, Muraoka Y, Fujii A, Naganawa H, Takita T. 1980. Chemistry of bleomycin. XXVII. Cleomycin, a new family of bleomycin-phleomycin group. J. Antibiotics 33, 1079-1082.
17. Takita T, Muraoka Y, Fujii A, Itoh H, Maeda K, Umezawa H. 1972. The structure of the sulfur-containing chromophore of phleomycin, and chemical transformation of phleomycin to bleomycin. J. Antibiotics 25, 197-199.
18. Umezawa H. 1976. Bleomycin: discovery, chemistry and action. GANN Monograph on Cancer Research, No. 19, pp.3-36, Tokyo, University of Tokyo Press.
19. Umezawa H, Takita T. 1980. The bleomycins: antitumor copper-binding antibiotics. Structure and Bonding 40, 73-99.
20. Umezawa Y, Morishima H, Saito S, Takita T, Umezawa H, Kobayashi S, Otsuka M, Narita M, Ohno M. 1980. Synthesis of the pyrimidine moiety of bleomycin. J. Am. Chem. Soc. 102, 6630-6631.
21. Takita T, Muraoka Y, Nakatani T, Fujii A, Iitaka Y, Umezawa H. 1978. Chemistry of bleomycin. XXI. Metal-complex of bleomycin and its implication for the mechanism of bleomycin action. J. Antibiotics 31, 1073-1077.
22. Sugiura Y, Muraoka Y, Fujii A, Takita T, Umezawa H. 1979. Chemistry of bleomycin. XXIV. Deamidobleomycin from view point of metal coordination and oxygen activation. J. Antibiotics 32, 756-758.
23. Sugiura Y, Suzuki T, Muraoka Y, Umezawa Y, Takita T, Umezawa H. 1981. Deglycobleomycin-iron complexes: Implications for iron-binding site and role of the sugar portion in bleomycin antibiotics. J. Antibiotics 34, 1232-1236.
24. Kuramochi H, Takahashi K, Takita T, Umezawa H. 1981. An active intermediate formed in the reaction of bleomycin-Fe(II) complex with oxygen. J. Antibiotics 34, 576-582.
25. Giloni L, Takeshita M, Johnson F, Iden C, Grollman P. 1981. Bleomycin-induced strand-scission of DNA. Mechanism of deoxyribose cleavage. J. Biol. Chem. 256, 8608-8615.
26. Burger RM, Peisach J, Horwitz SB. 1981. Activated bleomycin. A transient complex of drug, iron and oxygen that degrades DNA. J. Biol. Chem. 256, 11636-11644.
27. Kasai H, Naganawa H, Takita T, Umezawa H. 1978. Chemistry of bleomycin. XXII. Interaction of bleomycin with nucleic acids, preferential binding to guanine base and electrostatic effect of the terminal amine. J. Antibiotics 31, 1316-1320.
28. Povirk LF, Hogan M, Dattagupta N. 1979. Binding of bleomycin to DNA: Intercalation of the bithiazole rings. Biochemistry 18, 96-101.

29. Povirk LF. 1981. Copper (II) bleomycin, iron (III) bleo-
    mycin and copper (II) phleomycin: Comparative study of DNA
    binding. Biochemistry 20, 665-670.
30. Okubo H, Abe Y, Hori M, Asakura H, Umezawa H. 1981. A possi-
    ble role by bithiazole of bleomycin in causing double-strand
    scission of DNA. J. Antibiotics 34, 1213-1215.
31. Takahashi K, Yoshioka O, Matsuda A, Umezawa H. 1977. Intra-
    cellular reduction of the cupric ion of bleomycin copper
    complex and transfer or the cuprous ion to a cellular protein.
    J. Antibiotics 30, 861-869.
32. Umezawa H, Hori S, Sawa T, Yoshioka T, Takita T, Takeuchi T.
    1974. A bleomycin-inactivating enzyme in mouse liver. J.
    Antibiotics 27, 419-424.
33. Umezawa H, Takeuchi T, Hori S, Sawa T, Ishizuka M, Ichikawa
    T, Kanai T. 1972. Studies on the mechanism of antitumor
    effect of bleomycin on squamous cell carcinoma. J. Antibio-
    tics 25, 483-484.
34. Umezawa H, Takahashi Y, Fujii A, Saino T, Shirai T, Takita T.
    1973. Preparation of bleomycinic acid: Hydrolysis of bleo-
    mycin B2 by a Fusarium acylagmatine amidohydrolase. J. Anti-
    biotics 26, 117-119.
35. Takita T, Fukuoka T, Umezawa H. 1983. Chemical cleavage of
    bleomycin to bleomycinic acid and synthesis of new bleomycins.
    J. Antibiotics 26, 252-254.
36. Matsuda A, Yoshioka O, Ebihara K, Ekimoto H, Yamashita T,
    Umezawa H. 1978. The search for new bleomycins. Bleomycin
    Current Status and New Developments. pp.299-310. Academic
    Press.
37. Matsuda A, Yoshioka O, Takahashi K, Yamashita T, Ebihara K,
    Ekimoto H, Abe F, Hashimoto Y, Umezawa H. 1978. Preclinical
    studies on bleomycin-PEP (NK-631). Bleomycin: Current Status
    and New Developments, pp.311-332. Academic Press.
38. Noel JP. 1976. Radioactive metal-bleomycin complex for the
    diagnosis of cancer. Fundamental and Clinical Studies of
    Bleomycin (Monograph on Cancer Research No. 19), pp.301-316.
    Tokyo, University of Tokyo Press.
39. Oki T, Matsuzawa Y, Yoshimoto A, Numata K, Kitamura I, Hori
    S, Takamatsu A, Umezawa H, Ishizuka M, Naganawa H, Suda H,
    Hamada M, Takeuchi T. 1975. New antitumor antibiotics,
    aclacinomycins A and B. J. Antibiotics 28, 830-834.
40. Dantchev D, Paintrand M, Hayat M, Bourut C, Mathé G. 1979.
    Low heart and skin toxicity of a tetrahydropyranyl derivative
    of adriamycin (THP-ADM) as observed by electron and light
    microscopy. J. Antibiotics 32, 1085-1086.
41. Oki T, Yoshimoto A, Matsuzawa Y, Takeuchi T, Umezawa H. 1981.
    New anthracycline antibiotic, 2-hydroxyaclacinomycin A. J.
    Antibiotics 34, 916-918.
42. Takahashi Y, Naganawa H, Takeuchi T, Umezawa H. 1977. The
    structures of baumycins A1, A2, B1, B2, C1 and C2. J. Anti-
    biotics 30, 622-624.
43. Umezawa H, Takahashi T, Kinoshita M, Naganawa H, Masuda T,
    Ishizuka M, Tatsuta K, Takeuchi T. 1979. Tetrahydropyranyl
    derivatives of daunomycin and adriamycin. J. Antibiotics 32,
    1082-1084.

44. Umezawa H.   1972.   Enzyme Inhibitors of Microbial Origin.
    Tokyo, University of Tokyo Press.
45. Umezawa H.   1977.   Recent advances in bioactive microbial
    secondary metabolites.   Jap. J. Antibiotics 30 (Suppl.),
    138-163.
46. Umezawa H.   1976.   Structures and activities of protease
    inhibitors of microbial origin.   Methods in Enzymology,
    Vol. 45, pp.678-695.   Academic Press.
47. Umezawa H (ed.).   1981.   Small Molecular Immunomodifiers of
    Microbial Origin — Fundamental and Clinical Studies of
    Bestatin.   Tokyo, Japan Scientific Societies Press; Pergamon
    Press.
48. Ishizuka M, Iinuma H, Takeuchi T, Umezawa H.   1972.   Effect
    of diketocoriolin B on antibody formation.   J. Antibiotics
    25, 320-321.
49. Kunimoto T, Hori M, Umezawa H.   1973.   Mechanism of action
    of diketocoriolin B.   Biochim. Biophys. Acta 298, 513-525.
50. Ishizuka M, Takeuchi T, Umezawa H.   1981.   Studies on the
    mechanism of action of diketocoriolin B to enhance antibody
    formation.   J. Antibiotics 34, 95-102.
51. Aoyagi T, Suda H, Nagai M, Ogawa K, Suzuki J, Takeuchi T,
    Umezawa H.   1976.   Aminopeptidase activities on the surface
    of mammalian cells.   Biochim. Biophys. Acta 452, 131-143.
52. Umezawa H, Aoyagi T, Suda H, Hamada M, Takeuchi T.   1976.
    Bestatin, an inhibitor of aminopeptidase B, produced by
    actinomycetes.   J. Antibiotics 29, 97-99.
53. Aoyagi T, Tobe H, Kojima F, Hamada M, Takeuchi T, Umezawa H.
    1978.   Amastatin, an inhibitor of aminopeptidase A, produced
    by actinomycetes.   J. Antibiotics 31, 636-638.
54. Aoyagi T, Yamamoto T, Kojiri K, Kojima F, Hamada M, Takeuchi
    T, Umezawa H.   1978.   Forphenicine, an inhibitor of alkaline
    phosphatase produced by actinomycetes.   J. Antibiotics 31,
    244-246.
55. Umezawa H, Aoyagi T, Hazato T, Uotani K, Kojima F, Hamada M,
    Takeuchi T.   1978.   Esterastin, an inhibitor of esterase,
    produced by actinomycetes.   J. Antibiotics 31, 639-641.
56. Umezawa H, Aoyagi T, Uotani K, Hamada M, Takeuchi T, Takahashi
    S.   1980.   Ebelactone, an inhibitor of esterase produced by
    actinomycetes.   J. Antibiotics 33, 1594-1596.
57. Müller WEG, Zahn RK, Arendes J, Munsh N, Umezawa H.   1979.
    Activation of DNA metabolism in T cells by bestatin.   Bio-
    chem. Pharmacol. 28, 3131-3137.
58. Noma T, Yata J, Hoshi K, Ishii T.   1981.   The effect of
    bestatin on the lymphocyte functions.   J. Jpn. Soc. Cancer
    Ther. 16, 453-459 (in Japanese).